D1609038

ANTIGEN RETRIEVAL TECHNIQUES:

Immunohistochemistry and Molecular Morphology

Analytical Morphology and Molecular Pathology Series

JIANG GU AND GERHARD W. HACKER, *Series Editors*

Antigen Retrieval Techniques: Immunohistochemistry and Molecular Morphology
S.-R. Shi, J. Gu, and C.R. Taylor (Eds.)

Gold and Silver Staining Techniques
G.W. Hacker and J. Gu (Eds.)

Molecular and Analytical Morphology: Modern Protocols and Applications
G.W. Hacker and J. Gu (Eds.)

Other BioTechniques® Books Titles

Gene Cloning and Analysis by RT-PCR
P.D. Siebert and J.W. Larrick (Eds.)

Apoptosis Detection and Assay Methods
L. Zhu and J. Chun (Eds.)

Protein Staining and Identification Techniques
R.C. Allen and B. Budowle

Immunological Reagents and Solutions: A Laboratory Handbook
B.B. Damaj

Affinity and Immunoaffinity Purification Techniques
T.M. Phillips and B.F. Dickens

Yeast Hybrid Technologies
L. Zhu and G. Hannon (Eds.)

Viral Vectors: Basic Science and Gene Therapy
A. Cid-Arregui and A.M. García Carrancá (Eds.)

Ribozyme Biochemistry and Biotechnology
G. Krupp and R.K. Gaur (Eds.)

Bioinformatics: A Biologist's Guide to Biocomputing and the Internet
S. Brown

Gene Transfer Methods: Introducing DNA into Living Cells and Organisms
P.A. Norton and L.F. Steel (Eds.)

SNP and Microsatellite Genotyping: Markers for Genetic Analysis
A. Hajeer, J. Worthington, and S. John (Eds.)

ANTIGEN RETRIEVAL TECHNIQUES:
Immunohistochemistry and Molecular Morphology

Edited by

Shan-Rong Shi
University of Southern California Keck School of Medicine
Los Angeles, CA, USA

Jiang Gu
University of South Alabama
Mobile, AL, USA

Clive R. Taylor
University of Southern California Keck School of Medicine
Los Angeles, CA, USA

A BioTechniques® Books Publication
Eaton Publishing

Shan-Rong Shi, MD
Department of Pathology
University of Southern California Keck School of Medicine
HMR 310A, 2011 Zonal Ave.
Los Angeles, CA 90033

Jiang Gu, MD, PhD
Department of Biomedical Sciences
University of South Alabama
UCOM 6000
Mobile, AL 36688-0002

Clive R. Taylor, MD, PhD
Department of Pathology
University of Southern California Keck School of Medicine
HMR 204A, 2011 Zonal Ave.
Los Angeles, CA 90033

Library of Congress Cataloging-in-Publication Data

Antigen retrieval techniques : immunohistochemistry and molecular morphology / edited
by Shan-Rong Shi, Jiang Gu, Clive R. Taylor.
    p. ; cm. -- (Analytical morphology and molecular pathology series)
"A BioTechniques Books publication."
Includes bibliographical references and index.
ISBN 1-881299-43-0 (hardcover)
 1. Immunohistochemistry. I. Shi, Shan-Rong, 1936- II. Gu, Jiang. III. Taylor, C. R.
(Clive Roy) IV. Series.
 [DNLM: 1. Antigens--analysis. 2. Cytodiagnosis--methods. 3. Genetic Techniques. 4.
Immunohistochemistry--methods. 5. Pathology--methods. QW 573 A6297 2000]
QR183.6 .A58 2000
616.07'9-dc21

00-057816

ISBN 1-881299-43-0

Printed in the United States of America

9 8 7 6 5 4 3 2 1

Eaton Publishing
BioTechniques Books Division
154 E. Central Street
Natick, MA 01760
www.BioTechniques.com

Francis W. Eaton: *Publisher and President*
Stephen Weaver: *Director and Editor-in-Chief*
Christine McAndrews: *Managing Editor*
Sandy Lamont: *Production Manager*
Ken Strom: *Cover Designer*

Contributors

MATHILDE E. BOON • *Leiden Cytology and Pathology Laboratory, Leiden, The Netherlands*

GEORGIO CATTORETTI • *Department of Pathology, Columbia University College of Physicians and Surgeons, New York, NY, USA*

BENJAPORN CHAIWUN • *Department of Pathology, Chaingmai University, Thailand*

RICHARD J. COTE • *Department of Pathology, University of Southern California Keck School of Medicine, Los Angeles, CA, USA*

JULES M. ELIAS • *Department of Surgery, Oregon Health Sciences University, Portland, OR, USA*

PAUL EVERS • *Graduate School for Neurosciences Amsterdam, Netherlands Institute for Brain Research, Amsterdam, The Netherlands*

REAGIN FARLEY • *Department of Biomedical Sciences, University of South Alabama, Mobile, AL, USA*

QING FEI • *Department of Pathology, Columbia University College of Physicians and Surgeons, New York, NY, USA*

ALFRED CHRISTIAN FELLER • *Department of Pathology, Medical University of Luebeck, Luebeck, Germany*

JIANG GU • *Department of Biomedical Sciences, University of South Alabama, Mobile, AL, USA*

BRUNO GUHL • *Division of Cell and Molecular Pathology, Department of Pathology, University of Zürich, Zürich, Switzerland*

DEBRA HAWES • *Department of Pathology, University of Southern California Keck School of Medicine, Los Angeles, CA, USA*

KENJI KAWAI • *Department of Pathology, Tokai University School of Medicine, Tokai, Japan*

LAMBRECHT P. KOK • *Department of Biomedical Technology, University of Groningen, Groningen, The Netherlands*

FRANÇOISE LABAT-MOLEUR • *Laboratoire de Pathologie Cellulaire CHRU, Grenoble, France*

HUI Y. LAN • *Department of Medicine, Queen Mary Hospital, University of Hong Kong, Pokfulam, Hong Kong*

ANTHONY S.-Y. LEONG • *Hunter Area Pathology Services and The Discipline of Anatomical Pathology, University of Newcastle, Australia*

PAUL J. LUCASSEN • *Division of Medical Pharmacology, LACDR, Leiden University, Leiden, The Netherlands, and Institute Neurobiology, Faculty of Science, University of Amsterdam, Amsterdam, The Netherlands*

HARTMUT MERZ • *Department of Pathology, Medical University of Luebeck, Luebeck, Germany*

WIBKE MEYER • *Department of Pathology, Medical University of Leubeck, Luebeck, Germany*

ANKE MUELLER • *Department of Pathology, Medical University of Luebeck, Luebeck, Germany*

DAVID J. NIKOLIC-PATERSON • *Department of Nephrology and Monash University Department of Medicine, Monash Medical Centre, Clayton, Victoria, Australia*

ROBERT Y. OSAMURA • *Department of Pathology, Tokai University School of Medicine, Tokai, Japan*

KATHARINA OTTESEN • *Department of Pathology, Medical University of Luebeck, Luebeck, Germany*

LOUIS P. PERTSCHUK • *Department of Pathology, State University of New York Health Science Center at Brooklyn, and the Kings County Hospital Center, Brooklyn, NY, USA*

JÜRGEN ROTH • *Division of Cell and Molecular Pathology, Department of Pathology, University of Zürich, Zürich, Switzerland*

SHAN-RONG SHI • *Department of Pathology, University of Southern California Keck School of Medicine, Los Angeles, CA, USA*

YAN SHI • *Department of Pathology, University of Southern California Keck School of Medicine, Los Angeles, CA, USA*

JOHN W. STIRLING • *Department of Anatomical Pathology, SouthPath, Flinders Medical Centre, Bedford Park, Australia*

ALBERT J.H. SUURMEIJER • *Department of Pathology and Laboratory Medicine, University Hospital Groningen, Groningen, The Netherlands*

CLIVE R. TAYLOR • *Department of Pathology, University of Southern California Keck School of Medicine, Los Angeles, CA, USA*

JULIO F. TURRENS • *Department of Biomedical Sciences, University of South Alabama, Mobile, AL, USA*

HARRY B.M. UYLINGS • *Graduate School for Neurosciences Amsterdam, Netherlands Institute for Brain Research, Amsterdam, The Netherlands*

MENNO VAN LOOKEREN CAMPAGNE • *Department of Immunology, Genentech, South San Francisco, CA, USA*

MARTIN ZIAK • *Division of Cell and Molecular Pathology, Department of Pathology University of Zürich, Zürich, Switzerland*

YANMING ZHANG • *Department of Pathology, Medical University of Luebeck, Leubeck, Germany*

Preface

In response to the body of literature pertaining to use of the antigen retrieval (AR) technique in immunohistochemistry (IHC), which has been growing since 1991, we have attempted to summarize major achievements in this field. Our goal is to improve standardization and to further development and practical application of the method. The plan for editing such a book was enhanced by an international symposium on AR-IHC held at the Fifth Joint Meeting of the Japan Society of Histochemistry and Cytochemistry and the Histochemical Society in San Diego, July 25, 1998. The enthusiastic support of the leadership of the Histochemical Society, as well as that of speakers and audiences from Europe, Japan, the United States, and other countries, led us to believe in the need for this book at this time.

Antigen Retrieval Techniques is intended for clinical pathologists, research scientists, technicians, and graduate students who need to practice, standardize and develop the AR technique further in their work. Although the AR technique is a simple method, it is critical to use it in a scientific way, as described in this book.

We made a determined effort to review articles by Medline. It was not easy to collect all relevant publications because the term "antigen retrieval" has not been used consistently or uniformly. This book focuses on practical issues and on the development and application of the AR technique in histology and histopathology (morphology). It ignores similar methods applied to other fields in general immunology or Western blot technology.

We greatly appreciate the efforts of the contributors in writing the various chapters. Although some overlap exists, each chapter provides unique individual knowledge based on the expertise of the author. Some repetition of basic principles may be necessary when authors offer different points of view.

The editors wish to dedicate this book to the memory of Dr. Harold F. Schuknecht (1917–1996), a great teacher, surgeon, and scientist in clinical otology and otopathology, Harvard Medical School, for his excellent guidance and active support early in the development of the AR technique. It would not have been possible to develop the method without his kind help. We are indebted to Drs. Max L. Goodman (1932–1996), Atul K. Bhan, and Ben Z. Pilch and to Bruce Kaylor, technician, from the Department of Pathology, Massachusetts General Hospital, Harvard Medical School. We are also indebted to the Departments of Otolaryngology and Pathology, West China University of Medical Sciences (formerly Sichuan Medical College), Chengdu, China, for training and research over many years. To friends at the BioGenex Laboratories, San Ramon, California, we express our thanks for their help in development of the AR technique in early 1990.

Acknowledgment is made to the University Pathology Associates of the University of Southern California Keck School of Medicine for their support and all individuals working at the Immunohistochemical Lab of Pathology, particularly Dr. Richard J. Cote, Professor of Pathology and Urology, Lillian Young, Sandra Thu, Yan Shi, Donxing Liu, Camela Villajin-Busque, Maung Win, and Drs. S. Ashraf Imam, Nancy Barr, Debra Hawes, Sunanda Chatterjee, and Ram Datar for their help in daily clinical and research work. We wish to express our deep gratitude to The Histochemical Society, in particular Drs. Denis G. Baskin, Allen M. Gown, William L. Stahl, and Stephen W. Carmichael for their encouragement in sponsoring a symposium on AR-IHC in 1998, which greatly assisted the writing of this book. Appreciation is extended to Dr. Randall B. Widelitz for his enthusiastic help in preparing certain figures, and to Florence Miyagawa, Myrna Cisneros, and Rios Olga for their help in preparing manuscripts for this book.

The editors appreciate the active support of Stephen Weaver and Christine McAndrews of BioTechniques Books, Eaton Publishing. We are grateful for permission to reproduce illustrations and data from the *Journal of Histochemistry and Cytochemistry, Journal of Histotechnology, Biotechnic and Histochemistry, Applied Immunohistochemistry and Molecular Morphology, Aurix Nasas Larynx, Cell Vision, and Otolaryngology–Head and Neck Surgery.*

Shan-Rong Shi
Jiang Gu
Clive R. Taylor
May 2000

Contents

Overview: The Antigen Retrieval Technique for Immunohistochemistry: "Think Simple"

Clive R. Taylor[1], Shan-Rong Shi[1], and Jiang Gu[2]

[1]Department of Pathology, University of Southern California Keck School of Medicine, Los Angeles, CA; [2]Department of Biomedical Sciences, University of South Alabama, Mobile, AL, USA

It is our contention that other things being equal, simple techniques are better than complicated ones, for ease of performance, cost effectiveness, and reproducibility or standardization. In the history of scientific technology, in medicine as in other fields, many of the techniques in use today have evolved from an initial "immature" method that paradoxically may be both crude and complex at the same time, to an increasingly more refined approach that enhances performance through superior reagents and more efficient protocols, often employing automation. Typically this evolutionary process proceeds in fits and starts, does not follow a single sequence of thoughts or experiments, and may produce several alternative approaches, some of which, although pursued with great vigor by their respective champions, lead to blind alleys, before a clear winner emerges. The net result ideally fulfills the conditions outlined above (cost effectiveness, ease of performance, and standardization), and typically is simpler and often more elegant. However, the route to a simpler method is not always apparent early in the development of a technology, and often the reduction of complexity must await a better scientific understanding of the overall process, in both theory and practice. When seeking to improve a technology, the guiding philosophy therefore may be "Think simple."

The development of the antigen retrieval (AR) technique exemplifies this philosophy. As described in Chapter 1 of this book, this simple and effective method, just boiling archival deparaffinized tissue sections in water or buffer solution (7), was based on the industry and innovation of a group of scientists who explored the chemical reactions of formalin with proteins half a century ago (3–5). Without the long-neglected contribution of these pioneers, the simple AR concept might never have been developed.

Unfortunately, a number of different terms other than antigen retrieval have been

Antigen Retrieval Techniques
Edited by Shan-Rong Shi, Jiang Gu, and Clive R. Taylor
©2000 Eaton Publishing, Natick, MA

applied in the literature to this basic method, giving rise to a perception that the AR technique is more complicated than it is. These alternative terms have created much confusion, and a certain amount of obfuscation, rendering review of the literature for this book rather difficult. If we subscribe to the philosophy of simplification, we might start with the terminology. In the interest of simplicity we will present our conclusion, ahead of the argument, to spare those who would rather devote their time to information of practical as opposed to semantic value: "At this time, however, any new terminology, unless extremely well founded, seems likely to add confusion and to hamper access to the existing literature" (9). Thus antigen retrieval, having a clear priority, is preferred and used throughout this text.

Other terms, such as heat-induced epitope retrieval (HIER), have been advanced as alternatives in the literature, based as much on personal perception as on scientific reason. However, we recognize that unsubstantiated viewpoints will be encountered as long as we lack detailed scientific understanding of how AR works and indeed how formalin fixation per se works. Within this context, our rationale for the use of the term antigen retrieval is set forth below.

The development of the technique and the term antigen retrieval was based on review of the early biochemical studies on formalin-protein interactions reported by Fraenkel-Conrat and co-workers in the 1940s. It appeared probable to them, as to us, that reversal of the adverse effects of formalin fixation on the utility of molecules as injected antigens (i.e., as vaccines) was based on at least a partial reversal of the chemical modification of protein conformation induced by formalin fixation (discussed in detail in Chapter 1). It seemed logical, therefore, that retrieval (restoration, recovery) of antigenicity of proteins modified (or masked) by fixation in formalin might involve a return of structure toward the prefixation (or unfixed) state, a thought consistent with the general precept that antigen/antibody recognition is dependent on protein conformation (11,12). This concept is less easily applied to the consideration of separate antigenic determinants or epitopes, especially discontinuous epitopes (most antigenic determinants in cells and tissues are discontinuous epitopes), which consist of separated amino acid sequences that are spatially related because of a certain tertiary protein conformation. Restoration of the spatial relationships of amino acids constituting such an epitope only follows restoration of the overall protein conformation or the whole molecule, which arguably constitutes the antigen as a whole, or at least something more than the single epitope alone. In any event, for Fraenkel-Conrat and colleagues in their vaccine studies, this process was by definition restoration of antigenicity, since epitopes, although they can participate in an immune response, cannot induce one (i.e., antigens can serve as vaccines, and epitopes cannot). From this point of view, the term antigen retrieval appears appropriate in terms of historical accuracy and also to give proper precedence to foundation studies of more than half a century ago.

In addition, definitions of the terms antigen, antibody, and epitope (antigenic determinant) have been well documented, and the designation antigen–antibody has been widely used for many years to represent their basic interactions. The term "epitope" "corresponds to a cluster of amino acid residues that binds specifically to the binding site or paratope of an immunoglobulin molecule" or antibody (10). Thus, in contrast to *antigen–antibody*, the term *epitope* correlates with *paratope* rather than antibody. Furthermore, to be unreasonably pedantic (and invite all sorts of informed and uninformed comment) the concept of epitope "is not an intrinsic feature of a protein and does not exist independently of its paratope partner" (10). It follows that an epitope is

Table 1. Terms Used for the Antigen Retrieval Technique[a]

Terms	1966–1995	1995–1999 (August)
Antigen retrieval (AR)	120	221
Antigen unmasking	18	11
Epitope retrieval	3	32
Heat-induced epitope retrieval (HIER)	2[b]	5
Antigen recovery	27[b]	4
Antigen restoration	8[b]	0

[a]Number of Medline entries found.
[b]See discussion in text.

only a functional unit, not an intrinsic defined structural component of the protein—but then, of course, much the same may be argued for the term antigen, which ultimately is defined only by the ability of a molecule to elicit an immune response in an appropriate foreign environment, upon which it earns the title of antigen.

However, there are more practical reasons for preferring the term antigen retrieval. We are of the opinion, for reasons given below, that this term should include non-heating, in addition to the heating, methods. Within this single parameter, the term heat-induced or HIER is overly restrictive and not appropriate. Although HIER has the advantage of specifying the application of heat, it excludes all other approaches toward the issue of restoration of the ability of an antibody to produce a good immunostaining result in a fixed tissue section, with unfortunate results in the performance of literature searches. In general, changing the term antigen retrieval into HIER means changing a reasonable common term into an uncommon term.

The original terminology of AR has entered widespread, almost universal usage, and as such has clearly been accepted by most scientists. Other terms have appeared and have added little to the field, except confusion, as may be demonstrated by the brief survey of Medline given in Table 1.

The two HIER articles published during 1966 to 1995 are confusing for an unexpected reason; they have no connection with either antigens or epitopes but represent the names Mary Hier and Hier et al. (1,2). Thus far we have not encountered AR as an author, although he or she is probably putting pen to paper right now! As for the terms antigen recovery or antigen restoration, most articles in these categories are not related to the AR technique. These terms are used in immunology for a variety of purposes having to do with preparation and recovery of antigens in immunologic systems.

Unfortunately, many articles that do deal with use of the AR technique never mention the term but employ such nonspecific descriptions as microwave treatment. We have found it difficult to recover these articles by computer search, because the key word microwave causes the computer to regurgitate a thousand or more articles, most of which are not relevant. The use of the term antigen retrieval would at least render such articles available by search.

This book builds on the foundation of others; it recounts the latest in a series of endeavors designed to improve the quality and reliability of cell recognition in tissue sections. In a sense, AR rides the latest wave in the development of the art and science of histology, which began more than 100 years ago with the use of biological stains (dyes) and passed through the more specific phase of histochemical detection of enzymes, to the even more specific and more extensive application of immunohistochemical methods, to the beginnings of the age of molecular morphology (8). Throughout all these developments, fixatives and fixation have vexed pathologists, producing unknown alterations of protein structure or enzyme function that have thwarted generations of histochemists and immunohistochemists. Now AR offers some grounds for optimism, with benefits that appear to extend to in situ hybridization methods and into the molecular era.

Although the mechanism of AR-immunohistochemistry is still unclear, the successful application of the AR method has shed light on this issue. It is likely that hydrolysis of cross-linkages resulting from formalin-protein interactions during fixation of tissues may play a key role in understanding this mechanism, as discussed in some detail in Chapter 1. Analysis of the major factors that influence the effectiveness of AR and that are critical for establishing an optimal AR protocol to achieve maximal retrieval is the focus of Chapter 2.

In practice application of the high-temperature AR method shows significant variation in different fields of pathology. The principle fields are reviewed in succeeding chapters: diagnostic cytology (Chapter 3), TdT-mediated dUTP nick-end labeling (TUNEL; Chapter 4), immunoelectron microscopy (Chapter 5), in situ hybridization (Chapter 6), multiple immunostaining (Chapter 7), various specialized applications in the neurosciences (Chapter 8), detection of steroid hormone receptors (Chapter 9), experimental pathology using animal tissues (Chapter 10), demonstration of cell proliferation markers (Chapters 11 and 12), and tumor suppressor genes (Chapter 13). All these chapters are written by experts in their respective fields, each of whom has thereby contributed to the development and/or application of the AR technique. Further development and expanded application may involve even more scientific fields, as described in a recent article concerning enhancement of protein extraction for Western blot analysis from formalin-fixed, paraffin-embedded tissue sections by boiling a thick tissue section (50 µm) in lysis buffer containing 2% sodium dodecyl sulfate for 20 minutes (6). This is an interesting application of the heating AR method.

Combination of the AR technique with other methods of improving immunostaining results (such as enzyme digestion) and signal amplification is considered in Chapters 14 and 15.

The need to improve standardization of routine immunohistochemistry has been a critical issue for more than 20 years. It is easier said than done and is the topic of Chapter 16, which includes some practical approaches to the problem.

The nonheating AR methods (including enzyme digestion used alone or combined with the heating AR method) may be amenable to further development and are described in Chapters 17 and 18.

A summary of the AR technique (including protocols, technical tips, and trouble shooting) is included as an appendix for the reader's use in handling the daily practice of the AR technique.

REFERENCES

1.**Annas, G.J.** 1984. The case of Mary Hier: when substituted judgment becomes sleight of hand. Hastings Center Report *14*:23-25.
2.**D'Angelo, E.J.** 1981. Reversed cerebral asymmetries as a potential risk factor in autism: a reconsideration. Percept. Motor Skills *53*:101-102.
3.**Fraenkel-Conrat, H. and H.S. Olcott.** 1948. Reaction of formaldehyde with proteins. VI. Cross-linking of amino

groups with phenol, imidazole, or indole groups. J. Biol. Chem. *174*:827-843.

4. **Fraenkel-Conrat, H. and H.S. Olcott.** 1948. The reaction of formaldehyde with proteins. V. Cross-linking between amino and primary amide or guanidyl groups. J. Am. Chem. Soc. *70*:2673-2684.

5. **Fraenkel-Conrat, H., B.A. Brandon, and H.S. Olcott.** 1947. The reaction of formaldehyde with proteins. IV. Participation of indole groups. Gramicidin. J. Biol. Chem. *168*:99-118.

6. **Ikeda, K., T. Monden, T. Kanoh, M. Tsujie, H. Izawa, A. Haba, T. Ohnishi, M. Sekimoto, N. Tomita, H. Shiozaki, and M. Monden.** 1998. extraction and analysis of diagnostically useful proteins from formalin-fixed, paraffin-embedded tissue sections. J. Histochem. Cytochem. *46*:397-403.

7. **Shi, S.-R., R.J. Cote, and C.R. Taylor.** 1997. Antigen retrieval immunohistochemistry: past, present, and future. J. Histochem. Cytochem. *45*:327-343.

8. **Taylor, C.R. and R.J. Cote (Eds.).** 1994. Immunomicroscopy: A Diagnostic Tool for the Surgical Pathologist. 2nd ed. W.B. Saunders Co., Philadelphia.

9. **Taylor, C.R., S.-R. Shi, and R.J. Cote.** 1996. Antigen retrieval for immunohistochemistry. Status and need for greater standardization. Appl. Immunohistochem. *4*:144-166.

10. **Van Regenmortel, M.H.V.** 1994. The recognition of proteins and peptides by antibodies, p. 277-300. *In* C.J. van Oss and M.H.V. van Regenmortel (Eds.), Immunochemistry. Marcel Dekker, Inc., New York.

11. **Wilson, J.E.** 1991. The use of monoclonal antibodies and limited proteolysis in elucidation of structure-function relationships in proteins, p. 207-250. *In* C.H. Suelter (Ed.), Methods of Biochemical Analysis. John Wiley & Sons, New York.

12. **Wong, S.S. (Ed.).** 1991. Chemistry of Protein Conjugation and Cross-Linking, p. 1-48. CRC Press, Boca Raton.

Commentary: Immunohistochemistry: A Brief Historical Perspective

Jules M. Elias

Department of Surgery, Oregon Health Sciences University, Portland, OR, USA

This chapter is reprinted with permission from *The Journal of Histotechnology*, Special Issue: Diagnostic and Prognostic Immunopathology 22:163-167.

THE FIRST WAVE: TINCTORIAL STAINS

The past 50 years have witnessed the emergence of a remarkable diversity of methods for imparting color to particular cell and tissue elements. The history of staining begins with the development of general staining techniques that facilitated morphologic distinctions among different tissue components (e.g., nucleus vs. cytoplasm). The first dyes used by microscopists as stains were all natural dyestuffs. Best known among these is hematoxylin, sometimes alone or more often with the fluorescent dye eosin as a counterstain. An array of general tissue stains using hematoxylin was developed by Weigert, Heidenhain, Delafield, Harris, and Mayer at the end of the 19th century. The hematoxylin-eosin combination, commonly referred to as the H&E stain, is the most used general stain in surgical pathology. To this day, the periodic acid-Schiff stain, originally developed for demonstrating neutral mucopolysaccharides, is probably the most used special stain in surgical pathology. It has been used for classifying lipids and acute leukemia, for differentiating adenocarcinoma from squamous cell carcinoma, and for identifying certain fungi, fibrin, and Russell bodies, to name but a few of its applications. It was during this time that connective tissue stains more specialized in their application than H&E were developed. Although H&E is, in a sense, a special stain, the introduction of other tinctorial stains for the identification of tissue macromolecules was truly the first wave of special techniques embraced by histologists and pathologists. The number of special stains currently in use is in the thousands. Although the biochemical basis of most tinctorial methods was not understood, they were highly reproducible and provided a means of identifying carbohydrates, lipids, nucleic acids, pigments, metals, and microorganisms. The approach is now a common component in surgical pathology.

Antigen Retrieval Techniques
Edited by Shan-Rong Shi, Jiang Gu, and Clive R. Taylor
©2000 Eaton Publishing, Natick, MA

THE SECOND WAVE: HISTOENZYMOLOGY

In 1939, Gomori (15) and Takamatsu (25) simultaneously introduced a staining method for nonspecific alkaline phosphatase that launched a branch of histochemistry termed histoenzymology. Histoenzymology ushered in the second wave of special stains. The principle is simple. Frozen tissue sections are incubated at 37°C in a medium containing an appropriate substrate, and the released hydrolytic products are captured by heavy metal salts and deposited at sites of enzyme activity. Unlike tinctorial stains (except vital stains) that perform in routinely fixed tissue, histoenzymology, because it is based on the functional integrity of the enzyme of interest, demands the use of unfixed or mildly fixed fresh tissue sections. This second wave of special stains gave rise to the greatest number of publications in scientific and medical journals during the 1960s and 1970s. Histoenzymology was a remarkable achievement, as prior to this only biochemical measurement of serum enzymes was possible. However, it became immediately apparent that to achieve success in this field, the pathologist would have to have knowledge of both biochemistry and histochemistry. The study of the histochemical activity of an enzyme must be based on the properties of the enzyme that have been disclosed in detail by biochemical enzymology. Histoenzymology would eventually prove to be essential to modern hematologists and neuropathologists for the diagnosis of leukemia and skeletal muscle fiber typing, respectively (5,28).

Only a futurist could have foreseen that histoenzymology would eventually provide the basis for several major technologic advances, in particular, immunohistochemistry (IHC) and the first generation of molecular stains, in situ hybridization, and the polymerase chain reaction. In this setting, histoenzymology would be used to report the location of immune complexes or molecular probes in routine paraffin sections.

Interestingly, IHC provided another approach to histoenzymology based on the production of antibodies to particular enzymes, IHC users could expect to locate enzymes in routine paraffin sections (29). However, the use of IHC for enzyme detection is based on the integrity of the antigenicity of the enzyme, whereas classical histoenzymology is dependent on maintaining the integrity of the active site of the enzyme. Thus, IHC is not practical for measuring functional enzyme activity.

THE THIRD WAVE: IMMUNOHISTOCHEMISTRY

Histoenzymology provided a detection system for the third wave of special stains, namely, IHC. The ability to label antibodies directed against particular proteins with enzymes that can be visualized by ordinary brightfield microscopy has made IHC just another special stain in the eyes of the pathologist. As techniques for monoclonal antibody production improved, the number of specific antibodies increased logarithmically. This caused a quantum leap in the armamentarium of special stains available to the surgical pathologist. Stains for virtually any protein could be developed, predicated on the ability to produce specific antibodies directed against a particular protein. With the introduction of IHC, the practice of pathology would never be the same. The third wave of special techniques was truly a Toffler wave of immense proportions that continues to widen the horizons of the pathologist.

It was a seminal paper by Coons et al. in 1942, describing an immunofluorescence technique for detecting cellular antigens in tissue sections, that launched this third wave of special stains (7). The fluorescent antibody method provided, for the first time, a method for the specific identification of cells according to their antigenic makeup or cellular products. The procedure was highly successful in some areas of pathology and continues to be used in the study of renal and skin diseases (10,26). However, the need for fresh frozen sections and the concomitant poor morphologic details did little to enhance its popularity among surgical pathologists. Twenty-five years later, a revolution was launched with the simultaneous introduction of a peroxidase-labeled antibody method by Nakane (21) and by Avremeas (2). The final color reaction of this enzyme-labeled antibody method was mahogany brown, giving rise to the term "brown revolution." Because immunoperoxidase methods were more compatible with the basic substrates of surgical pathology (namely formalin-fixed, paraffin-embedded tissue specimens) it soon became the most popular marker in IHC. The use of hematoxylin as a counterstain enabled pathologists to use established morphologic criteria in the context of IHC. Immunoenzyme methods were considered to be more sensitive than immunofluorescence, because the fixed ratio of fluorescein to protein (antibody) did not permit amplification of the signal, whereas the enzymatic (peroxidase) reaction could be amplified by increasing the time of development.

The immunoperoxidase method provided the soil for subsequent developments aimed at the "indirect" amplification of the target protein of cells and tissues. The development of the immunoglobulin bridge method by Mason et al. (18) was followed by the more popular peroxidase anti-peroxidase (PAP) method from Sternberger et al. (24), both with multilayers of immunoglobulins used to boost sensitivity by providing a greater number of horseradish peroxidase (HRP) molecules. The latter technique was unique in that HRP was attached to its specific antibody by an antigen (HRP)-antibody (anti-HRP antibody), thereby avoiding the loss of enzyme activity associated with chemical conjugation methods used for HRP-labeled antibody methods. By using multilayers of immunoglobulins, the PAP method increased the sensitivity of IHC significantly while lowering background noise (nonspecific staining). The PAP method dominated IHC for over a decade until the extraordinarily high affinity of avidin for biotin was used to link reactants in multistep staining procedures. The subsequent avidin-biotin complex (ABC) method developed by Hsu et al. (17) was purported to amplify the target to levels greater than all previous immunoenzyme methods. Biotin, a low-molecular-weight vitamin, is easily attached to second-layer antibodies and provides a bridge for the addition of avidin that is chemically conjugated to HRP. Both the PAP method and the ABC method use the location of the peroxidase moiety for detection of the site of the antibody-antigen reaction in the tissue section. Put another way, the amount of protein available for binding by the primary antibody (the ultimate source of increased sensitivity) is not altered by this improvement in IHC.

Just when it was presumed that the limits of target detection sensitivity had been reached, a new innovation in IHC, a tyramine amplification system, was introduced by Adams in 1992 (1). The tyramine method is based on the HRP-catalyzed deposition of biotinylated tyramine at sites of immunoreactivity (4). HRP reacts with hydrogen peroxide and the phenolic moieties of tyramide to produce a quinone-like structure bearing a radical on the C2 group. This intermediate tyramide then binds to electron-rich aromatic amino acids on the sample surface in close proximity to the HRP. As this reaction is very short-lived, deposition occurs only in the location at which it is generated or in immediate proximity to this site. The numerous biotin-conjugated tyramides can be detected with an avidin-conjugate (27). The tyramine method purportedly allowed an increase in sensitivity of up to 1000-fold compared with the ABC proce-

9

dures (20). However, other investigators reported that the tyramine method of target amplification increased sensitivity only in the range of 5-fold to 50-fold (23).

Thus, for several decades, the main focus of IHC research was to devise techniques for the "indirect" amplification of target proteins by means of signal amplification. By increasing the amount of final colored reaction product produced by enzyme reporter molecules, the detection of smaller amounts of target proteins or those that are weakly expressed was possible. An increase in the number of HRP reporter molecules was looked on as the best means of increasing IHC sensitivity. Greater amounts of enzyme label was the focus of the developers of the bridge and PAP methods, as well as of the avidin-biotin methods. The tyramine-HRP method, described as the catalyzed reporter deposition technique (CARD), also used signal amplification to increase IHC sensitivity; a hapten (e.g., biotin) is deposited that, in turn, serves as the nidus for avidin-conjugate (HRP) binding. It is the efficiency of hapten deposition that boosts signal amplification to new heights. Because both specific and nonspecific (background) IHC signals are greatly amplified with CARD amplification it is essential that appropriate positive and negative controls be used to aid in the interpretation of staining.

ANTIGEN RESTORATION

Over the past 50 years, investigators have pursued signal amplification as the best means to increase the sensitivity of IHC. Target amplification was not given due consideration because of the protein denaturing effects of formalin fixation. However, lurking in the background was the knowledge that the denaturing effects of formalin fixation could be reversed by various treatments (10). Simply bathing deparaffinized sections in a cold 20% sucrose-saline solution could, over several days, restore a certain amount of immunoreactivity. However, despite these manipulations, the nature of the antigen, in particular its ability to withstand fixation and embedding, continued to interfere with achieving optimal detection of many protein antigens. Consequently, many protocols have been developed to overcome the limitations imposed by aldehyde fixation and by other effects due to exposure to organic solvents and embedding in paraffin. Historically, pretreatment of routine paraffin sections with proteases was used to unmask immunoreactive protein antigens altered by either fixation or embedding media (paraffin or plastic) (8). Enzymatic treatment with proteolytic enzymes presumably breaks the formalin-induced methylene cross-links in the antigenic molecules, restoring their immunoreactivity. The duration of digestion is dependent on the length of time a tissue is exposed to aldehyde fixation, which directly impacts on the extent of antigenic masking of the protein antigen. According to Battifora, "The most common cause of poor reproducibility in immunohistologic studies is the unpredictable alteration of antigenic sites that is introduced by tissue fixation and processing" (3).

Proteolytic enzyme pretreatment is still useful for particular protein antigens and has recently gained new status for use with carbohydrate antigens. Pretreatment of paraffin sections with N-glycanase F to remove N-glycosidically linked oligosaccharides results in a dramatic increase in specificity and intensity of immunogold labeling for sugar moieties present on O-glycosidically linked oligosaccharides (16). Prior to the introduction of enzyme digestion of aldehyde-fixed sections, pretreatment with a 30% sucrose solution or postfixation of formalin-fixed paraffin sections in acetic acid was used to enhance immunoreactivity of certain antigenic determinants (9).

Early attempts to use enzyme digestion to restore the antigenicity of protein targets reversing the denaturing effects of chemical fixation in neutral buffered formaldehyde (NBF) were not widely appreciated. Since overfixation of tissue in NBF causes formation of excess aldehyde cross-links that mask proteins, methods that unmask these proteins would "directly" amplify the signal. Isolated reports in the 1970s indicated that proteolytic digestion could unmask immunoreactive sites altered by NBF fixation (6,9). Enzyme digestion schemes that were suitable to particular proteins were developed. It soon became apparent that not all proteins benefit from protease digestion, which could actually lower immunoreactivity of particular proteins. Others showed that pretreatment of sections in chloroform was more effective than protease digestion for the demonstration of particular membrane antigens (11). Although other approaches toward restoration of antigenicity were examined, proteolytic enzyme digestion was considered the state of the art for restoring immunoreactivity for over a decade.

At present, IHC procedures are regarded as the method of choice for solving most diagnostic problems in surgical pathology. As with all other technical innovations, there are pitfalls and limitations associated with IHC. A significant limitation is that small amounts of antigens may not be detectable, particularly after prolonged formalin fixation. This could severely limit retrospective studies (e.g., autopsy specimens) that employ newly developed antibodies. At present, the most widely used antigen retrieval technique in IHC for diagnostic pathology is high-temperature microwave heating of sections. In 1991, Shi and coworkers (22) introduced antigen retrieval systems that employed high-temperature microwave treatment in heavy metal solutions as a means of overcoming the deleterious effects of formaldehyde fixation. The use of high temperature to undo the masking effects of aldehyde interaction with tissue proteins caused a dramatic change in the attitude of users of IHC. Increases in sensitivity could now be achieved by raising the amount of available target to new heights, thereby significantly lowering the amount of primary antibody needed to form in situ immune complexes. Thus, not only was sensitivity increased but the specificity was increased as well, as the risk of nonspecific background staining and/or biological cross-reactivity with shared epitopes was greatly diminished by using highly diluted primary antibodies. IHC staining reactions with many antibodies benefit from pretreatment of sections with high temperature using a variety of heating devices, including microwaves, autoclaves, steamers, or pressure cookers (19). Enzymatic digestion is ineffective in restoring overfixation-caused loss of vimentin immunoreactivity but is extremely enhanced by microwave irradiation. Nonetheless, for particular antigens, enzymatic treatment is still desirable. Various investigators combined enzyme digestion with microwave treatment to improve immunoreactivity further above that of either approach used separately (14).

Lack of standardization continues to hamper IHC (13). Conceptually, in the absence of biochemical analysis, positive IHC staining reflects only the presence of the "putative" antigen of interest. Assuming that reliable positive controls exhibit an acceptable reaction, it is difficult to interpret negative IHC staining in a test section. This result may simply be a reflection of the inability of the primary antibody to reach its antigen binding site. The coupling of the antibody to the epitope of the antigen of interest relies on the maintenance of the three-dimensional structural integrity of the antigen. The denaturation of proteins by aldehyde-based fixatives alters the structural integrity of these antigenic epitopes.

Nonspecific staining can render interpretation of IHC results difficult. Classically, inconsistencies of IHC results have been attributed to nonspecific reactions due to (*i*) nonspecific binding of antibodies and reagents, (*ii*) cross-reacting natural antibodies, and (*iii*) the existence of the same or similar epitopes on different antigens (biologic cross-reactivity). These inconsistencies of IHC results were detected in both frozen and paraffin sections, but the complete or partial loss of IHC staining due to inter-molecular and intramolecular cross-linkages of tissue proteins after exposure to alde-hyde-containing fixatives is limited to the latter. The early observation that unfixed cryostat sections of fresh frozen tissue were necessary for IHC staining of some anti-gens, as particular proteins were partially or completely ablated in formaldehyde-fixed paraffin-embedded sections, set the stage for future efforts to overcome this seri-ous limitation. The use of antigen restoration techniques, often in combination with protease digestion, has had a dramatic positive impact on the limits of IHC sensitivi-ty. In effect, the use of both ends of the sensitivity spectrum to increase sensitivity (signal and target amplification) has indeed brought forth a new level of interest in IHC. It is currently the major special stain used in surgical pathology.

SUMMARY

What began as a spectrum of tinctorial techniques to introduce color into biologic material followed by microscopic observation has not changed with the development of histoenzymology, IHC, and molecular stains. Each of the subsequent staining waves was designed for the easy detection of a final colored reaction product at the anatomic site of interest. Each subsequent wave enlarged the number of specific chemical groupings or specific compounds that could be demonstrated in routine paraffin sections, while at the same time increasing signal amplification. It was the work of Shi and coworkers in developing antigen restoration methods that finally attacked the amplification of the target. The use of antigen resortation techniques, often in combination with protease digestion, has had a dramatic impact on the per-ceived limits of IHC sensitivity. In effect, the use of both signal and target amplifica-tion methods had, indeed, brought a new level of interest to surgical pathology. No longer is overfixation in aldehyde-containing fixatives a limiting factor in the demon-stration of most tissue proteins. If present trends continue, IHC will surpass tinctori-al stains in usage and will become the major special stain used in surgical pathology.

With increased sensitivity of IHC, the responsibility of users of these methods in a clinical setting increases. Technologic advances notwithstanding, it is essential that pathologists and histologists alike become thoroughly familiar with the biology of the disease entity being studied. Knowing what biologic questions to ask will make more efficient use of these stains in the clinical setting. Just as with histoenzymology, the use of IHC in the clinical arena demands an understanding of the biology of the pro-teins detected; for example, the use of antibodies to the oncoprotein p53 to make prognostic predictions of patient outcome requires a full understanding of the role of this protein in the biology of disease (12). With the introduction of in situ molecular methods that depend on the use of IHC enzyme detection systems for the location of molecular probes, we are reminded once again that history, given enough time, will eventually repeat itself.

REFERENCES

1.**Adams, J.C.** 1992. Biotin amplification of biotin and horseradish peroxidase signals in histochemical stains. J. Histochem. Cytochem. *40*:577-580.

2.**Avremeas, S.** 1971. Coupling of enzymes to proteins with glutaraldehyde. Use of the conjugates for the detection of antigens and antibodies. Immunohistochemistry 6:394.

3.**Battifora, H.** 1991. Assessment of antigen damage in immunohistochemistry. Am. J. Clin. Pathol. 96:669.

4.**Bobrow, M.N., K.J. Shaughnessy, and G.J. Litt.** 1989. Catalyzed reported deposition, a novel method of signal amplification. Application to immunoassays. J. Immunol. Methods 125:279.

5.**Bonilla, E. and D.L. Schotland.** 1970. Histochemical diagnosis of muscle phosphofructokinase deficiency. Arch. Neurol. 22:8.

6.**Brozman, M.** 1978. Immunohistochemical analyses of formaldehyde and trypsin- or pepsin-treated material. Acta Histochem. 63:251.

7.**Coons, A.H., H.J. Creech, R.N. Jones, and E. Berliner.** 1942. The demonstration of pneumococcal antigen in tissues by the use of fluorescent antibody. J. Immunol. 45:159.

8.**Denk, G.S. and E.H. Beutner.** 1974. Effect of formaldehyde, glutaraldehyde and sucrose on the tissue antigenicity. Int. Arch. Allergy 47:562.

9.**Denk, H., T. Radaszkiewcz, and E. Weirich.** 1977. Pronase pretreatment of tissue sections enhances sensitivity of the unlabeled antibody technique (PAP). J. Immunol. Methods 15:163.

10.**Elias, J.M.** 1982. The renal biopsy. *In* Principles and Techniques in Diagnostic Histopathology. Developments in Immunohistochemistry and Enzyme Histochemistry. Noyes Publications, Park Ridge, NJ.

11.**Elias, J.M.** 1990. Immunohistopathology: A Practical Approach to Diagnosis. ASCP Press, Chicago.

12.**Elias, J.M.** 1999. The p53 dilemma—a case of too much too soon? J. Histotechnol. (In press).

13.**Elias, J.M., A.M. Gown, R.M. Nakamura, D.C. Wibur, G.E. Herman, E.S. Jaffe, H. Battifora, and D.J. Brigati.** 1989. Special report: quality control in immunohistochemistry. Am. J. Clin. Pathol. 92:836-843.

14.**Elias, J.M., B. Rosenberg, M. Margiotta, and C. Kutcher.** 1999. Antigen restoration of MIB-1 immunoreactivity in breast cancer: combined use of enzyme predigestion and low temperature for improved measurement of proliferation indexes. J. Histotechnol. (In press).

15.**Gomori, G.** 1939. Microtechnical demonstration of phosphatase in the tissue sections. Proc. Soc. Exp. Biol. Med. 42:23.

16.**Guhl, B., M. Ziak, and J. Roth.** 1998. Unconventional antigen retrieval for carbohydrate and protein antigens. Histochem. Cell Biol. 110:603.

17.**Hsu, S.M., L. Raine, and H. Fanger.** 1981. Use of avidin-biotin-peroxidase complex (ABC) in immunoperoxidase techniques: a comparison between ABC and unlabeled antibody (PAP) procedures. J. Histochem. Cytochem. 29:577-580.

18.**Mason, T.E., R.F. Phifer, S.S. Spicer, R.A. Swallow, and R.B. Dreskin.** 1969. An immunoglobulin-enzyme bridge method for localizing tissue antigens. J. Histochem. Cytochem. 17:563-569.

19.**McNicol, A.M. and J.A. Richmond.** 1998. Optimizing immunohistochemistry: antigen retrieval and signal amplification. Histopathology 12:97.

20.**Merz, H., R. Malisius, S. Mannweiler, et al.** 1995. Immunomax. A maximized immunohistochemical method for the retrieval and enhancement of hidden antigens. Lab. Invest. 73:149-156.

21.**Nakane, P.K.** 1968. Simultaneous localization of multiple tissue antigens using the peroxidase-labeled antibody method: a study on pituitary glands of rat. J. Histochem. Cytochem. 16:557-560.

22.**Shi, S.R., M.E. Key, and K.L. Kalra.** 1991. Antigen retrieval in formalin-fixed, paraffin-embedded tissues: an enhancement method for immunohistochemical staining based on microwave oven heating of tissue sections. J. Histochem. Cytochem. 39:741.

23.**Speel, E.J.M., A.H.N. Hopman, and P. Komminoth.** 1999. Amplification methods to increase the sensitivity of in situ hybridization: play card (s). J. Histochem. Cytochem. 47:281.

24.**Sternberger, L.A., P.H. Hardy, J.J. Cuculis, and H.G. Meyer.** 1970. The unlabeled antibody enzyme method of immunocytochemistry. Preparation and properties of soluble antigen-antibody complex (horseradish peroxidase-antihorseradish peroxidase) and its use in identification of spirochetes. J. Histochem. Cytochem. 18:315-333.

25.**Takamatsu, H.** 1939. Histologische und biochemische studien uber die phosphatase, histochemische untersuchungsmethodik der phosphatase und deren vereilung in verschiedenden chemische untersuchhungsmethodik der phosphatase und deren vereilung in verschiedenen organen und geweben. Trns. Soc. Pathol. Jpn. 29:492.

26.**Taylor, C.R.** 1983. Immunoenzyme techniques and their application to diagnostic studies. Ann. NY Acad. Sci. 420:115.

27.**Totos, G., A. Thakhi, C. Hauser-Kronberger, and R.R. Tubbs.** 1997. Catalyzed reporter deposition: a new era in molecular and immunomorphology-Nanogold-Silver staining and colorimetric detection and protocols. Cell Vision 4:433.

28.**Yam, L.T., C.Y. Li, and W.H. Crosby.** Cytochemical identification of monocytes and granulocytes. Am. J. Clin. Pathol. 55:283.

29.**Yaziji, H., A.J. Janckila, S.C. Lear, et al.** 1995. Immunohistochemical detection of tartrate-resistant acid phosphatase in non-hematopoietic human tissues. Am. J. Clin. Pathol. 104:397.

Section I

Basic Information

Development of the Antigen Retrieval Technique: Philosophical and Theoretical Bases

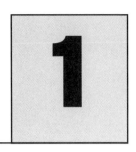

Shan-Rong Shi[1], Jiang Gu[2], Julio F. Turrens[2], Richard J. Cote[1], and Clive R. Taylor[1]

[1]*Department of Pathology, University of Southern California Keck School of Medicine, Los Angeles, CA, and* [2]*Department of Biomedical Sciences, University of South Alabama, Mobile, AL, USA*

INTRODUCTION

The observation of natural phenomena, both macroscopically and (more recently) microscopically, has long provided the basis for studies of living organisms. From the beginning, a major aim of biomedical research has been the correlation of structure with function, in order to understand how organs, tissues, and cells work under various conditions and when they are normal versus abnormal. The development of morphologic methods has been closely correlated with developments in other basic sciences, especially chemistry and physics. In particular, the term morphology increasingly has been used to mean microscopic observation, with greater use of the light microscope and the introduction of the microtome and biologic stains in the 19th century. The discovery of cells was followed by the beginning of histology (Malpighi, 1628–1694), and the publication of *Cellularpathologie* by Rudolf Virchow in 1860 may be regarded as the beginning of modern "morphology" (81). In the 20th century, morphology was further revolutionized by advances in physics (resulting in ultrastractural morphology by electron microscopy), chemistry (resulting in histochemistry and enzyme histochemistry), immunology (resulting in immunohistochemistry), and molecular biology (resulting in in situ hybridization) (Figure 1).

In light of the rapid advances in contemporary morphology, several new terms, (functional, analytical, and molecular morphology) have been introduced, signifying the potential to gain deeper insight into structure–function correlations. The unique

Antigen Retrieval Techniques
Edited by Shan-Rong Shi, Jiang Gu, and Clive R. Taylor
©2000 Eaton Publishing, Natick, MA

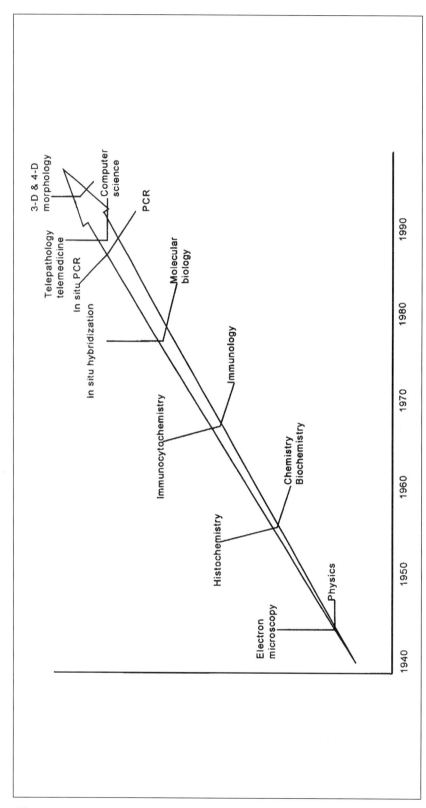

Figure 1. Diagram illustrating the characteristics of advances in morphologic science. The lower right half below the arrow bar describes the major developments in other disciplines. The upper left half presents the corresponding developments of morphologic techniques that were derived from the other scientific disciplines. The years are presented in chronologic order by the horizontal line. In summary, major advancements in other scientific disciplines have led to invention of new morphologic techniques. Each new technique in turn results in a wave of morphologic discoveries because of the visualization of new elements or new prospects of a known element. Reprinted with permission from Reference 23a.

advantage of morphology is the ability to localize sharply natural phenomena, normal or abnormal, into exact compartments of cells or tissues, providing insight for studies of functions of cells and tissues and contributing to an understanding of the mechanisms of diseases. The basic philosophy of the morphologist is not only that "seeing is believing" but also that "seeing is the source of thinking," which is in essence the approach used by an experienced pathologist to make an accurate diagnosis by histopathologic observation. In an editorial, Brigati (6) offered a negative response to the question, "Will the histopathology laboratory surrender its paraffin blocks to the molecular biologist?" and in counterpoint predicted that "The day is coming when someone somewhere will see one point mutation in a cell with a light microscope."

Immunohistochemistry (IHC) has a long history, from the moment that Coons et al. (11) developed an immunofluorescence technique to detect bacteria in 1941. However, immunofluorescence techniques did not lend themselves well to the examination of routine hematoxylin and eosin (H&E) formalin paraffin sections, and 30 years passed without the method finding broad diagnostic application. In the early 1970s, extensive efforts were made to render immunoperoxidase methods applicable to routine formalin-fixed, paraffin-embedded tissues, through a series of technical developments including increasingly sensitive detection systems, and the later additional various pretreatments prior to the immunostaining procedure (77,78).

The philosophy underlying the application of IHC for routine formalin-fixed tissues was emphasized by Taylor et al. (80) in 1981. However, early IHC methods, including initial unmasking procedures such as the enzymatic digestion, while widely applied, failed to give satisfactory IHC staining of many antigens, as pointed out by Leong et al. (34). A particular drawback of enzymatic digestion was that it was difficult to standardize and control the optimal digestion conditions for individual tissue sections when they were stained with different antibodies. These difficulties in standardization provided a powerful incentive for the development of a new technique, the requirements being that it should be more widely applicable and easier to use than enzymatic digestion. In addition, any new method should enhance immunohistochemical staining of routine paraffin sections in a reproducible and reliable manner. The application of IHC to routinely processed tissues represented a new era for the demonstration of antigens in the types of processed tissues that abound in university pathology laboratories, thereby allowing pathologists to correlate immunologic findings directly with traditional cytologic and histologic criteria (79). It also provided the impetus for development of an antigen retrieval (AR) technique by another of the authors. The first seeds in the development of a retrieval approach for routinely processed celloidin-embedded human temporal bone sections sprouted in the early 1980s, when Shi studied under Dr. Schuknecht's guidance at the Eastern National Temporal Bone Bank in Boston. Subsequent attempts to perform IHC study on archival human temporal bone sections were actively supported by Dr. Shuknecht in the early 1990s.

A key question for the development of the AR technique was whether the cross-linkages of protein caused by formalin fixation are reversible or irreversible. The answer was in essence already available in the literature through the studies of Fraenkel-Conrat and co-workers published in the1940s (17–19). Their work indicated that hydrolysis of cross-linkages between formalin and protein may be limited under usual laboratory conditions by certain amino acid side chains, such as imidazol and indol. However, these cross-linkages could be disrupted by high-temperature heating (above 100°C) or strong alkaline treatment. These observations formed the basis for the development of AR in both heating and nonheating methods, the latter involving immersion of celloidin-embedded human temporal bone sections in sodium hydroxide-methanol solutions prior to immunostaining (56,57). The high-temperature heating AR technique has since been adopted universally as a simple, effective, and reliable pretreatment for routine IHC in surgical pathology as well as analytical morphology (5,7,9,10,12,21,35,62,71,72,82,84,88). The following description focuses on several key points of development of the AR technique on the basis of chemical modification of protein conformation.

FORMALIN FIXATION

As a fixative for tissue, formalin is prepared from a commercial formalin concentrate (100% formalin), which is a 37% to 40% solution of formaldehyde (HCHO), by dilution to a 10% solution, i.e., 3.7% to 4% formaldehyde. Ferdinand Blum recommended the use of formalin fixation, considering it superior to other methods available at the time (1893) (16,54). Formalin has several advantages over alcohol and other precipitative (non-cross-linking) fixatives, particularly the superior preservation of morphologic detail. In marked contrast to the prevailing scientific consensus prior to 1974 (77), many antigens are in fact demonstrable in routine paraffin sections in spite of (or perhaps because of!) formalin fixation. Quick and effective fixation of fresh tissue is necessary if antigens are to be fixed in situ, prior to autolytic changes. Formalin-induced modification of protein, a special form of cross-linking (90), is an efficient process to retain an antigen in its original location of tissue, as exemplified by immunohistochemical detection of estradiol in paraffin tissue sections (29). Although the exact mechanism of formalin fixation is still unknown, the chemical process leading to protein fixation by formalin appears to involve multiple reactions among formaldehyde, various amino acid residues, and even peptide bonds. To understand the complexity of this process, one must first look at the variety of reactions in which aldehydes and ketones may participate.

Chemistry of Aldehydes

Aldehydes and ketones are organic compounds in which a carbon atom (C) is covalently bound to oxygen (O) through two bonds (carbonyl group). Since O atoms tend to attract electrons, the presence of a double bond between C and O displaces the electrons on the C atom toward the O atom. The loss of electron density creates an area of positive charge density on the C atom, generated by the positive charges in the nucleus, and therefore makes this C atom a target for reactions termed nucleophilic additions. The simplest of these reactions involves the reversible hydration of a carbonyl to form a gem-diol (C atom with two hydroxyl groups bound to it). In the case of formaldehyde, the product is called methylene glycol (reaction 1):

$$H_2C = O + H_2O \leftrightarrow H_2C(OH)_2 \qquad [1]$$

The proportion of molecules in the gem-diol configuration varies with the chemical nature of the aldehyde or ketone. In the case of diluted formaldehyde (10% formalin, a 4% solution of formaldehyde), practically all molecules are present as gem-diols instead of free aldehydes. A similar reaction to that shown in reaction [1] leads to the formation of hemiacetals (reaction 2) or hemiketals (reaction 3) when an alcohol reacts with an aldehyde or a ketone, respectively:

$$RHC = O + R'OH \leftrightarrow RH\ C \diagup^{OH}_{\diagdown OR'} \qquad [2]$$

$$RRC = O + R'OH \leftrightarrow RR\ C \diagup^{OH}_{\diagdown OR'} \qquad [3]$$

The formation of hemiketals or hemiacetals may involve different reactive groups within a single molecule as it is observed in the formation of cyclic derivatives from sugars in water (e.g., glucose, Figure 2). In the case of sugars, the tendency to form these cyclic structures is so strong that in most cases the proportion of molecules in the openchain form is less than 1%.

At acidic pH these hemiacetals and hemiketals may continue reacting with alcohols producing acetals and ketals (for aldehydes and ketones, respectively) by forming ether derivatives through a reaction in which the second alcohol group also participates (reactions 4 and 5):

$$RHC = O + 2\ R'OH \leftrightarrow RH\ C \diagup^{OR'}_{\diagdown OR'} + H_2O \qquad [4]$$

$$RRC = O + 2\ R'OH \leftrightarrow RR\ C \diagup^{OR'}_{\diagdown OR'} + H_2O \qquad [5]$$

Another common reaction involving carbonyl-containing molecules is the formation of imine-derivatives or Schiff bases through their reaction with primary amines. In most cases, unless followed by complex intramolecular rearrangements, these reactions are also fully reversible (reaction 6).

$$RHC = O + R'NH_2 \leftrightarrow RHC = NR' + H_2O \qquad [6]$$

An example of Schiff base formation that is of clinical relevance is the glycosylation of basic residues in hemoglobin (HbAIC), as observed in diabetic patients. In this case, excessive levels of blood glucose favor its reaction with amino groups from amino acid side chains (i.e., lysine). The imines resulting from this reaction are rearranged (Amadori rearrangement) into stable adducts that become useful markers of hyperglycemia over time.

Another reaction that is relevant to the chemistry of protein fixation involves the interaction of the carbonyl-containing compounds formaldehyde and secondary amines. Known as the Mannich reaction, this is a more complicated, multistep interaction, which involves first a reaction between formaldehyde and an amine to produce an iminium ion (reaction 7):

$$H_2C = O + RR'NH_2^+ \leftrightarrow RR'HN^+ - CH_2OH \leftrightarrow H_2C = N^+RR' + H_2O \qquad [7]$$
$$\text{iminium ion}$$

In a second part of the reaction, the iminium ion may react with another carbonyl-containing molecule to form an intermediate product. For the second reaction to occur, the carbonyl-containing molecule must be in an enol configuration (reaction 8):

$$RC = OCH_3 \leftrightarrow R - COH = CH_2 \qquad [8]$$
$$\text{(ketone)} \qquad \text{(enol)}$$

In the final step of the Mannich reaction, the iminium ion (reaction 7) and the enol (reaction 8) react together to produce a stable product (reaction 9) (Figure 3):

$$H_2C = N^+RR' + R - COH = CH_2 \leftrightarrow RC = O - CH_2CH_2NRR' + H^+ \qquad [9]$$

Possible Reactions between Formaldehyde and Proteins

The amino acid side chains in proteins include many groups that may react with aldehydes or ketones in reactions similar to those mentioned above. For example, several basic amino acids contain primary amines (i.e., lysine), imidazol groups (histidine), and guanidinium groups (arginine). Other amino acids such as serine and tyrosine contain alcohol groups. Other reactive groups include the carbonyls of amides, such as those observed in peptide bonds and in the side chains of glutamine and asparagine. Another important carbonyl is also found in the amino acid tyrosine, which is actually an enol in equilibrium with its ketone configuration (Figure 4).

With this wide variety of potential reactive components, it is difficult to predict the exact products of the interaction of formalin with a tissue containing a multiplicity of proteins (amino acid chains). For example, serine could react with formaldehyde to produce hemiacetals (Figure 5). Lysine would react, forming Schiff bases (50). Amides and guanidyl derivatives become more reactive with formaldehyde in the presence of primary amines, suggesting the participation of a Mannich mechanism (18). Therefore, it is difficult to predict whether the reaction between formaldehyde with even a single amino acid such as lysine will: *(i)* produce a Schiff base (Figure 6A), *(ii)* form a bridge between lysine and serine (Figure 6C), or *(iii)* produce a cross-linked derivative with groups in the peptide bond (Figure 6D); tissues contain numerous lysine groups (Figure 6B), as well as numerous other amino acids.

In summary, although a vast amount of literature exists on the subject of protein modification by formaldehyde, there is no clear consensus as to which are the predominant molecular species resulting from the fixation of proteins in tissues by formaldehyde (50). However, there is no doubt that some of the cross-linked adducts are very stable and remain irreversibly changed even after extensive washing (at room

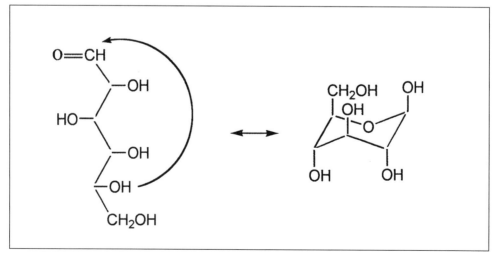

Figure 2. Spontaneous conversion of glucose to a hemiacetal.

temperature), while others revert under varying conditions to free formaldehyde and the amino acid (50).

Cross-linking: a special form of chemical modification. As described, the exact chemical reactions of formalin-induced modification of protein during fixation of tissue are very complicated and still unknown. Nevertheless, it is generally accepted that cross-linking between protein end groups is the essential feature of formalin fixation. In this context, cross-linking may be regarded as a special form of chemical modification of protein (90) and may be defined as a process involving the joining of two molecular components by covalent or other bonds, achieved by the use of cross-linking reagents, such as tissue fixatives.

The basic chemical reactions in the process of tissue fixation have been divided into two stages: the primary reaction is an addition reaction between an amine and an aldehyde (e.g., formalin) or ketone (e.g., acetone) [formaldehyde at its regular concentration in water (4%) occurs as a methylene glycol—$CH_2 (OH)_2$—as well as part free HCHO, and reacts with primary amino groups such that $R\text{-}NH_2 + HCHO \rightarrow R\text{-}NH\text{-}CH_2OH$], followed by a secondary condensation reaction as follows: $R\text{-}NH\text{-}CH_2OH + H_2N\text{-}CO\text{-}R' \rightarrow R\text{-}NH\text{-}CH_2\text{-}NH\text{-}CO\text{-}R' + H_2O$.

As stated above, both aldehydes and ketones are carbonyl compounds that can

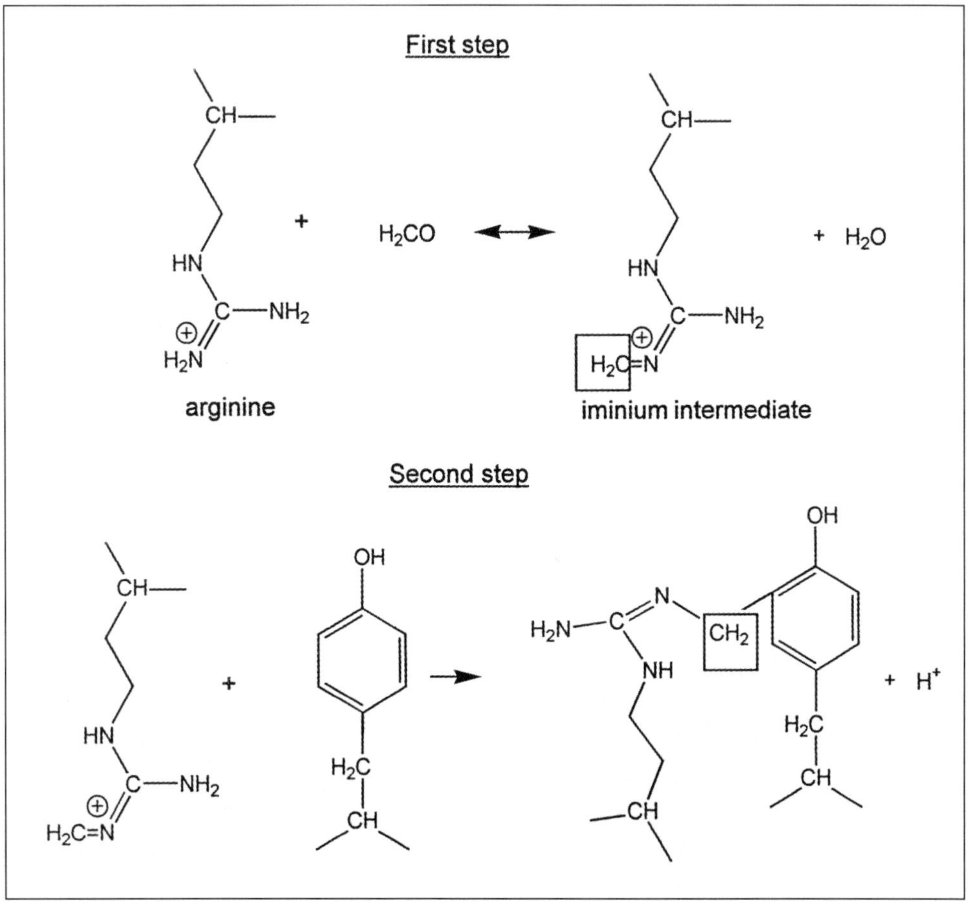

Figure 3. Mannich reaction among arginine, formaldehyde, and tyrosine.

react with the amino groups of proteins to form Schiff bases (reaction 6) (90). This type of reaction of acetone may be used to explain the beneficial effects of AR-IHC for those tissues fixed in fixatives other than formalin (e.g., in acetone) (21,49).

In simple terms, while not proved, it seems most likely that the chemical reaction of proteins and formaldehyde in tissue will follow basically the same pattern demonstrated in test tubes, providing a potentially useful avenue for future studies of the effects of fixation and its reversal upon antigenicity.

FEATURES OF FORMALIN FIXATION

Time, Temperature, and pH Dependence: Clock Reaction

Numerous studies have demonstrated that formalin fixation is a slow process, measured in hours for the usual tissue block; for this reason it has been termed a clock reaction. The slow process of protein-formaldehyde reaction may result from several conditions:

1. Formaldehyde in solution in water is readily hydrated to form a glycol called methylene glycol [$CH_2(OH)_2$], and cross-link formation may rely on a reconversion of methylene glycol to formaldehyde, because the primary covalent chemical reaction of fixation depends on free formaldehyde being present (16).
2. Complete formalin fixation also requires that the secondary condensation reaction occur, and this is a variable, complex, and time-, pH-, and temperature-dependent process.
3. There are also the simple but important physical limitations of the size of the tissue block, the tissue density (permeability), and the rate of penetration of the formalin solution, all of which vary.

Fox et al. (16) investigated this clock reaction based on fixation of frozen sections of rat kidney by ^{14}C formaldehyde. They found that formladehyde binding to tissue

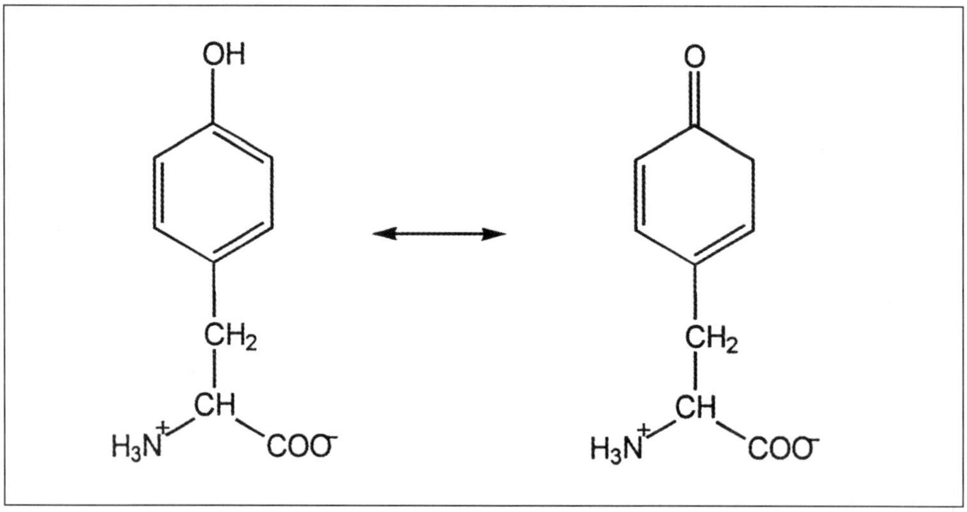

Figure 4. Two possible configurations of the amino acid tyrosine. Although the aromatic ring stabilizes the alcohol configuration, this structure is in a dynamic equilibrium called tautomerization with the ketone form. The ketone and enol form are known as tautomers.

sections increased with time until the maximum (equilibrium) was reached. The time required to reach equilibrium was shorter (18 h) at higher temperature (37°C) than at lower temperature (24 h at 25°C). Based on this conclusion and physical limitations, a thinner tissue specimen (2 mm) is recommended for more uniform fixation in formalin. Also, from these types of observations, rapid fixation protocols, using formalin, have been developed using higher temperatures, induced by conventional heating methods (45) or microwave heating (31).

The pH is also an important factor in formalin fixation, because formalin selectively reacts with uncharged primary amino groups, which are influenced by pH. Traditionally, neutral buffered formalin around pH 7.0 has been used for tissue fixation. It is known that more amino groups are discharged at higher pH; thus more formalin-induced cross-links may be produced at higher pH as a consequence of the greater abundance of uncharged amino groups. However, acidic formalin solution has been recommended for rapid fixation of certain small molecules, such as estradiol, as described below (29). For some antigens, pH may also affect the retention of either acidic or basic molecules in situ within the tissues during formalin fixation. For example, Larsson (33) found that gastrin-17 molecules are readily extracted from tissue when basic or neutral formalin are used as fixative, while such molecules are retained in situ by acidic formalin fixation. Therefore, concerning application of AR technique, the critical issues during formalin fixation of tissue include the possible extraction or dislocation of antigens, as well as the degree to which masking occurs during fixation. According to experiments reported by Fraenkel-Conrat and Olcott (18), the optimal pH value for

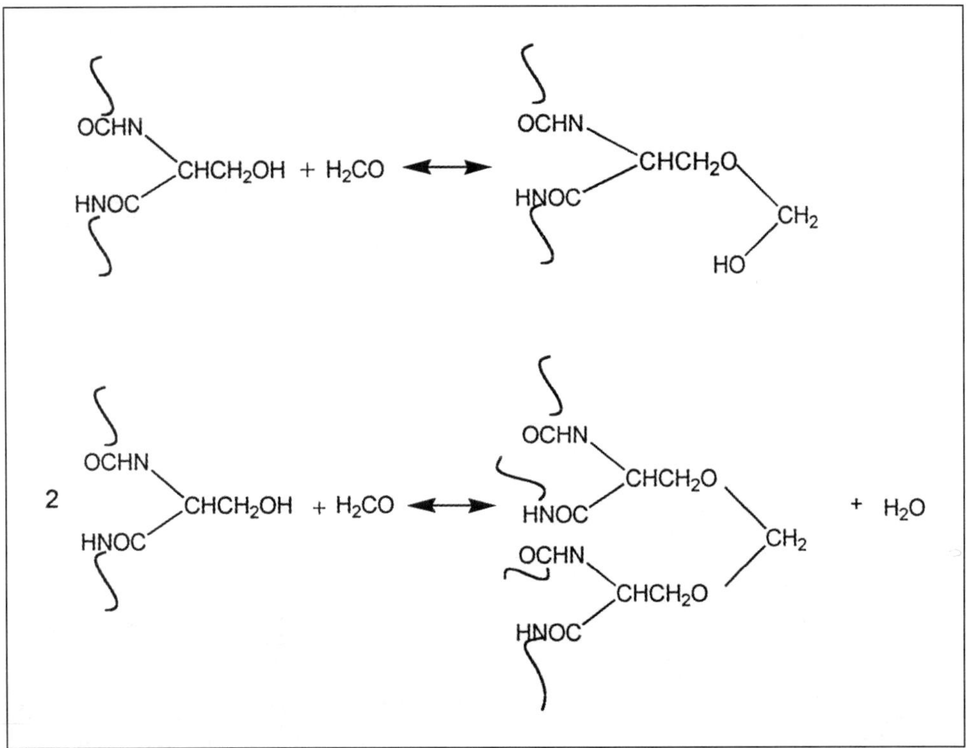

Figure 5. Top: Reaction between serine and formaldehyde (hemicetal). Bottom: Cross-linking between two serine molecules (acetol).

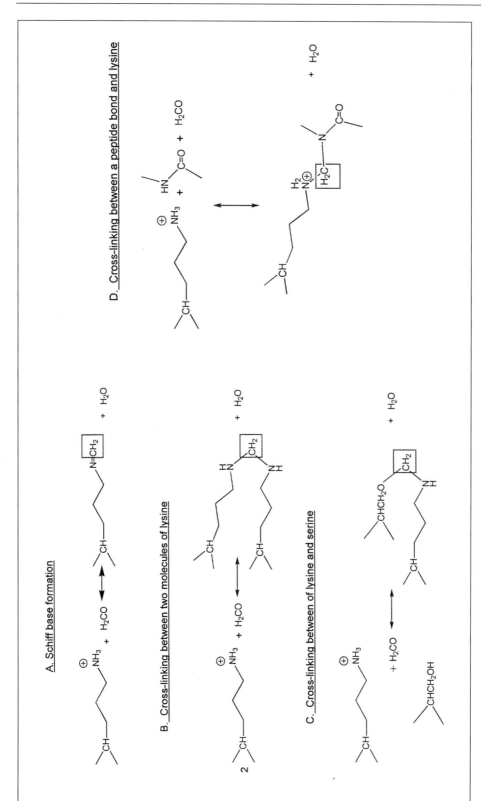

Figure 6. Reaction between lysine and formaldehyde.

completion of condensation and cross-linking of proteins during formalin fixation may be different for various side chains of amino acids. For example, a condensation reaction involving alanine and acetamide occurs readily at high pH (above pH 11), whereas a range of pH 3.2 to 7.6 is favorable for amines and amides in most circumstances. In spite of these known exceptions, neutral buffered formalin has been applied for tissue fixation for many years and seems to be satisfactory for most antigens.

Another possible advantage of using neutral buffered formalin may be attributed to the fact that an irreversible cross-link of formalin-tryptophane (in gramicidin) is much less readily formed in neutral or acidic solution than in alkaline solution (17). The effect of formalin on many proteins may therefore be influenced by monitoring the pH value (50).

In our studies of AR-IHC under the influence of pH, we have demonstrated that different groups of antigens correlated with three patterns of AR-IHC using different AR solutions at various pH values (see Chapter 2). In light of the data showing that formalin–protein reactions are pH dependent, these differences may be explained on the basis of protein structure.

Influence of Fixation on Antigenicity: Masking Effects

It has long been accepted that formalin fixation results in variable loss of antigenicity, otherwise known as a masking effect. Antigens may be divided on this basis into two main groups: formalin-sensitive and formalin-resistant. More antigens are in the formalin-sensitive group, displaying reduced immunoreactivity after formalin fixation. The possible mechanism with respect to selective masking effects of formalin fixation for different epitopes of different antigens may be attributed to cross-linking of critical side chains of amino acids, with subtle alteration in the overall three-dimensional shape of the molecule, as described previously and as demonstrated by studies using ^{14}C formaldehyde to localize the major reaction sites of protein structures. For example, Hua et al. (25) studied the binding of H-2K^b-specific monoclonal antibodies to formalin-fixed splenic or tumor cells and demonstrated that the loss of antigenicity, as detected by three of nine antibodies tested, correlated with the modification of protein (antigen) structure occurring as a consequence of formalin-induced alteration of lysine 89. Their conclusion was confirmed by comparative observation of mutant H-2K^{bm3} cells, which have alanine substituted for lysine 89, resulting in loss of reactivity with the same three antibodies. This study was based on brief and weak formalin fixation (1% formaldehyde for 15 min). It was recognized that different results might have been obtained with longer times of fixation, which would allow secondary condensation reactions to occur, as described previously.

Advantages and Drawbacks of Formalin as a Fixative

A long history of use of formalin as a standard tissue fixative has revealed the following advantages:

1. Formalin fixation provides good preservation of morphology for a variety of tissues without significant detriment, even after extending period of fixation in 10% formalin for years. "Good" is a somewhat subjective term encompassing the various artifactual changes that result in presentation of the morphologic features that "please" the pathologist, based on previous experience and the manner of fixation/processing to which the pathologist has become accustomed.

2. Formalin is economical, much less expensive than most alternatives.
3. Formalin fixation can "sterilize" tissue specimens in a more reliable way than precipitating fixatives, particularly in the case of a virus.
4. Carbohydrates are better preserved by formalin fixation (91).
5. Formalin fixation provides better preservation of many antigens in situ, avoiding the leaching out of proteins that may occur with other fixatives. It is known that many low-molecular-weight proteins or peptides are extracted by non-cross-linking fixatives such as alcohol- or methanol-based solutions but are well preserved in tissue by formalin in the form of cross-linked derivatives (33). Traditionally, non-cross-linking precipitating fixatives have been recommended to replace aldehyde fixation in order to retain the immunoreactivity of some larger proteins such as intermediate filaments and immunoglobulins.

Thus, formalin may be regarded as a satisfactory fixative for both morphology and immunohistochemistry providing that AR can be successfully employed to recover these antigens that are diminished or lost. In 1997, Prento and Lyon (53) compared the performance of six commercial fixatives that have been offered as "formalin substitutes" with the performance of formalin. They concluded that the best immunostaining was obtained by combining formalin fixation with the AR technique and that none of the six proposed substitutes for formalin were adequate for histopathology (i.e., they did not give the good morphology to which the pathologist had become accustomed).

A recent study of immunohistochemical localization of estradiol in formalin-fixed, paraffin-embedded tissue sections demonstrated the necessity of formaldehyde fixation in IHC for some antigens (29). Jungblut and Sierralta (29) found that estradiol could be demonstrated in situ as a nuclear staining pattern only if the estradiol had been covalently bound by the Mannich reaction during fixation in acetic acid–formaldehyde.

Thus formalin-induced cross-linking of protein appears to serve as an efficient means of in situ preservation of antigen in most circumstances, despite the simultaneous masking of antigenicity.

Based on this observation, the development of a simple AR method to unmask antigenicity would be helpful, not only for performing retrospective studies on routinely processed paraffin sections, but also to allow retention of the traditional standard formalin fixation method for tissues worldwide. This latter issue is of some importance, since enormous effort has been expended in searching for alternative fixatives to replace formalin, in an attempt to achieve better preservation of antigenicity for IHC and good morphology. However, as noted above, these efforts have been uniformly unsuccessful; the ideal fixative for IHC, applicable to all antigens, may never be found (33,81). Indeed, formalin may be the prefered fixative for most antigens, because of superior preservation of both morphology and antigenicity. It may be advantageous to continue using formalin as the standard fixative, while developing improved (in terms of universal application and reliability) techniques and standardization for AR.

DEVELOPMENT OF ANTIGEN RETRIEVAL

Basic Source: Fraenkel-Conrat and Co-Workers in the 1940s

At the Western Regional Research Laboratory, Albany, California, Fraenkel-Conrat and co-workers (17–19) conducted a series of studies of formaldehyde–protein reactions under a variety of experimental conditions in the1940s. They demonstrated that formalin-induced cross-linking resulted in an increase of the average molecular weights of salmine and other proteins (18). They also showed that cross-links occurring between aminomethylol groups and phenol, imidazole, or indole groups in Mannich reactions (19) lead to the formation of stable compounds with formaldehyde (17). In addition, they showed that the cross-links of the Mannich reaction are different from other cross-links such as amino, amide, and guanidyl linkages, in terms of regular hydrolysis, in that they can be reversed by heat or alkaline treatment.

High-Temperature Heating Method

The high-temperature heating method is a simple procedure that requires boiling of formalin-fixed, deparaffinized tissue sections in water or various solutions. It was developed in 1990 and published in 1991 (56). The most important factor emphasized in the first article was high-temperature heating using either microwave or conventional heating methods. Metal solutions of 1% zinc sulfate and saturated lead thiocyanate, as well as distilled water, were tested as AR solutions. Use of a metal salt solution was based on previous studies of zinc formalin fixative (28). The major results of this first article were the following: *(i)* a protocol was presented for the microwave heating AR method (see Appendix); *(ii)* among 52 monoclonal and polyclonal antibodies tested, 39 demonstrated a significant increase in immunostaining, 9 showed no change, and 4 showed reduced immunostaining; certain antibodies that were unreactive with formalin-fixed tissues gave excellent staining after AR heating; *(iii)* conventional heating by immersing slides in boiling water may also yield improved immunostaining, although microwave heating in distilled water or metal solution appeared to be superior; *(iv)* the dramatic effect of AR-IHC could be achieved using archival paraffin sections fixed in formalin for as long a period as 2 years; and *(v)* the specificity of AR-IHC was reliable,—no false positive results were found.

Nonheating Method of Alkaline Treatment

A nonheating AR method that simply requires immersing slides in a strong alkaline solution (NaOH–methanol) was developed for immunostaining on formalin-fixed, routinely acid-decalcified, celloidin-embedded human temporal bone sections in 1991 and published in 1992 (57). A total of 60 formalin-fixed and routinely processed celloidin-embedded human temporal bone tissues were tested using 15 monoclonal antibodies. Results showed strong positive staining for seven monoclonal antibodies, moderate positive staining for four antibodies, and weak positive staining for one antibody. Three antibodies showed negative results. There was no significant difference in immunoreactivity among sections from different blocks, regardless of the fixative and stored time, which ranged from less than 1 year to 30 years. The specificity of this nonheating method was demonstrated by negative control groups. There was sharp immunolocalization of keratin, vimentin, neurofilament, muscle-specific actin, S-100 protein, neuron specific enolase, and glial fibrillary acidic protein. Similar results have subsequently been documented in other studies (see Chapter 18). In 1993, a combined technique was described, combining nonheating and heating AR methods, for enhancement of AR-IHC for numerous antibodies (see Chapters 14 and 18). The dramatic results of strong alkaline treatment, in AR-IHC may be attributed to reversal of the Mannich reaction of formalin–tryptophan by strong alkaline treatment as described above.

Various Modifications

Since the publication of the AR technique in 1991, many investigators have devoted resources and effort to find a chemical that may significantly improve the efficiency of AR-IHC, resulting in a plethora of detailed reports (5,10,15,24,27,32,40,52,58, 59,61,62,64,66,84). However, no single chemical has been identified as an essential component of the AR process to date (30,62–64,66,68,84). In addition to microwave and conventional heating methods (56), Shin et al. (69) described a hydrated autoclaving method to enhance immunoreactivity of tau protein in brain tissue fixed in formalin, with good results. Subsequently, domestic pressure cookers and steamers were applied for high-temperature heating procedures with some success (46,83).

As a simple and extremely effective technique, heat-induced AR was consequently applied in pathology and other fields of morphology and has attracted worldwide attention. In 1991, Greenwell et al. (23) published an article concerning the use of AR-IHC for immunostaining of proliferating cell nuclear antigen (PCNA) in archival formalin fixed, paraffin-embedded rodent tissues, immediately after the microwave heating AR technique was documented. They used exactly the same AR protocol as described above, employing a lead thiocyanate solution and achieved excellent results for PCNA immunostaining in animal tissues. The increase in staining intensity resulting from the use of metal salt AR solutions has subsequently been demonstrated in several studies (62,84). The only article (41) that reported a poor result was based on inappropriate comparisons, as analyzed in detail elsewhere (63). In this study, Momose et al. (41) attempted to document their conclusion that the original 1991 AR technique was not superior to enzyme digestion for immunostaining of 17 antibodies. However, their comparison was based on different antibodies, different clones, and/or different sources of reagents, and only three antibodies (vimentin, AE1, and PSA) were the same as those tested by the original article. Of the three antibodies, only AE1 showed a significantly different result, which might have been caused by use of the multi-tissue block in their test that was made of formalin-fixed tissues stored in 70% alcohol for a longer time (4). A major drawback of metal salts, particularly lead salts, is the potentially toxic effect, as noted by Suurmeijer and Boon (71). It is therefore better to avoid lead or other toxic metal salts if other solutions may serve with equal effect in AR-IHC staining.

The use of citrate buffer solution for AR heating method was documented by Cattoretti et al. (8), Gown et al. (21), Leong et al. (35), Taylor et al. (82), Suurmeijer and Boon (71), Swanson (73), Cuevas et al. (12), and others (64). Cattoretti et al. (9) extended their investigation to 256 antibodies using citrate buffer of pH 6.0 as the AR solution with the microwave heating protocol previously documented (56). Meanwhile, the effectiveness of several chemicals, (such as urea, glycine-HCl buffer, Tris-HCl, phosphate buffer, periodic acid, aluminum chloride, and other metals as well as detergent solutions) have been documented (62–64,84). In addition, several commercial AR solutions such as TUF have been developed. It seems that chemicals have been credited as the major factors that influence the effect of AR-IHC. This is a particularly interesting issue with regard to commercial products, the chemical nature of which is generally kept secret.

Facing an anarchy of different or unknown AR solutions, a critical issue must be addressed in order to standardize the AR technique, i.e., what are the major factors that influence the effect of AR-IHC? As previously emphasized in the literature (5,26,38, 62–64,84), heating appears to be the most important factor, based on the following facts:

1. A significant enhancement of immunohistochemical staining can be achieved

by using high-temperature heating of the routinely processed paraffin-embedded tissue sections in pure distilled water (30,48,56).

2. Higher temperature in general yields better results (5,26,62–64,84). Our recent study demonstrated that an optimal result of AR-IHC is correlated with the product of heating temperature (T) × time of AR heating treatment (t) (65).

3. Equivalent intensities of IHC staining can be obtained using different buffers as AR solutions if the pH value of the solutions is monitored in a comparable manner; thus the chemical composition per se is not a necessary factor for satisfactory results (14,60).

4. No AR effect can be demonstrated following immersion of the paraffin sections in citrate buffer solution without heating.

These critical points have subsequently been demonstrated by numerous studies (see Chapter 2).

The use of various buffer solutions as AR solutions has provided food for thought. A hypothesis was proposed by our group in 1993, that the effect of AR-IHC may be influenced by the pH value of the AR solution to a greater degree than the chemical components of the AR solution. We performed a study concerning the influence of pH on AR-IHC, with results supporting the hypothesis that the pH value was more critical than the chemical composition of the buffer solution (see Chapter 2). Evers and Uylings (14) also found that AR-IHC is pH and temperature dependent at the same time. They tested two antibodies, MAP-2 and SMI-32, and indicated that the optimal values were pH 4.5 for MAP-2 and pH 2.5 for SMI-32. In addition, they demonstrated that the use of 4% $AlCl_3$ as the AR solution for SMI-32 could achieve a similar result to that obtained by using a citrate buffer of pH 2.5. They concluded that it was not important what kind of solution was used as long as the pH was at an appropriate level.

Although chemical components of the AR solution may play roles as cofactors, as recently documented by Pileri et al. (Reference 52; EDTA-NaOH solution of pH 8.0 always yields stronger intensity of AR-IHC than citrate buffer of pH 6.0 or Tris-HCl buffer of pH 8.0), there are no specific chemicals that must be present for a satisfactory result (30,62–64,66,69,84).

Demonstration of the two major factors that influence the effect of AR-IHC provides a basis for establishing a test battery approach, by which optimal protocols may be validated for maximal retrieval of AR-IHC. Furthermore, with this method, standardization of AR-IHC on routinely processed tissues may be achievable (see Chapter 16 and Appendix for details).

In summary, development of the AR technique is predicated on an approach of rendering archival formalin-fixed, paraffin-embedded tissues suitable for IHC. Achieving this goal has proved to be a critical issue in contemporary morphology (77–80), with far-reaching changes in the practice of diagnostic surgical pathology and research.

MECHANISM OF EFFECT OF ANTIGEN RETRIEVAL

The mechanism of AR is not yet clear at this time. Several hypotheses have been proposed, including the following:

• Loosening or breaking of the cross-linkages caused by formalin fixation (57,62).

• Protein denaturation based on the observation that some antigens or endogenous enzymatic activities may be lost after heating AR treatment (9).

- Multiple pathways, including breaking of cross-linkages, extraction of diffusible blocking proteins, precipitation of proteins, and rehydration of the tissue sections, which allows better penetration of antibody and increased accessibility to epitopes (71).

- In addition to the multiple-pathway hypothesis, mobilization by microwave energy of the last traces of paraffin, which may not have been extractable by standard techniques, thereby inproving antibody penetration (21).

- Hydrolysis of Schiff bases (70).

- Removal of cage-like calcium complexes, which might be bound to protein during formalin fixation. Removal may be effected by heating and calcium chelation for antigen retrieval (43).

- Heat-induced reversal of various chemical modifications of protein structure that occur during formalin fixation (62).

The hypothesis of the heat-induced reversal of chemical modifications produced by formalin is based on an essential principle of immunology that antigen–antibody recognition is protein structure dependent. Antibodies recognize specific epitopes localized in a particular spatial configuration within the protein molecule. This is particularly true for discontinuous antigenic determinants, which are composed of residues from different parts of the amino acid sequence (2,3). Conformational changes of protein structure caused by formalin fixation may mask the antigenicity in tissue. The AR method may lead to a restoration of the original protein structure (induced by high-temperature heating or other nonheating procedures such as strong alkaline treatment) and reestablishment of the three-dimensional structure of protein in its native condition, or very close to that state (Figure 7).

In other words, the mechanism of AR-IHC appears to involve a restoration of the structure of fixed proteins through a series of conformational changes, including the possible breakage of formalin-induced cross-linkages, the whole process being driven by thermal energy from the heat source through a process of hydrolysis of the formalin-induced cross-linking (3,51,55,86,89,90). The term denaturation is not appropriate to express this process, as an initial denaturation has already occurred during formalin fixation of the tissue; in a sense AR unfixes the tissue, returning proteins toward the unfixed state. The term renaturation may be more appropriate, in terms of restoration of structure, if not function. Because antigen–antibody recognition is solely based on reciprocity of protein structures, further studies concerning the mechanism of AR-IHC may be focused on studying the alterations of protein structure taking place during fixation and unfixation or retrieval, based on recent studies showing variable results using different AR combination protocols (39,62,74–76,85).

The exact chemical reaction involved in this modification–restoration mechanism is not clear and in all probability may differ for different proteins (antigens) according to their amino acid composition and tertiary folding characteristics. The most likely process that would restore part of the native configuration of a formalin-modified antigen is the hydrolysis of some of the cross-linkages and other formalin adducts that resulted from formalin-protein fixation. As observed earlier (reactions 4–7), water is a common product in these reactions, and many of them are fully reversible by slight changes in pH or increases in temperature. In support of this hypothesis, as noted previously, there is evidence that extending washing of formalin-fixed tissue in water may in same instances reverse the loss of immunoreactivity (i.e., give an AR effect) (50). These two variables (heat and low pH), which work in many ways against the preservation of native structures, contribute to the effectiveness of the AR technique. Indeed, it may be that the AR technique takes advantage of the fact that formalin-induced cross-linking protects the natural protein structure from complete denaturation and paradoxically allows fixed proteins to survive the vigorous heating of the microwave AR method.

The reason why the same retrieval protocol works for some proteins but not others, even though they may be located in the same cellular compartment, is not clear, but some of the following considerations may be included: *(i)* protein may be extracted (leached out) from the tissue during inappropriate fixation or subsequent processing, particularly during dehydration by alcohol; *(ii)* a wide variety of different chemical modifications and different cross-linkages inevitably occur in structurally different proteins, and not all are reversible by AR to the same degree; and *(iii)* structural factors may confer rigidity on some proteins, preventing irreversible denaturation during the vigorous heating of the AR process or by extremes of pH. This hypothesis is based on previous study for native proteins. Rigid protein motifs (i.e., β-barrels, membrane channels, etc.) are more likely to withstand aggressive AR treatment than soluble, globular structures that have an overall similar amino acid composition (through obviously different sequences). For example, the protein Cu-Zn superoxide dismutase (an enzyme in which the active site is protected by a β-barrel structure) is highly resistant to denaturation by heating probably because of its high rigidity (20).

Recently, Morgan et al. (43,44) proposed a hypothesis concerning the mechanism of AR that focused on the binding of calcium ions to proteins during formalin fixation. This proposal was based on experiments showing that a negative immunostaining result for monoclonal antibody MIB-1 was produced by using a solution of $CaCl_2$ with citrate buffer for heating the paraffin sections. They concluded that calcium complex formation with proteins in formalin-fixed tissue may mask antigens and that the release of calcium from this cage-like calcium complex may require a considerable amount of energy, such as high-temperature heating and calcium chelation by citrate. Our own observations suggest that this calcium-induced effect is seen for some antigens but may not be sufficient to explain the loss of immunoreactivity for many others and thus is unlikely to represent the general mechanism of AR-IHC.

We recently performed a study of calcium-induced modification of thrombospondin (TSP) and Ki-67, by IHC staining on frozen tissue sections using seven monoclonal antibodies to TSP and Ki-67 (67). This experiment was based on a series of biochemical studies published 10 years previously by Dixit et al. (13). Our experiments involved incubation of frozen sections with solutions of 50 mM $CaCl_2$, and/or 10 mM EDTA at 4°C overnight, prior to immunostaining. We found that calcium-induced modification of protein structure appeared to occur, as evidenced by loss of IHC staining for both TSP and MIB-1 after calcium incubation (Figure 8B, C, and F). Among the reagents tested, only calcium chloride gave reduced IHC staining (Figure 8A, E vs. B, C, and F). This calcium-induced modification of protein conformation could be reversed (and staining restored) by sequential incubation with EDTA following calcium incubation (Figure 8D and H), a finding consistent with the earlier biochemical studies showing calcium-induced modification of protein conformation (13,89). The very same monoclonal antibodies to TSP (A6.1 and D4.6) tested by the biochemists were tested by us, with similar results (13). Not surprisingly, we noted that not all antigens are affected by calcium in the same manner, an observation supported by others. For example, Wakabayashi et al. (87) found that detectable antigen-antibody immunoreactivity of protein C could only be achieved in the presence of calcium, the exact reverse of its effect in TSP.

Summary

The chemical reaction of formalin fixation is a complicated process, as demonstrated by serial studies of protein chemistry. Cross-linking is the essential feature of formalin fixation. The AR technique is a heat-induced remodification of formalin-induced modification of protein conformation, and hydrolysis of cross-linking resulting from formalin fixation may play an essential role in such remodification.

CONCLUSION AND FUTURE PROSPECTS

Extensive use of AR-IHC has dramatically increased the range and variety of antibodies that are applicable to routinely processed archival tissues. On the other hand, the widespread use of AR has raised questions for further investigations. Current major issues include the following:

1. There is a pressing need for standardization of the AR technique, which is

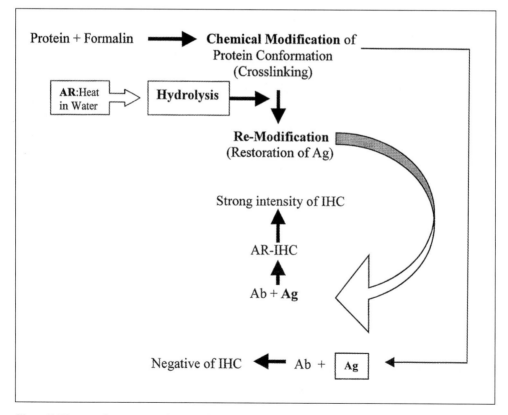

Figure 7. Diagram of our suggested mechanism of AR-IHC. AR, antigen retrieval; IHC, immunohistochemistry; Ag, antigen; Ag in square, formalin-modified antigen, which can not be recognized by antibody, resulting in negative immunostaining. Hydrolysis of the cross-linking induced by high-temperature heating tissue section in water may be the key role played by the AR technique. Modified with permission from Reference 62.

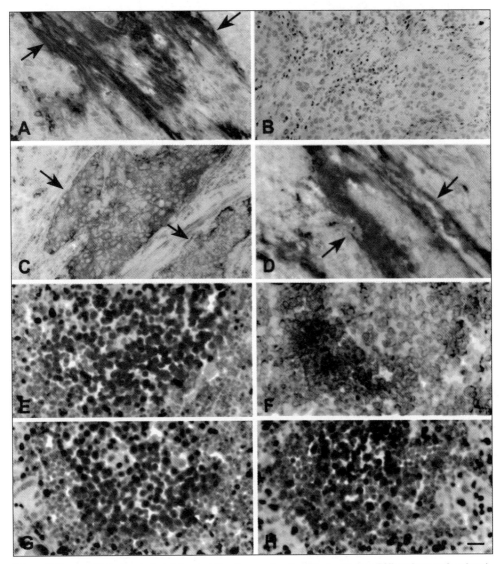

Figure 8. Immunohistochemical staining results of monoclonal antibody Ab-3 to TSP and monoclonal antibody MIB-1 on frozen tissue sections of bladder cancer and lymph node. The effects of pretreatment with $CaCl_2$ of TSP (A–D), and the monoclonal antibody MIB-1 on frozen sections of lymph node showing similar effects of $CaCl_2$ (E–H). (A) Frozen section fixed in 10% neutral buffered formaldehyde (NBF) for 10 min showed strong TSP labeling of extracellular pattern (arrows): no pretreatment (positive control). (B) Frozen section incubated with 50 mmol/L $CaCl_2$ at 4°C overnight, then fixed in 10% NBF. A negative staining result was demonstrated in 50% of total area in the section. (C) Frozen section incubated with $CaCl_2$ at 4°C overnight, and then fixed in 10% NBF. An altered pattern of staining showing cytoplasmic staining of cancer cells (arrows) was showed in 40% of the total area in the tissue section for Ab-3. Such an altered pattern was demonstrated in 4/7 antibodies. (D) Frozen tissue section incubated with 20 mmol/L EDTA after overnight incubation with 50 mmol/L $CaCl_2$ and fixed in 10% NBF for 10 minutes. Restoration of extracellular positive staining (arrows) was demonstrated. (E) Frozen tissue section of lymph node was incubated in distilled water at 4°C overnight and then fixed in acetone, showing strong MIB-1 nuclear staining of the germinal center. (F) Frozen section incubated with 50 mmol/L $CaCl_2$ at 4°C overnight and then fixed in acetone showed a negative result. (G) Frozen section incubated with 20 mmol/L EDTA at 4°C overnight and then fixed in acetone showed slightly decreased nuclear staining. (H) Frozen section incubated with 20 mmol/L EDTA after overnight incubation with 50 mmol/L $CaCl_2$ at 4°C and fixed in acetone showed partial restoration of nuclear staining of MIB-1. AEC was used as chromogen, and hematoxylin was used as the counterstain. Original magnification × 100. Scale bar = 50 μm (A–D) × 200; 25 μm (E–H). Reprinted with permission from Reference 67. **(See color plate A1).**

35

discussed at length in Chapter 16.

2. Further development of the AR technique in order to retrieve most, if not all, antigens masked by formalin fixation is clearly a desirable goal. While it is theoretically possible that all altered antigens may be restored by optimal AR treatment, we are short of this goal in practice, and the prospect of a single universally applicable and effective universal or PAN-AR method seems remote.

3. In some measure, the difficulties inherent in the development of a broadly applicable AR method stem from our ignorance of the mechanism of action of AR (22), which in turn is rooted in our relative lack of understanding of the basis of action of formalin fixation. Basic research is called for here, as proposed previously (67), regarding the detection of molecular alterations of protein based on chemical modification, in the fond hope that this may be of some service to investigators interested in the detection of subtle changes in molecular structure by light microscopy using previous studies as a basis (1,36,37,42,47,67,90). This is an exceedingly complex area of protein chemistry, but complexity has not deterred research in other areas.

4. Finally, as widespread use of AR has changed the degree to which many antigens can be demonstrated in fixed tissues, we must carefully evaluate all the pre-AR literature and the newer results of AR-IHC based on clinical, biochemical, and molecular biologic data.

REFERENCES

1. **Asaga, H. and T. Senshu.** 1993. Combined biochemical and immunocytochemical analyses of postmortem protein deimination in the rat spinal cord. Cell Biol. Int. *17*:525-532.
2. **Atassi, M.Z.** 1975. Antigenic structure of myoglobin: the complete immunochemical anatomy of a protein and conclusions relating to antigenic structures of proteins. Immunochemistry *12*:423-438.
3. **Barlow, D.J., M.S. Edwards, and J.M. Thornton.** 1986. Continuous and discontinuous protein antigenic determinants. Nature *322*:747-748.
4. **Battifora, H.** 1986. The multitumor (sausage) tissue block: novel method for immunohistochemical antibody testing. Lab. Invest. *55*:244-248.
5. **Boon, M.E. and L.P. Kok.** 1995. Breakthrough in pathology due to antigen retrieval. Mal. J. Med. Lab. Sci. *12*:1-9.
6. **Brigati, D.J.** 1991. Editorial. Will the histopathology laboratory surrender its paraffin blocks to the molecular biologist? J. Histotechnol. *14*:217-218.
7. **Brown, R.W. and R. Chirala.** 1995. Utility of microwave-citrate antigen retrieval in diagnostic immunohistochemistry. Mod. Pathol. *8*:515-520.
8. **Cattoretti, G., M.H.G. Becker, G. Key, M. Duchrow, C. Schluter, J.Galle, and J.Gerdes.** 1992. Monoclonal antibodies against recombinant parts of the Ki-67 antigen (MIB 1 and MIB 3) detect proliferating cells in microwave-processed formalin-fixed paraffin sections. J. Pathol. *168*:357-363.
9. **Cattoretti, G., S. Pileri, C. Parravicini, M.H.G. Becker, S. Poggi, C. Bifulco, G. Key, L. D'Amato, E. Sabattini, E. Feudale, et al.** 1993. Antigen unmasking on formalin-fixed, paraffin-embedded tissue sections. J. Pathol. *171*:83-98.
10. **Cattoretti, G. and A.J.H. Suurmeijer.** 1995. Antigen unmasking on formalin-fixed paraffin-embedded tissues using microwaves: a review. Adv. Anat. Pathol. 2:2-9.
11. **Coons, A.H., H.J. Creech, and R.N. Jones.** 1941. Immunological properties of an antibody containing a fluorescent group. Proc. Soc. Exp. Biol. Med. *47*:200-202.
12. **Cuevas, E.C., A.C. Bateman, B.S. Wilking, P.A. Johnson, J.H. Williams, A.H.S. Lee, D.B. Jones, and D.H. Wright.** 1994. Microwave antigen retrieval in immunocytochemistry: a study of 80 antibodies. J. Clin. Pathol. *47*:448-452.
13. **Dixit, V.M., N.J. Galvin, K.M. O'Rourk, and W.A. Frazier.** 1986. Monoclonal antibodies that recognize calcium-dependent structures of human thrombospondin. Characterization and mapping of their epitopes. J. Biol. Chem. *261*:1962-1966.
14. **Evers, P. and H.B.M. Uylings.** 1994. Microwave-stimulated antigen retrieval is pH and temperature dependent. J. Histochem. Cytochem. *42*:1555-1563.
15. **Evers, P. and H.B.M. Uylings.** 1994. Effects of microwave pretreatment on immunocytochemical staining of vibratome sections and tissue blocks of human cerebral cortex stored in formaldehyde fixative for long periods. J.

Neurosci. Methods *55*:163-172.

16. **Fox, C.H., F.B. Johnson, J. Whiting, and P.P. Roller.** 1985. Formaldehyde fixation. J. Histochem. Cytochem. *33*:845-853.
17. **Fraenkel-Conrat, H., B.A. Brandon, and H.S. Olcott.** 1947. The reaction of formaldehyde with proteins. IV. Participation of indole groups. Gramicidin. J. Biol. Chem. *168*:99-118.
18. **Fraenkel-Conrat, H. and H.S. Olcott.** 1948. The reaction of formaldehyde with proteins. V. Cross-linking between amino and primary amide or guanidyl groups. J. Am. Chem. Soc. *70*:2673-2684.
19. **Fraenkel-Conrat, H. and H.S. Olcott.** 1948. Reaction of formaldehyde with proteins. VI. Cross-linking of amino groups with phenol, imidazole, or indole groups. J. Biol. Chem. *174*:827-843.
20. **Getzoff, E.D., J.A. Tainer, M.M. Stempien, G.I. Bell, and R.A. Hallewell.** 1989. Evolution of CuZn superoxide dismutase and the Greek key β-barrel structural motif. Proteins *5*:322-336.
21. **Gown, A.M., N. de Wever, and H. Battifora.** 1993. Microwave-based antigenic unmasking. A revolutionary new technique for routine immunohistochemistry. Appl. Immunohistochem. *1*:256-266.
22. **Gown, A.M. and H. Yaziji.** 1998. Mechanisms of heat-induced epitope retrieval: the role of divalent metal ion chelation. J. Histochem. Cytochem. *46*:A14.
23. **Greenwell, A., J.F. Foley, and R.R. Maronpot.** 1991. An enhancement method for immunohistochemical staining of proliferating cell nuclear antigen in archival rodent tissues. Cancer Lett. *59*:251-256.
23a. **Gu, J.** 1997. Computerized three- and four-dimensional modeling of biomedical images for morphologists and pathologists. Cell Vision *4*:6-15.
24. **Hazelbag, H.M., L.J.C.M. vd Broek, E.B.L. van Dorst, G.J.A. Offerhaus, G.J. Fleuren, and P.C.W. Hogendoorn.** 1995. Immunostaining of chain-specific keratins on formalin-fixed, paraffin-embedded tissues: a comparison of various antigen retrieval systems using microwave heating and proteolytic pre-treatments. J. Histochem. Cytochem. *43*:429-437.
25. **Hua, C., C. Langlet, M. Buferne, and A.M. Schmitt-Verhulst.** 1985. Selective destruction by formaldehyde fixation of an H-2K[b] serological determinant involving lysine 89 without loss of T-cell reactivity. Immunogenetics *21*:227-234.
26. **Igarashi, H., H. Sugimura, K. Maruyama, Y. Kitayama, I. Ohta, M. Suzuki, M. Tanaka, Y. Dobashi, and I. Kino.** 1994. Alteration of immunoreactivity by hydrated autoclaving, microwave treatment, and simple heating of paraffin-embedded tissue sections. APMIS *102*:295-307.
27. **Imam, S.A., L. Young, B. Chaiwun, and C.R. Taylor.** 1995. Comparison of 2 microwave based antigen retrieval solutions in unmasking epitopes in formalin-fixed tissue for immunostaining. Anticancer Res. *15*:1153-1158.
28. **Jones, M.D., P.M. Banks, and B.L. Caron.** 1981. Transition metal salts as adjuncts to formalin for tissue fixation. Lab. Invest. *44*:32A.
29. **Jungblut, P.W. and W.D. Sierralta.** 1998. Identification of target cells by immunohistochemical detection of covalently rearranged estradiol in rehydrated paraffin sections. Histochem. Cell Biol. *109*:295-300.
30. **Katoh, A. and S. Breier.** 1994. Nonspecific antigen retrieval solutions. J. Histotechnol. *17*:378-378.
31. **Kok, L.P. and M.E. Boon (Eds.).** 1992. Microwave Cookbook for Microscopists. Art and Science of Visualization. 3rd ed., p. 150-163. Coulomb Press, Leyden.
32. **Kwaspen, F., F. Smedts, J. Blom, A. Peonk, M.-J. Kok, M. Vaan Dijk, and F. Ramaekers.** 1995. Periodic acid as a nonenzymatic enhancement technique for the detection of cytokeratin immunoreactivity in routinely processed carcinomas. Appl. Immunohistochem. *3*:54-63.
33. **Larsson, L.-I.** 1988. Immunocytochemistry: Theory and Practice. Chapter 2, p. 41-170. Fixation and tissue pretreatment. CRC Press, Boca Raton.
34. **Leong, A.S.-Y., J. Milios, and C.G. Duncis.** 1988. Antigen preservation in microwave-irradiated tisses: a comparison with formaldehyde fixation. J. Pathol. *156*:275-282.
35. **Leong, A.S.-Y. and J. Milios.** 1993. An assessment of the efficacy of the microwave antigen-retrieval procedure on a range of tissue antigens. Appl. Immunohistochem. *1*:267-274.
36. **Lillie, R.D.** 1958. Acetylation and nitrosation of tissue amines in histochemistry. J. Histochem. Cytochem. *6*:352-362.
37. **Lillie, R.D. and H.M. Fullmer (Eds.).** 1976. Histopathologic Technic and Practical Histochemistry. 4th ed., p. 226-326. McGraw-Hill Book Co, New York.
38. **Lucassen, P.J., R. Ravid, N.K. Gonatas, and D.F. Swaab.** 1993. Activation of the human supraoptic and paraventricular nucleus neurons with aging and in Alzheimer's disease as judged from increasing size of the Golgi apparatus. Brain Res. *632*:105-113.
39. **MacDonald, G., P. Dillman, and I. Shirley.** 1995. Evaluation of six histological fixatives using image analysis to measure reaction product concentration. J. Histotechnol. *18*:119-125.
40. **Merz, H., O. Rickers, S. Schrimel, K. Orscheschek, and A.C. Feller.** 1993. Constant detection of surface and cytoplasmic immunoglobulin heavy and light chain expression in formalin-fixed and paraffin-embedded material. J. Pathol. *170*:257-264.
41. **Momose, H., P. Mehta, and H. Battifora.** 1993. Antigen retrieval by microwave irradiation in lead thiocyanate. Appl. Immunohistochem. *1*:77-82.
42. **Montero, C. and D.I. Segura.** 1989. Histochemical blockade of the antigen-antibody reaction using immunoperoxidase demonstration of lysozyme in Paneth cells and lamina propria mononucleocytes of human small intestine as a model system. J. Histochem. Cytochem. *37*:1063-1068.

43.**Morgan, J.M., H. Navabi, K.W. Schimid, and B. Jasani.**1994. Possible role of tissue-bound calcium ions in citrate-mediated high-temperature antigen retrieval. J. Pathol. *174*:301-307.

44.**Morgan, J.M., H. Navabi, and B. Jasani:** 1997. Role of calcium chelation in high-temperature antigen retrieval at different pH values. J. Pathol. *182*:233-237.

45.**Ni, C., T.C. Chang, S.S. Searl, E. Coughlin-Wilkinson, and D.M. Albert.** 1981. Rapid paraffin fixation for use in histologic examinations. Ophthalmology *88*:1372-1376.

46.**Norton, A.J., S. Jordan, and P. Yeomans.** 1994. Brief, high-temperature heat denaturation (pressure cooking): a simple and effective method of antigen retrieval for routinely processed tissues. J. Pathol. *173*:371-379.

47.**Olcott, H.S. and H. Fraenkel-Conrat.** 1947. Specific group reagents for proteins. Chem. Rev. *41*:151-197.

48.**O'Reilly, P.E., S.S. Raab, T.H. Niemann, J.R. Rodgers, and R.A. Robinson.** 1997. p53, proliferating cell nuclear antigen, and Ki-67 expression in extrauterine leiomyosarcomas. Mod. Pathol. *10*:91-97.

49.**Oyaizu, T., S. Arita, T. Hatano, and A. Tsubura.** 1996. Immunohistochemical detection of estrogen and progesterone receptors performed with an antigen-retrieval technique on methacarn-fixed paraffin-embedded breast cancer tissues. J. Surg. Res. *60*:69-73.

50.**Pearse, A.G.E. (Ed.).** 1968. Histochemistry, Theoretical and Applied. 3rd ed., Vol. 1, Chapter 5. The chemistry of fixation, p. 70-86. Little, Brown & Company, Boston.

51.**Perutz, M.F. (Ed.).** 1992. Protein Structure, New Approaches to Disease and Therapy, p. 41-59. W.H. Freeman and Company, New York.

52.**Pileri, S.A., G. Roncador, C. Ceccarelli, M. Piccioli, A. Briskonatis, E. Sabattini, S. Ascani, D. Santini, P.P. Piccaluga, O. Leone, et al.** 1997. Antigen retrieval techniques in immunohistochemistry: comparison of different methods. J. Pathol. *183*:116-123.

53.**Prento, P. and H. Lyon.** 1997. Commercial formalin substitutes for histopathology. Biotechnol. Histochem. *72*:273-282.

54.**Puchtler, H. and S.N. Meloan.** 1985. On the chemistry of formaldehyde fixation and its effects on immunohistochemical reactions. Histochemistry *82*:201-204.

55.**Scheraga, H.A.** 1971. Theoretical and experimental studies of conformations of polypeptides. Chem. Rev. *71*:195-217.

56.**Shi, S.-R., M.E. Key, and K.L. Kalra.** 1991. Antigen retrieval in formalin-fixed, paraffin-embedded tissues: an enhancement method for immunohistochemical staining based on microwave oven heating of tissue sections. J. Histochem. Cytochem. *39*:741-748.

57.**Shi, S.-R., C. Cote, K.L. Kalra, C.R. Taylor, and A.K. Tandon.** 1992. A technique for retrieving antigens in formalin-fixed, routinely acid-decalcified, celloidin-embedded human temporal bone sections for immunohistochemistry. J. Histochem. Cytochem. *40*:787-792.

58.**Shi, S.-R., B. Chaiwun, L. Young, R.J. Cote, and C.R. Taylor.** 1993. Antigen retrieval technique utilizing citrate buffer or urea solution for immunohistochemical demonstration of androgen receptor in formalin-fixed paraffin sections. J. Histochem. Cytochem. *41*:1599-1604.

59.**Shi, S.-R., B. Chaiwun, L. Young, A. Imam, R.J. Cote, and C.R. Taylor.** 1994. Antigen retrieval using pH 3.5 glycine-HCl buffer or urea solution for immunohistochemical localization of Ki-67. Biotech. Histochem. *69*:213-215.

60.**Shi, S.-R., A. Imam, L. Young, R.J. Cote, and C.R. Taylor.** 1995. Antigen retrieval immunohistochemistry under the influence of pH using monoclonal antibodies. J. Histochem. Cytochem. *43*:193-201.

61.**Shi, S.-R., R.J. Cote, L. Young, S.A. Imam, and C.R. Taylor.** 1996. Use of pH 9.5 Tris-HCl buffer containing 5% urea for antigen retrieval immunohistochemistry. Biotech. Histochem. *71*:190-196.

62.**Shi, S.-R., R.J. Cote, and C.R. Taylor.** 1997. Antigen retrieval immunohistochemistry: past, present, and future. J. Histochem. Cytochem. *45*:327-343.

63.**Shi, S.-R., R.J. Cote, L.L. Young, and C.R. Taylor.** 1997. Antigen retrieval immunohistochemistry: practice and development. J. Histotechnol. *20*:145-154.

64.**Shi, S.-R., J. Gu, K.L. Kalra, T. Chen, R.J. Cote, and C.R. Taylor.** 1997. Chapter 1. Antigen retrieval technique: a novel approach to immunohistochemistry on routinely processed tissue sections, p. 1-40. *In* J. Gu (Ed.), Analytical Morphology: Theory, Applications & Protocols. Eaton Publishing, Natick, MA.

65.**Shi, S.-R., R.J. Cote, B. Chaiwun, L.L. Young, Y. Shi, D. Hawes, T. Chen, and C.R. Taylor.** 1998. Standardization of immunohistochemistry based on antigen retrieval technique for routine formalin-fixed tissue sections. Appl. Immunohistochem. *6*:89-96.

66.**Shi, S.-R., R.J. Cote, and C.R. Taylor.** 1998. Antigen retrieval immunohistochemistry used for routinely processed celloidin-embedded human temporal bone sections: standardization and development. Auris Nasus Larynx *25*:425-443.

67.**Shi, S.-R., R.J. Cote, D. Hawes, S. Thu, Y. Shi, L.Young, and C.R. Taylor.** 1999. Calcium-induced modification of protein conformation demonstrated by immunohistochemistry: what is the signal? J. Histochem. Cytochem. *47*:463-469.

68.**Shi, Y., G.-D. Li, and W.-P. Liu.** 1997. Recent advances of the antigen retrieval technique. Linchuang yu Shiyan Binglixue Zazhi (J. Clin. Exp. Pathol.) *13*:265-267 (in Chinese).

69.**Shin, R.-W., T. Iwaki, T. Kitamoto, and J. Tateishi.** 1991. Hydrated autoclave pretreatment enhances TAU immunoreactivity in formalin-fixed normal and Alzheimer's disease brain tissues. Lab. Invest. *64*:693-702.

70.**Shiurba, R.A., E.T. Spooner, K. Ishiguro, M. Takahashi, R. Yoshida, T.R. Wheelock, K. Imahori, A.M.**

Cataldo, and R.A. Nixon. 1998. Immunocytochemistry of formalin-fixed human brain tissues: microwave irradiation of free-floating sections. Brain Res. Brain Res. Protocols 2:109-119.

71. **Suurmeijier, A.J.H. and M.E. Boon.** 1993. Notes on the application of microwaves for antigen retrieval in paraffin and plastic tissue sections. Eur. J. Morphol. *31*:144-150.

72. **Swanson, P.E.** 1993. Editorial. Methodologic standardization in immunohistochemistry. A doorway opens. Appl. Immunohistochem. *1*:229-231.

73. **Swanson, P.E.** 1994. Microwave antigen retrieval in citrate buffer. Lab. Med. *25*:520-522.

74. **Szekeres, G., J. Audouin, and A. Le Tourneau.** 1994. Is immunolocalization of antigens in paraffin sections dependent on method of antigen retrieval? Appl. Immunohistochem. *2*:137-140.

75. **Szekeres, G., Y. Lutz, A.L. Tourneau, and M. Delaage.** 1994. Steroid hormone receptor immunostaining on paraffin sections with microwave heating and trypsin digestion. J. Histotechnol. *17*:321-324.

76. **Szekeres, G., A. Le Tourneau, J. Benfares, J. Audouin, and J. Diebold.** 1995. Effect of ribonuclease A and deoxyribonuclease I on immunostaining of Ki-67 in fixed-embedded sections. Pathol. Res. Pract. *191*:52-56.

77. **Taylor, C.R. and J. Burns.** 1974. The demonstration of plasma cells and other immunoglobulin containing cells in formalin-fixed, paraffin-embedded tissues using peroxidase labelled antibody. J. Clin. Pathol. *27*:14-20.

78. **Taylor, C.R.** 1979. Immunohistologic studies of lymphomas: new methodology yields new information and poses new problems. J. Histochem. Cytochem. *27*:1189-1191.

79. **Taylor, C.R.** 1980. Immunohistologic studies of lymphoma: past, present and future. J. Histochem. Cytochem. *28*:777-787.

80. **Taylor, C.R. and G. Kledzik.** 1981. Immunohistologic techniques in surgical pathology. A spectrum of new special stains. Hum. Pathol. *12*:590-596.

81. **Taylor, C.R. and R.J. Cote (Eds.).** 1994. Immunomicroscopy: A Diagnostic Tool for the Surgical Pathologist. 2nd ed. W.B. Saunders Co., Philadelphia.

82. **Taylor, C.R., S.-R. Shi, B. Chaiwun, L. Young, S.A. Imam, and R.J. Cote.** 1994. Strategies for improving the immunohistochemical staining of various intranuclear prognostic markers in formalin-paraffin sections: androgen receptor, estrogen receptor, progesterone receptor, p53 protein, proliferating cell nuclear antigen, and Ki-67 antigen revealed by antigen retrieval technique. Hum. Pathol. *25*:263-270.

83. **Taylor, C.R., S.-R. Shi, C. Chen, L. Young, C. Yang, and R.J. Cote.** 1996. Comparative study of antigen retrieval heating methods: microwave, microwave and pressure cooker, autoclave, and steamer. Biotech. Histochem. *71*:263-270.

84. **Taylor, C.R., S.-R. Shi, and R.J. Cote.** 1996. Antigen retrieval for immunohistochemistry. Status and need for greater standardization. Appl. Immunohistochem. *4*:144-166.

85. **Tesch, G.H., M. Wei, Y.-Y. Ng, R.C. Atkins, and H.Y. Lan.** 1995. Enhancement of immunodetection of cytokines and cytokine receptors in tissue sections using microwave treatment. Cell Vision 2:435-439.

86. **Vasquez, M., G. Nemethy, and H.A. Scheraga.** 1994. Conformational energy calculations on polypeptides and proteins. Chem. Rev. *94*:2183-2239.

87. **Wakabayashi, K., Y. Sakata, and N. Aoki.** 1986. Conformation-specific monoclonal antibodies to the calcium-induced structure of protein C. J. Biol. Chem. *261*:11097-11105.

88. **Werner, M., R. von Wasielewski, and P. Komminoth.** 1996. Antigen retrieval, signal amplification and intensification in immunohistochemistry. Histochem. Cell Biol. *105*:253-260.

89. **Wilson, J.E.** 1991. The use of monoclonal antibodies and limited proteolysis in elucidation of structure-function relationships in proteins, p. 207-250. *In* C.H. Suelter (Ed.), Methods of Biochemical Analysis. John Wiley & Sons, New York.

90. **Wong, S.S. (Ed.).** 1991. Chemistry of Protein Conjugation and Cross-Linking, p. 1-48. CRC Press, Boca Raton.

91. **Yokoo, H. and Y. Nakazato.** 1996. A monoclonal antibody that recognizes a carbohydrate epitope of human protoplasmic astrocytes. Acta Neuropathol. *91*:23-30.

Major Factors Influencing the Effectiveness of Antigen Retrieval Immunohistochemistry

2

Benjaporn Chaiwun[1], Shan-Rong Shi[2], Richard J. Cote[2], and Clive R. Taylor[2]

[1]Department of Pathology, Chiangmai University, Thailand, and [2]Department of Pathology, University of Southern California Keck School of Medicine, Los Angeles, CA, USA

INTRODUCTION

Following its introduction in the early 1990s (37), the antigen retrieval (AR) technique has been widely used to enhance the value of immunohistochemistry (IHC) for both routine surgical pathology and research, including retrospective studies on archival, formalin-fixed, paraffin-embedded tissue. This technique has provided improved reliability and reproducibility of IHC staining. However, a universal AR method that could be applied for all antibodies has not yet been developed, and different variations of the AR technique (using different AR solutions, different heating temperatures, and different heating durations) have been used in different laboratories. Exploratory studies have been performed in an effort to improve the standarization of AR for use on archival tissues. In this context, understanding the major factors that influence the effectiveness of AR-IHC is a critical issue.

As previously described in Chapter 1, the AR technique was developed on the basis of biochemical studies of formalin–protein reactions carried out by Fraenkel-Conrat and co-workers in the 1940s (8–10). Two separate approaches to AR were examined, namely, high-temperature heating and strong alkaline treatment. There was an initial misconception that the chemical composition of the AR solution was the critical factor in effectiveness, resulting from the availability of commercial AR reagents such as metal salt solutions. Subsequently, numerous studies of AR-IHC have demonstrated that the heating conditions, temperature, and time are the most important factors in successful AR for most antigens.

Antigen Retrieval Techniques
Edited by Shan-Rong Shi, Jiang Gu, and Clive R. Taylor
©2000 Eaton Publishing, Natick, MA

HEATING CONDITIONS

As noted previously, the AR-IHC heating method is based on biochemical studies of Fraenkel-Conrat and co-workers (8–10), who documented that the chemical reactions occurring between protein and formalin may be reversed (at least in part) by high-temperature heating or strong alkaline hydrolysis. We demonstrated that the use of conventional heating at 100°C may achieve similar results to those obtained by microwave (MW) heating and also that distilled water could be used as the AR solution, albeit with slightly less effect (37). Subsequently, several publications have reported similar results using conventional heating (16,20,21,54). Malmstrom et al. (28) performed AR-IHC on proliferating cell nuclear antigen (PCNA; PC10 and 19F4) using distilled water as the AR solution with routinely processed paraffin sections of urinary bladder carcinoma and obtained good results.

The chemical reactions occurring during the formalin fixation process remain obscure. Studies of the mode of action of the AR technique may improve our understanding of how formaldehyde produces cross-linkages and may shed light on the exact mechanism of cross-linking of proteins. Mason and O'Leary (29) demonstrated that the process of cross-linking does not result in discernable alteration of the protein secondary structure, at least as determined by calorimetric and infrared spectroscopic investigation. However, they noted that significant denaturation of unfixed purified proteins occurred at temperature ranges from 70° to 90°C, whereas similar temperatures had virtually no adverse effect on formalin-fixed proteins (i.e., formalin-fixed proteins are more heat stable). Thus, the AR heating technique, employing high-temperature heating of tissue sections fixed in formalin, may exploit the fact that the cross-linkage of protein produced by formalin fixation may protect formalin-modified epitopes from denaturation during the heating phase. Although the mechanism of action of the AR technique is not clear, it appears unlikely, based on the above observation, that "protein denaturation alone is the mechanism," as advocated by Cattoretti et al. (2).

In our original article, we found significantly different intensities of immunostaining between formalin-fixed and alcohol-fixed tissue sections after AR treatment (37). This observation is in accordance with Suurmeijer and Boon's (48) data stating that AR was effective in formalin-fixed tissues, but much less effective in alcohol-fixed tissues. Igarashi et al. (16) conducted a careful study using four heating methods, as described below, and obtained very good retrieval by heating alcohol-fixed tissues that had been postfixed with formalin, suggesting that the existence of cross-linkages is a precondition for any effective enhancement of staining by the AR method.

The fact that high temperature is an important factor in AR-IHC has been demonstrated in a variety of studies. Lucassen et al. (27) studied AR-IHC of a monoclonal antibody to the antigen MG-160, a sialoglycoprotein of the medial cisternae of the Golgi apparatus, using different heating temperatures, and emphasized the importance of temperature during MW-AR treatment. Kawai et al. (20) found that heating at 90°C for 10 minutes was more effective than heating at 60°C for 120 minutes; however, overnight heating at 60°C gave a satisfactory AR effect for PCNA and p53 IHC staining. Igarashi et al. (16) studied the AR heating technique using 56 antibodies and several heating methods, including hydrated autoclaving (121°C, 2 atm for 20 min), MW oven heating (100°C for 10 min), conventional heating in distilled water (60°C overnight), and conventional heating in 20% $ZnSO_4$ (90°C for 10 min). They found that higher temperature heating (by MW or autoclave) was superior for most antibodies tested, although a few antibodies (HHF35 and CGA7) gave better results at

Table 1. Correlation of Heating Temperature and Heating Time in High-Temperature Heating Antigen Retrieval[a]

Heating time	Temperature (°C)				
(min)	100	90	80	70	60
5	++	+	-	-	-
5 × 2	+++	++	-	-	-
5 × 3	+++	++	-	-	-
5 × 4	++++	+++	±	-	-
5 × 6	++++	++++	++	+	-
5 × 8	NT	NT	+++	+	±
5 × 10	NT	NT	++++	+	±
5 × 12	NT	NT	NT	++	+
5 × 14	NT	NT	NT	++	+
5 h	NT	NT	NT	+++	+
10 h	NT	NT	NT	++++	++

[a]The monoclonal antibody MIB-1 was applied to routinely processed archival paraffin sections of tonsils from two cases. All tests were repeated twice and examined independently by three authors. Both the microwave oven and the water bath were used for heating tissue sections before immunostaining. NT, no test. Reprinted with permission from Reference 42.

60°C overnight. Our experience also indicates an inverse correlation between heating temperature and heating time, as expressed by the formula:

$$AR = T \times t \qquad\qquad [1]$$

where AR is the optimal AR-IHC result, T is the temperature of AR heating, and t is the time of AR heating treatment.

Recently, we conducted an experiment to study further the correlation between the heating temperature and the heating time, under a variety of different heating conditions. Our conclusion was based on careful comparison of different heating temperatures ranging from 60° to 100°C with heating times ranging from 5 minutes to 10 hours, using an MW oven, conventional heating (water bath and hot plate), pressure cooker, or autoclave (Table 1). A similarly strong intensity of AR-IHC staining could be generated by the following heating conditions ($T \times t$): 100°C × 20 minutes, 90°C × 30 minutes, 80°C × 50 minutes, and 70°C × 10 hours (40,42,54). Shibuya et al. (43) also determined that the intensity of AR-IHC may be dependent on both the heating temperature and time. Furthermore, Munakata and Hendricks (32) demonstrated that an extended heating time may be required to obtain an optimal AR-IHC result for tissue sections "overfixed" in formalin.

In our recent observations (unpublished data), different antibodies [AE1, CAM 5.2, PCNA (PC-10), and vimentin] were tested on tissue sections following fixation in 10% neutral buffered formalin (NBF) for 1, 7, 14, and 30 days, with MW-AR pretreatment using different AR solutions (distilled water, 5% urea, citrate buffer, lead thiocyanate, and pH 3.5 glycine-HCl solutions) and different heating times [ranging from 5 to 120 min (5 min × 24). We found no significant difference in IHC staining results among the different AR solutions, except with distilled water, which showed slightly less IHC staining quality than the other solutions. These studies also confirmed that the longer the heating time, the better the IHC staining results with all AR solutions [again, except distilled water, which tended to decrease the staining intensity slightly of some antibodies when the tissues were heated for an extended period (120 min)]. We concluded that the optimal IHC staining intensity could be obtained at heating times of 10 minutes (5 min × 2) to 20 minutes (5 min × 4) for most formalin-sensitive antigens and for tissue fixed in formalin for different durations.

Our experience of extending heating times up to 30 minutes and beyond (in 5-min increments) indicates that two cycles of 5 minutes in an MW oven at a high power setting are suitable for most commonly used antibodies. Although absolute maximal or optimal staining may be achieved using 20 minutes for some antibodies, the difference in quality is not sufficient to warrant routine use of the 20-minute heat exposure. For any individual antibody, an optimal AR protocol may be established by using a test battery method, as described in the Appendix. Interestingly, the AR procedure has no adverse effects either on IHC staining intensity (for both formalin-sensitive and formalin-resistant antigens) or on morphology, even though the tissues were heated for long periods (120 min). Recently, lower temperature heating (below boiling conditions, around 90°C) has been recommended for AR-IHC. In this case, a longer heating time is required to reach the optimal heating condition (see Appendix). Suurmeijer and Boon (47) found that repeating the boiling cycles was more effective than extending the boiling time of a single cycle when using the AR technique (i.e., three MW cycles of 5 min was superior to using the MW continuously for 15 min). Emanuels et al. (5) reported a modified MW heating program that included 3 minutes of heating, followed by 5 minutes of cooling, repeating the cycle one to six times to avoid drying the sections, but we see no reason for recommending this approach above the more commonly employed 2 × 5-minute exposure described previously.

pH OF THE ANTIGEN RETRIEVAL SOLUTION

The pH value of the AR solution is also an important factor. Recently, we tested the hypothesis that the pH of the AR solution may influence the quality of immunostaining by using seven different AR buffer solutions (acetate, citrate, phosphate, Tris-HCl, sodium diethylbarbiturate-HCl, sodium phosphate-citric acid, and dimethylglutaric acid-NaOH buffers) at a series of different pH values ranging from 1.0 to 10.0 (38). We evaluated the staining of monoclonal antibodies to cytoplasmic antigens [AE1, HMB45, neuron-specific enolase (NSE)], nuclear antigens [MIB-1, PCNA, estrogen receptor (ER)], and cell surface antigens [MT-1, L26, epithelial membrane antigen (EMA)] on routinely formalin-fixed, paraffin-embedded sections under different pH conditions with MW-AR heating for 10 minutes. The pH value of the AR buffer solution was carefully measured before, immediately after, and 15 minutes after the AR procedure. From this study, we drew the following conclusions:

1. There were three types of patterns reflecting the influence of pH. First (type A), several antigens (L26, PCNA, AE1, EMA, and NSE) showed no significant variation using AR solutions with pH values ranging from 1.0 to 10.0; second (type B), other antigens (MIB-1, ER) showed a dramatic decrease in the intensity of the AR-IHC staining at middle range pH values (pH 3.0–6.0) but strong AR-IHC results above and below these critical zones; and third (type C), still other antigens (MT1, HMB45) showed negative or weak focally positive immunostaining with a low pH (1.0–2.0) but excellent results in the high pH range (Figures 1 and 2).

2. Among the seven buffer solutions at any given pH value, the intensity of AR-IHC staining was similar, with the single exception that Tris-HCl buffer tended to produce better results at higher pH compared with other buffers.

3. Optimization of the AR system should include optimization of the pH of the AR solution.

4. A high-pH AR solution, such as Tris-HCl or sodium acetate buffer at pH 8.0–9.0, may be suitable for most antigens. This conclusion has been supported by several recent studies. For example, Pileri et al. (34) revealed that stronger intensity of AR-IHC may be achieved using AR solution at higher pH value, particularly using EDTA-NaOH at pH 8.0, and Evers and Uylings (7) obtained the best immunostaining results on formalin-overfixed brain tissues using Tris-HCl buffer at pH 9.0.

5. Low-pH AR solutions are most useful for nuclear antigens such as retinoblastoma protein (RB), ER protein, and androgen receptor.

6. Focal weak false-positive nuclear staining may be found when using low-pH AR solution [the use of negative control slides is important to exclude this possibility (38,52)].

Evers and Uylings (6) also found that the AR-IHC is pH and temperature dependent. They tested two antibodies, MAP-2 and SMI-32, and indicated that the optimal pH values were pH 4.5 for MAP-2, and pH 2.5 for SMI-32. In addition, they demonstrated that the use of 4% aluminum chloride as the AR solution for SMI-32 could achieve a similar result to that obtained using citrate buffer of pH 2.5, from which

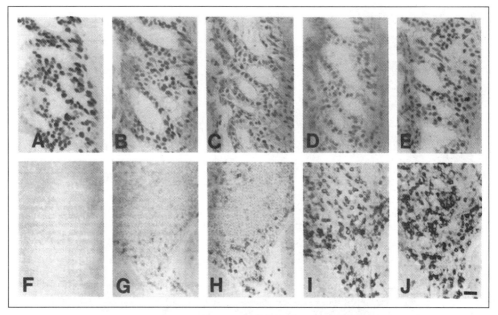

Figure 1. Comparisons of the intensity of AR immunostaining in routinely formalin-fixed, paraffin-embedded tissue sections. (A–E) A monoclonal antibody (mAb) to ER in breast tissue. (F–J) mAb MT1 in lymph node. Sodium diethylbarbiturate-HCl (SDH) buffer was utilized as the AR solution for both antibodies. (A–E) The pH values of the AR solution were pH 2.0, 3.0, 4.0, 6.0, and 8.0, which correspond to staining intensities of ++++, +++, +, ++, and +++, respectively, for ER with a type B pattern. (F–J) A type C pattern with SDH as the AR solution of pH 2.0, 3.0, 4.0, 6.0, and 8.0 and staining intensities of -, +, ++, +++, and ++++, respectively, for MT1. Some nuclei showed very weak false nuclear staining in F. Diaminobenzidine (DAB) was the chromogen, and hematoxylin was the counterstain. Original magnification 100×. Bar = 20 μm. Reprinted with permission from Reference 38. **(See color plate A2).**

they concluded that it is not important what kind of solution is used as long as the pH is at an appropriate level.

MOLARITY OF THE SOLUTION

Suurmeijer and Boon (47) tested the effect of molarity using an aluminum chloride solution with concentrations of 0.5%, 1%, 2%, and 4% for AR-IHC staining of vimentin on routinely processed paraffin tissue sections. They found that the optimal staining for vimentin in 10 different tissue components was achieved with 4% aluminum chloride. Suurmeijer (46) compared AR results with the use of 0.01 mol/L and 0.3 mol/L aluminum chloride and found that different antigens showed significantly different responses to changes in molarity.

CHEMICAL COMPOSITION OF THE SOLUTION

In our initial studies of the AR technique, we used a metal salt in the AR solution and obtained good results for several antibodies tested. The use of metal salt solutions was based on earlier studies concerning zinc–formalin fixation of tissue sections (19). We speculated that the metal salt solution might effectively influence the struc-

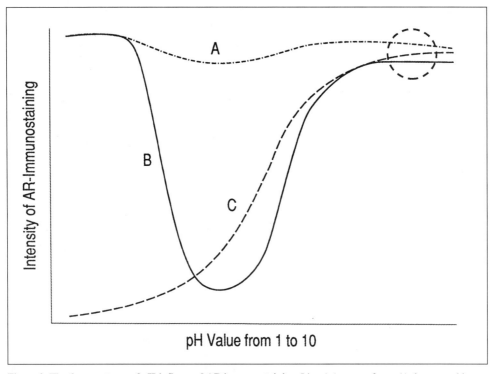

Figure 2. The three patterns of pH-influenced AR immunostaining. Line A (pattern of type A) shows a stable pattern of staining with only a slight decrease in staining intensity between pH 3.0 and 6.0. Line B (pattern of type B) shows a dramatic decrease in staining intensity between pH 3.0 and 6.0. Line C (pattern of type C) exhibits an ascending intensity of AR immunostaining that correlated with an increasing pH value of the AR solution. Circle (right) indicates the advantage of using an AR solution of higher pH value. Reprinted with permission from Reference 38.

ture of protein by playing a role in refixation of the retrieved antigens. The increase of immunostaining intensity resulting from the use of metal salt AR solutions has subsequently been demonstrated by several studies (12,13,21,27,30,33,44,45,47,53). However, a major drawback of using metal salts, particularly lead salts, is the potential toxic effect, as mentioned by Suurmeijer and Boon (47). It is therefore better to avoid using lead or other toxic metal salts if other solutions may serve with equal effect in the AR procedure. It should also be noted that some authors (31) reported poor AR-IHC staining results with the use of metal salt solutions, based on inappropriate comparative studies, as discussed elsewhere (41).

From our more recent studies regarding AR-IHC under the influence of pH (38), we found that while the pH is critical, the chemical composition of the AR solution may, in some instances, also play a role as a cofactor. For example, for antibodies to RB protein, including a polyclonal antibody (RB-WL-1) and a monoclonal antibody (PMG3-245; BioGenex, San Ramon, CA, USA), we found that a better staining result was obtained using acetate buffer solution at pH 1.0 to 2.0 with MW heating at 100°C for 10 minutes, compared with citrate buffer at the same pH value. Imam et al. (17) reported that the use of a glycine-HCl solution at pH 3.6 as the AR solution yielded stronger immunostaining with antibodies to some antigens (such as androgen receptor, ER, Ki-67, MIB-1, EMA, MT-1, and actin) compared with that obtained using citrate buffer as the AR solution, raising the possibility that the chemical composition of glycine-HCl may play a role in AR treatment. Another example of the possible influence of chemical components in the AR solution was provided by Hazelbag et al. (14), who demonstrated that a simple detergent solution could yield the same AR immunostaining result as obtained using the commercial AR solution known as target unmasking fluid (TUF; Kreatech Biotechnology, Amsterdam, The Netherlands) for a variety of antibodies to keratin.

The potential functions of chemical components in the AR solution include: *(i)* secondary fixation after unfixation by high-temperature heating; *(ii)* stabilization of antigens during heating or strong alkaline hydrolysis; *(iii)* maintenance of optimal molarity; and *(iv)* as unknown cofactors in reconfiguring the unfixed protein, thereby recovering antigenicity. Analysis of these separate factors may allow development of new AR solutions applicable to those cell surface antigens that do not respond well to current retrieval methods. For example, we recently tested the influence of different chemicals in AR and found that a mixed AR solution of Tris-HCl at pH 9.5 with 5% urea may yield stronger staining intensity for some antigens (39). Similarly, Kwaspen et al. (22) reported the use of 1% periodic acid as an AR solution for MW-AR-IHC to study keratin expression on archival tissue sections, providing strong positive staining.

COMMENTS

In conclusion, major factors that influence the results of AR-IHC staining include heating temperature and heating time (heating condition $T \times t$) and the pH value of the AR solution. The chemical component and molarity of the AR solution are cofactors that may also influence the effectiveness of AR-IHC in certain instances.

In a broad sense, factors that influence AR-IHC may be grouped into three categories, pre-AR treatment (formalin fixation and processing of the tissue into sections), AR treatment, and post-AR treatment (immunostaining).

Several other factors, apart from the AR process itself, may also play a role in the

Table 2. Immunostaining Intensity of Different Antibodies on Tissues Fixed in Formalin for Different Durations without AR Pretreatment[a]

Fixation time (days)	Primary Antibody			
	AE1	CAM 5.2	PCNA	Vimentin
1	++	++++	++/+++	++
7	++/+	++++	++	+
14	+	++++	++	+
30	-	+++/++++	-	-

[a]Immunostaining intensities are graded as - to ++++, representing negative to strongest intensity of staining. (Frozen sections were used as a standard for the strongest intensity, as ++++). PCNA, proliferating cell nuclear antigen.

success of the procedure. These factors include fixation (type and duration of fixative), type of epitopes (antigens) or antibodies, and dehydration (especially in incompletely fixed tissues) in pre-AR treatments, and ease of detection and signal amplification procedures in post-AR treatments.

Pre-Antigen Retrieval Treatment

Fixation

Common fixatives used in histopathology are divided into two groups: coagulant fixatives, such as ethanol, and cross-linking fixatives, such as formaldehyde. Both types of fixative can cause changes in the steric configuration of proteins, which may mask antigenic sites (epitopes) and adversely affect antibody binding. It has been well recognized that cross-linking fixatives alter the IHC results of a significant number of antigens, whereas coagulant fixatives (especially ethanol) have been reported to preserve immunoreactivity, for at least some antigens, better than cross-linking fixatives (3,11,26,37). In most surgical pathology laboratories, the fixative used is 10% NBF (a cross-linking fixative), for which the immunostaining intensity is known to be fixation–time-dependent for many antigens (1,26,42). Moreover, there are reports that the longer the fixation time, the more vigorous the retrieval procedure required (32,53). However, most antigens masked by formalin fixation have been shown to be retrievable by various AR methods, as is discussed below. Finally, it is worthy of note that, because of the adverse effects of 10% NBF on IHC staining, many other fixatives have been proposed (4,51), but none have proved to be satisfactory (35). Thus, there appears to be a role for the AR procedure, for the foreseeable feature.

Type of Antigen (Epitope)/Antibody

As mentioned earlier, fixatives (especially cross-linking fixatives) frequently alter protein structure with adverse effects on IHC staining. Immunohistochemical protocols employing polyclonal antibodies are often less affected than those employing monoclonal antibodies, because polyclonal antibodies recognize multiple epitopes, not all of which are equally impaired by the fixation process (24). However, there are also several reports of formalin-resistant epitopes detected by monoclonal antibodies (3,8,15,25,26,36), and indeed, attempts have been made specifically to develop and screen for monoclonal antibodies that are effective in formalin–paraffin sections.

In general, it is difficult to predict, either on theoretical grounds or from prior experience, whether a particular newly developed monoclonal antibody will successfully detect its corresponding antigen (epitope) in formalin–paraffin sections. In practice, each antibody must be tested and evaluated experimentally. One study in our laboratories (B. Chaiwun, unpublished observation) illustrates these points. We performed IHC staining using four different monoclonal antibodies, including AE1 (Signet, Dedham, MA, USA), CAM 5.2 (Becton-Dickinson, San Jose, CA, USA), anti-PCNA (PC-10) (Dako, Carpinteria, CA, USA), and anti-vimentin (Dako) on tissues that were fixed in 10% NBF for 1, 7, 14, and 30 days. IHC stains were performed without AR pretreatment, and parallel frozen tissue sections were stained in every case, serving as intensity reference standards. We found three patterns of antigen masking and retrieval (unmasking) results, as shown in Table 2 and Figure 3. These findings suggest that it may be possible to classify antigens into three broad categories (highly formalin-sensitive epitopes, moderately formalin-sensitive epitopes, and formalin-resistant epitopes), providing some guidance as to whether AR pretreatment may be needed for a particular individual antibody. However, as noted above, the final decisions as to whether to employ AR is always based on observed staining results.

Highly Formalin-Sensitive Epitopes

Antibodies to these highly formalin-sensitive epitopes yielded weak IHC staining even when the tissues were fixed in formalin for only 24 h. The staining intensities were dramatically decreased in tissues fixed for longer periods. Negative IHC staining was obtained in tissue fixed for 30 days (vimentin, AE-1).

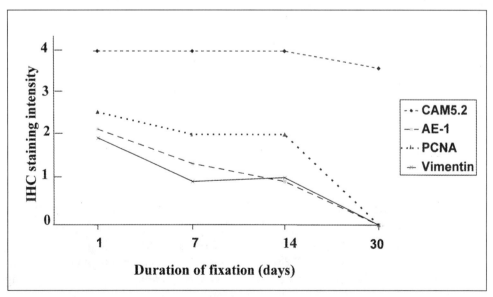

Figure 3. The three patterns of IHC staining intensity of epitopes in tissue fixed in formalin for different durations (see Table 2).

Moderately Formalin-Sensitive Epitopes

Antibodies to these moderately formalin-sensitive epitopes yielded slightly reduced IHC staining when the tissue was fixed in formalin for 24 hours and showed a gradual decrease in staining intensity as the tissues were fixed for longer periods in formalin. Negative IHC staining was obtained in tissue fixed for 30 days (PCNA).

Formalin-Resistant Epitopes

Formalin-resistant epitopes revealed excellent IHC staining intensity throughout different durations of formalin fixation, ranging from 1 to 30 days (CAM 5.2). This type of epitope needs no AR pretreatment for IHC staining.

Indeed, the hypothetical mechanism of AR (as proposed in Chapter 1) suggests the possibility that heat-induced AR applied to formalin-resistant epitopes may itself have adverse consequences. In general, high-temperature heating (in AR) is a process of correction or reversal of the formalin-induced modification of protein conformation. As previously mentioned, the AR technique exploits the formalin-induced modification of protein structure, whereby modified proteins resist denaturation by the intense heating of the AR process. If an epitope of a certain protein is formalin resistant, it may mean that there has been no significant modification of the epitope-associated protein structure during formalin fixation. Under these circumstances, the high-temperature heating may denature this unchanged protein structure and produce a poor immunostaining result.

Dehydration: Before Embedding

Although less critical than other steps, inappropriate dehydration has been demonstrated to decrease the IHC staining intensity in some antigens, especially in tissue incompletely fixed by formalin (18,23,24). One proposed mechanism is that the incompletely fixed tissue may be postfixed by ethanol, and possibly extracted during the dehydration sequence. This phenomenon may also account for relatively weak IHC staining, either with or without AR pretreatment, of some antibodies in the central portion of formalin-fixed, paraffin-embedded tissue sections, which may reflect incomplete penetration of the formalin into the tissue center.

Because each step in the fixation process cannot be controlled, and detailed fixation times are not available for each formalin-fixed paraffin tissue sections other approaches have been explored to achieve optimal IHC staining (42,49,50). Recognizing that heating temperature, heating time, and pH of the AR solution are the key variables, a simple approach has been devised to standardize these factors, as exemplified by the use of a test battery (see Appendix).

Treatment after Antigen Retrieval

The effectiveness and quality of the immunohistochemical staining procedure performed after AR treatment, will clearly affect the apparent success of AR. If the immunostaining protocol per se is poor, then, however effective the recovery of antigen, the overall result must also be poor. In brief, two critical issues should be kept in mind with regard to the immunostaining procedure to achieve satisfactory results:

1. After AR treatment, the sensitivity or ease of detection of many antigens in for-

malin–paraffin tissue sections is significantly increased, sometimes approximating that of frozen tissue sections. Under these circumstances, further dilution of the primary antibody may be necessary to reduce background staining.

2. AR heating treatment may be combined with signal amplification procedures to improve the intensity of staining for certain antigens, such as leukocyte surface antigens that show very weak or negative staining results (see Chapter 14 and Appendix).

A satisfactory IHC result requires a complete plan of standardization not only for the AR procedure itself, but also for the other factors described above including the fixation and immunostaining protocols, all of which affect the overall result.

REFERENCES

1. **Battifora, H. and M. Kopinski.** 1986. The influence of protease digestion and duration of fixation on the immunostaining of keratins. A comparison of formalin and ethanol fixation. J. Histochem. Cytochem. *34*:1095-1100.
2. **Cattoretti, G., S. Pileri, C. Parravicini, M.H.G. Becker, S. Poggi, C. Bifulco, G. Key, L. D'Amato, E. Sabattini, E. Feudale et al.** 1993. Antigen unmasking on formalin-fixed, paraffin-embedded tissue sections. J. Pathol. *171*:83-98.
3. **Cuevas, E.C., A.C. Bateman, B.S. Wilkins, P.A. Johnson, J.H. Willams, A.H.S. Lee, D.B. Jones, and D.H. Wright.** 1994. Microwave antigen retrieval in immunocytochemistry: a study of 80 antibodies. J. Clin. Pathol. *47*:448-452.
4. **Dapson, R.W.** 1993. Fixation for the 1990's: a review of needs and accomplishments. Biotech. Histochem. *65*:75-82.
5. **Emanuels, A., H. Hollema, A. Suurmeyer, and J. Koudstaal.** 1994. A modified method for antigen retrieval MIB-1 staining of vulvar carcinoma. Eur. J. Morphol. *32* (Suppl 2-4):335-337.
6. **Evers, P. and H.B.M. Uylings.** 1994. Microwave-stimulated antigen retrieval is pH and temperature dependent. J. Histochem. Cytochem. *42*:1555-1563.
7. **Evers, P. and H.B.M. Uylings.** 1997. An optimal antigen retrieval method suitable for different antibodies on human brain tissue stored for several years in formaldehyde fixative. J. Neurosci. Methods *72*:197-207.
8. **Fraenkel-Conrat, H., B.A. Brandon, and H.S. Olcott.** 1947. The reaction of formaldehyde with proteins. IV. Participation of indole groups. Gramicidin. J. Biol. Chem. *168*:99-118.
9. **Fraenkel-Conrat, H. and H.S. Olcott.** 1948. Reaction of formaldehyde with proteins. The cross linking of amino groups with phenol, imidazole, or indole groups. J. Biol. Chem. *174*:827-843.
10. **Fraenkel-Conrat, H. and H.S. Olcott.** 1948. The reaction of formaldehyde with proteins. V. Cross-linking between amino and primary amide or guanidyl groups. J. Am. Chem. Soc. *70*:2673-2684.
11. **Gown, A.M., N. de Wever, and H. Battifora.** 1993. Microwave based antigenic unmasking. A revolutionary new technique for routine immunohistochemistry. Appl. Immunohistochem. *1*:256-266.
12. **Greenwell, A., J.F. Foley, and R.R. Maronpot.** 1991. An enhancement method for immunohistochemical staining of proliferating cell nuclear antigen in archival rodent tissues. Cancer Lett. *59*:251-256.
13. **Gu, J., M. Forte, H. Hance, N. Carson, C. Xenachis, and R. Rufner.** 1994. Microwave fixation, antigen retrieval and accelerated immunocytochemistry. Cell Vision *1*:76-77.
14. **Hazelbag, H.M., L.J.C.M. van den Broek, E.B.L. van Dorst, G.J.A. Offerhaus, G.J. Fleuren, and P.C.W. Hogendoorn.** 1995. Immunostaining of chain-specific keratins on formalin-fixed, paraffin-embedded tissues: a comparison of various antigen retrieval systems using microwave heating and proteolytic pre-treatments. J. Histochem. Cytochem. *43*:429-437.
15. **Hoyt, J.W., A.M. Gown, D.K. Kim, and M.S. Berger.** 1995. Analysis of proliferative grade in glial neoplasms using antibodies to the Ki-67 defined antigen and PCNA in formalin fixed deparaffinized tissues. J. Neurooncol. *24*:163-169.
16. **Igarashi, H., H. Sugimura, K. Maruyama, Y. Kitayama, I. Ohta, M. Suzuki, M. Tanaka, Y. Dobashi, and I. Kino.** 1994. Alteration of immunoreactivity by hydrated autoclaving, microwave treatment, and simple heating of paraffin-embedded tissue sections. APMIS *102*:295-307.
17. **Imam, S.A., L. Young, B. Chaiwun, and C.R. Taylor.** 1995. Comparison of two microwave based antigen-retrieval solutions in unmasking epitopes in formalin-fixed tissue for immunostaining. Anticancer Res. *15*:1153-1158.
18. **Jaarsma, P.** 1992. Dehydration and immunohistochemistry. Histochem. J. *24*:493.
19. **Jones, M.D., P.M. Banks, and B.L. Caron.** 1981. Transition metal salts as adjuncts to formalin for tissue fixation. Lab. Invest. *44*:32A.
20. **Kawai, K., A. Serizawa, T. Hamana, and Y. Tsutsumi.** 1994. Heat-induced antigen retrieval of proliferating

cell nuclear antigen and p53 protein in formalin-fixed, paraffin-embedded sections. Pathol. Int. *44*:759-764.

21. **Kawai, K., S. Umemura, and Y. Tsutsumi.** 1994. Antigen retrieval by heating treatment. Saibo *26*:152-157.

22. **Kwaspen, F., F. Smedts, J. Blom, A. Peonk, M.-J. Kok, M. Van Dijk, and F. Ramaekers.** 1995. Periodic acid as a nonenzymatic enhancement technique for the detection of cytokeratin immunoreactivity in routinely processed carcinomas. Appl. Immunohistochem. *3*:54-63.

23. **Larsson, L.I.** 1988. Immunocytochemistry: Theory and Practice. Ch. 2, p. 41-74. CRC Press, Boca Raton.

24. **Larsson, L.I.** 1993. Tissue preparation methods for light microscopic immunohistochemistry. Appl. Immunohistochem. *1*:2-16.

25. **Layfield, R., K. Bailey, J. Lowe, R. Allibone, R.J. Mayer, and M. Landon.** 1996. Extraction and protein sequencing of immunoglobulin light chain from formalin-fixed cerebrovascular amyloid deposits. J. Pathol. *180*:455-459.

26. **Leong, A.S.Y. and P.N. Gilham.** 1989. The effects of progressive formaldehyde fixation on the preservation of tissue antigens. Pathology *21*:266-268.

27. **Lucassen, P.J., R. Ravid, N.K. Gonatas, and D.F. Swaab.** 1993. Activation of the human supraoptic and paraventricular nucleus neurons with aging and in Alzheimer's disease as judged from increasing size of the Golgi apparatus. Brain Res. *632*:105-113.

28. **Malmstrom, P.-U., K. Wester, J. Vasko, and C. Busch.** 1992. Expression of proliferative cell nuclear antigen (PCNA) in urinary bladder carcinoma. Evaluation of antigen retrieval methods. APMIS *100*:988-992.

29. **Mason, J.T. and T.J. O'Leary.** 1991. Effects of formaldehyde fixation on protein secondary structure: a calorimetric and infrared spectroscopic investigation. J. Histochem. Cytochem. *39*:225-229.

30. **Merz, H., O. Rickers, S. Schrimel, K. Orscheschek, and A.C. Feller.** 1993. Constant detection of surface and cytoplasmic immunoglobulin heavy and light chain expression in formalin-fixed and paraffin-embedded material. J. Pathol. *170*:257-264.

31. **Momose, H., P. Mehta, and H. Battifora.** 1993. Antigen retrieval by microwave irradiation in lead thiocyanate. Appl. Immunohistochem. *1*:77-82.

32. **Munakata, S. and J.B. Hendricks.** 1993. Effect of fixation time and microwave oven heating time on retrieval of the Ki-67 antigen from paraffin-embedded tissue. J. Histochem. Cytochem. *41*:1241-1246.

33. **Pavelic, Z.P., L.G. Portugal, M.J. Gootee, P.J. Stambrook, C. Smith, R.E. Mugge, L. Pavelic, K. Wilson, C.R. Buncher, Y.Q. Li et al.** 1993. Retrieval of p53 protein in paraffin-embedded head and neck tumor tissues. Arch. Otolaryngol. Head Neck Surg. *119*:1206-1209.

34. **Pileri, S.A., G. Roncador, C. Ceccarelli, M. Piccioli, A. Briskomatis, E. Sabattini, S. Ascani, D. Santini, P.P. Piccaluga, O. Leone et al.** 1997. Antigen retrieval techniques in immunohistochemistry: comparison of different methods. J. Pathol. *183*:116-123.

35. **Prento, P. and H. Lyon.** 1997. Commercial formalin substitutes for histopathology. Biotech. Histochem. *72*:273-282.

36. **Rugtveit, J., H. Scott, T.S. Halstensen, J. Norstein, and P. Brandtzaeg.** 1996. Expression of the L1 antigen (calprolectin) by tissue macrophages reflects recent recruitment from peripheral blood rather than upregulation of local synthesis: implications for rejection diagnosis in formalin-fixed kidney specimens. J. Pathol. *180*:194-199.

37. **Shi, S.-R., M.E. Key, and K.L. Kalra.** 1991. Antigen retrieval in formalin-fixed, paraffin-embedded tissues. An enhancement method for immunohistochemical staining based on microwave oven heating of tissue reactions. J. Histochem. Cytochem. *39*:741-748.

38. **Shi, S.-R., S.A. Imam, L. Young, R.J. Cote, and C.R. Taylor.** 1995. Antigen retrieval immunohistochemistry under the influence of pH using monoclonal antibodies. J. Histochem. Cytochem. *43*:193-201.

39. **Shi, S.-R., R.J. Cote, L. Young, S.A. Imam, and C.R. Taylor.** 1996. Use of pH 9.5 Tris-HCl buffer containing 5% urea for antigen retrieval immunohistochemistry. Biotech. Histochem. *71*:190-196.

40. **Shi, S.-R., R.J. Cote, C. Yang, C. Chen, H.J. Xu, W.F. Benedict, and C.R. Taylor.** 1996. Development of optimal protocol for antigen retrieval: a "test battery" approach exemplified with reference to the staining of retinoblastoma protein (pRB) in formalin-fixed paraffin sections. J. Pathol. *179*:347-352.

41. **Shi, S.-R., R.J. Cote, and C.R. Taylor.** 1997. Antigen retrieval immunohistochemistry: practice and development. J. Histotechnol. *20*:145-154.

42. **Shi, S.R., R.J. Cote, B. Chaiwun, L.L. Young, Y. Shi, D. Hawes, T. Chen, and C.R. Taylor.** 1998. Standardization of immunohistochemistry based on antigen retreival technique for routine formalin-fixed tissue sections. Appl. Immunohistochem. *6*:89-96.

43. **Shibuya, M., H. Utsunomiya, and R.Y. Osamura.** 1993. Immunohistochemical determination of the proliferating cells with monoclonal antibody MIB-1 on paraffin-embedded section—using antigen retrieval method. Byori-to-Rinsho *11*:373-377.

44. **Siitonen, S.M., O.P. Kallioniemi, and J.J. Isola.** 1993. Proliferating cell nuclear antigen immunohistochemistry using monoclonal antibody 19A2 and a new antigen retrieval technique has prognostic impact in archival paraffin-embedded node-negative breast cancer. Am. J. Pathol. *142*:1081-1089.

45. **Spires, S.E., C.D. Jennings, E.R. Banks, D.P. Wood, D.D. Davey, and M.L. Cibull.** 1994. Proliferating cell nuclear antigen in prostatic adenocarcinoma: correlation with established prognostic indicators. Urology *43*:660-666.

46. **Suurmeijer, A.J.H.** 1994. Optimizing immunohistochemistry in diagnostic tumor pathology with antigen

retrieval. Eur. J. Morphol. *32* (Suppl 2-4):325-330.

47.**Suurmeijer, A.J.H. and M.E. Boon.** 1993. Notes on the application of microwaves for antigen retrieval in paraffin and plastic tissue sections. Eur. J. Morphol. *31*:144-150.

48.**Suurmeijer, A.J.H. and M.E. Boon.** 1993. Optimizing keratin and vimentin retrieval in formalin-fixed, paraffin-embedded tissue with the use of heat and metal salts. Appl. Immunohistochem. *1*:143-148.

49.**Taylor, C.R.** 1994. An exaltation of experts: concerted efforts in the standardization of immunohistochemistry (perspectives in pathology). Hum. Pathol. *25*:2-11.

50.**Taylor, C.R.** 1994. The current role of immunohistochemistry in diagnostic pathology. Adv. Pathol. Lab. Med. *7*:59-105.

51.**Taylor, C.R. and S.R. Shi.** 1994. Fixation, processing, special applications, p. 42-70. *In* C.R. Taylor and R.J. Cote (Eds.), Immunomicroscopy: A Diagnostic Tool for the Surgical Pathologist. W.B. Saunders, Philadelphia.

52.**Taylor, C.R., S.-R. Shi, B. Chaiwun, L. Young, S.A. Imam, and R.J. Cote.** 1994. Standardization and reproducibility in diagnostic immunohistochemistry. Hum. Pathol. *25*:1107-1109.

53.**Taylor, C.R., S.R. Shi, B. Chaiwun, L. Young, S.A. Imam, and R.J. Cote.** 1994. Strategies for improving the immunohistochemical staining of various intranuclear prognostic markers in formalin-paraffin sections: androgen receptor, estrogen receptor, progesterone receptor, protein, proliferating cell nuclear antigen, and Ki-67 antigen revealed by antigen retrieval techniques. Hum. Pathol. *25*:263-270.

54.**Taylor, C.R., S.R. Shi, C. Chen, L. Young, C. Yang, and R.J. Cote.** 1996. Comparative study of antigen retrieval heating methods: microwave, microwave and pressure cooker, autoclave, and steamer. Biotech. Histochem. *71*:263-270.

Section II

Development and Expanding Application

The MIB-1 Method for Fine-Tuning Diagnoses in Cervical Cytology

3

Mathilde E. Boon,[1] Lambrecht P. Kok,[2] and Albert J.H. Suurmeijer[3]

[1]Leiden Cytology and Pathology Laboratory, Leiden, [2]Department of Biomedical Technology, University of Groningen, Groningen, and [3]Department of Pathology and Laboratory Medicine, University Hospital Groningen, Groningen, The Netherlands

INTRODUCTION

While traveling during the past few years in developed and developing countries, we observed that antigen retrieval (AR) is widely used in diagnostic pathology practice. Of all markers used, MIB-1 (Ki-67) is the most prominent. It allows the pathologist to identify the proliferating cells much more easily than the traditional method used since the beginning of this century (i.e., counting mitotic figures to estimate the biologic potential of the tumor). The mitotic figures as seen in hematoxylin and eosin (H&E) sections represent only the tip of the iceberg. In MIB-1-stained sections, many more cells prove to be cycling cells. Therefore, it is not surprising that, particularly in tumor pathology, MIB-1 staining has become state of the art. In all pathology laboratories, whether in India or in the United States, the MIB-1 method can easily be performed on histologic and cytologic samples.

Thanks to recent developments, for the price of a local phone call, every pathologist can do a fascinating search through the literature, making use of the facilities that the internet provides. The authors of this chapter recently searched the MIB-1 literature using the free access to MEDLINE (PubMed) provided by the U.S. National Library of Medicine. In total, we found some 600 MIB-1 papers. Virtually all of these papers were published in the past five years (1994–1998), after the key publi-

Antigen Retrieval Techniques
Edited by Shan-Rong Shi, Jiang Gu, and Clive R. Taylor
©2000 Eaton Publishing, Natick, MA

Table 1. Correlation of MIB-1 Labeling with Other Prognosticators

Prognosticator	Reference	Material studied
Metallothioneins	17	Benign, CIN, SCC
Transcription factors	14	Benign, CIN
Topoisomerase II-α	13	Benign, CIN, SCC
Laminin receptor	2	Benign, CIN, SCC
p53	3	SCC
p53	10	SCC before and after chemotherapy

CIN, cervical intraepithelial neoplasia; SCC, squamous cell carcinoma.

cation of Cattoretti et al. (6) when the AR period for MIB-1 began. Almost one-quarter of these papers were published in 1998. Our main interest was cervical pathology; thus, we further narrowed down our search by the additional key word cervix. We ended up with 20 publications, which were reviewed for this chapter. This method of searching the literature was determined to be reliable, in that it listed all of our own MIB-1 papers among the search results.

MIB-1 AND OTHER PROGNOSTICATORS

As with other tumor sites, MIB-1 labeling correlates with prognosis (10–12,13, 19,22). Therefore, it is to be anticipated that the percentage of MIB-1-positive nuclei in tissue sections is in accordance with those of other prognosticators. This is indeed the case, as can be seen in Table 1. McCluggage et al. (17) reported that overexpression of metallothioneins in cervical lesions appears to occur at some point along the spectrum of high-grade cervical intraepithelial neoplasia (CIN) and may be related to cell proliferation. The transcription factors Skn-1, Oct-1, and AP2 and the novel proliferation marker topoisomerase II-α are also related to MIB-1 labeling of CIN lesions (13). Laminin plays an important role during the progression of solid tumors; therefore, Al-Saleh et al. (2) investigated the 67-kDa laminin receptor and MIB-1 staining of cervical lesions. They found that there was a positive correlation between expression of the 67-kDa laminin receptor and MIB-1 protein for each type of lesion studied. Thus, both prognosticators are valuable for cervical lesion studies. Positive correlations were also found for the well-established prognosticator p53, with MIB-1 labeling in sections of squamous cell carcinoma (SCC) (3,10). Of special interest are the publications of the group in Ancona (Italy), investigating these markers before and after chemotherapy, and, accordingly, differentiating good from poor responders (9). These authors also used MIB-1 staining to evaluate a group with a known poor prognosis [i.e., young women with SCC (12)]. They established that, for this group, the MIB-1 indices are higher than for older patients having a better prognosis.

As can be argued, cytology is not a good method of establishing MIB-1 staining of the parent tumor in cases of SCC; therefore, cytologic samples cannot be used to prognosticate SCC patients. However, CIN lesions are different, in that their cytology contains the cell population on which prognostic analysis can be safely used. Therefore, it is important to know that, for CIN lesions, MIB-1 labeling correlates with other prognosticators (2,13,14,17).

Table 2. Benign and (Pre)Malignant MIB-1-Positive Cells in Cervical Smears

Type of cell	Nuclear shape	Exfoliation pattern
Histiocytes	Bean shape	Rows and streaks
Lymphoid cells	Round	Starry sky pattern
Herpes virocytes	Nuclear molding	Single giant cells
Benign reserve cells	Oval, often damaged	Rows and small clumps, epithelial fragments
Benign endocervical cells	Oval	Single or small clusters
(Pre)malignant cells, CIN, and SCC	Variable	Single and many epithelial fragments
AIS and AC	Variable	Single and in many epithelial fragments

CIN, cervical intraepithelial neoplasia; AIS, adenocarcinoma in situ; SCC, squamous cell carcinoma; AC, adenocarcinoma.

MIB-1-POSITIVE STAINING OF VARIOUS CELL TYPES IN CERVICAL SMEARS

We established that only a few types of benign cells, including herpes virocytes and cells from lymph follicles (follicular cervicitis), which morphologically are easily recognizable, stain heavily for MIB-1. In addition, cells from tissue repair display some positive staining, mainly located in and around the nucleolus. Completely atrophic smears also contain MIB-1-positive cells. Occasionally, a few cylindrical endocervical cells and reserve cells stain positive, but most negative smears lack positive cell populations. In contrast, smears from patients with dysplasia, carcinoma in situ (CIS), or invasive carcinoma contain many epithelial fragments with heavily positive-staining nuclei (5). For the proper classification of MIB-1-positive cells, nuclear shape and exfoliation patterns are important (Table 2).

Only those cells present in epithelial fragment smears can be used to compare the staining results of smears and histologic sections. In benign squamous and metaplastic epithelium, only a few basal cells stain positive (1,8,21), and accordingly, in the corresponding epithelial fragments in the smear, one will only find a few MIB-1-positive nuclei, located mainly on one side of the fragment. Condyloma express MIB-1-positive nuclei higher up in the epithelium (18), as do the corresponding epithelium fragments in the smear. Koilocytotic cells may or may not stain positive in histologic sections (25), and the same is true for the corresponding smears. For human papillomavirus (HPV)-induced cervical lesions, MIB-1 staining correlates with CIN grade (1,11,22) and not with HPV type (1,11,25).

It is amply documented that MIB-1 labeling correlates strongly with CIN grade (1,2,13,14,21,22); this phenomenon can also be seen in the epithelial fragments of the corresponding smears. Clinical applications are presented in this chapter. The labeling of benign cervical epithelium is low and exclusively basely located, and, accordingly, no MIB-1-positive cells exfoliate from the surface (Figure 1). In CIS, labeling is also found on the surface of the epithelium; thus, exfoliating MIB-1-positive cells appear (Figure 1).

Correlating MIB-1 staining of SCC in histology and cytology proves to be highly problematic because, in cytology, one is often confronted with the necrotic surface of the carcinoma lacking MIB-1 staining. It is reported that in histologic sections, the maximal level of MIB-1 labeling is found in invasive carcinoma (13), whereas we have encountered smears from SCC completely lacking MIB-1-positive nuclei but containing cells recognizable morphologically as malignant. In other words, MIB-1 staining of smears from SCC is of limited value.

For glandular endocervical carcinomas [adenocarcinoma (AC)], we are not confronted with the problems of a necrotic surface. Thus, for these lesions, the MIB-1 staining in histology (7,15,24) and cytology are similar, as is the case for the glandular in situ cases [adenocarcinoma in situ (AIS)]. Applications for diagnostic practice are presented in this chapter.

ANTIGEN RETRIEVAL OF ARCHIVAL CERVICAL SMEARS

During AR, the Papanicolaou stain is removed from the smear. After AR, the

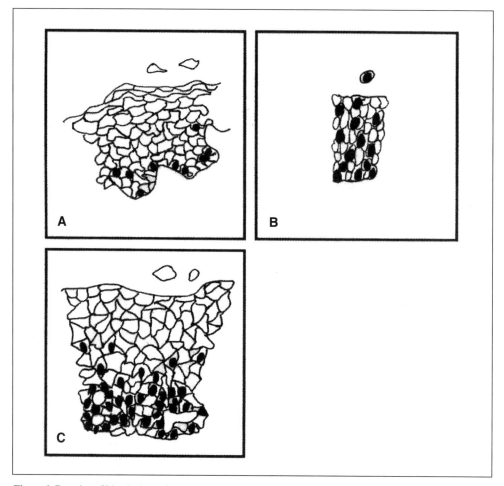

Figure 1. Drawing of histologic sections showing MIB-1-positive nuclei distribution. (A) Normal epithelium (no MIB-1-positive exfoliating cells). (B) CIS (MIB-1-positive exfoliating cells). (C) Invasive SCC (note the necrotic surface and no MIB-1-positive exfoliating cells).

smear can be stained for MIB-1 following the standard streptavidin-biotin (SAB) protocol using an antisera dilution of 1:300. After immunostaining, the slides are counterstained with Gill hematoxylin. MIB-1-positive nuclei are brown; MIB-1-negative nuclei and (to a lesser extent) cytoplasm are blue. If desired, the MIB-1 smear can be counterstained by the Papanicolaou method; the cytoplasm thus appears in the characteristic turquoise-to-red color range.

Prior to MIB-1 staining, the smears are treated as follows:
1. The smear is placed in a plastic jar containing 10 mmol/L citrate buffer, pH 6.0.
2. The jar is placed in a microwave oven and brought to boiling for 20 minutes. Care should be taken that the smears stay submerged in the citrate buffer.
3. The slides are allowed to cool slowly in the citrate buffer.
4. The slides are rinsed in Tris-buffered saline (TBS; 0.05 mol/L Tris, 0.15 mol/L NaCl) for 2 minutes.

This method can be used on archival smears. Prior destaining might result in a negative MIB-1 signal and is thus not advised (23). Both wet-fixed and air-dried smears can be used. We noted that partly air-dried cells in smears fixed with an alcohol containing spray fixative also stain beautifully for MIB-1.

VISUALIZING NORMAL AND ABNORMAL PROLIFERATING RESERVE CELLS

Primitive or reserve cells can be identified by their high nuclear/cytoplasmic (N/C) ratio, the 25- to 55-μm^2 nuclear area, and a cytoplasm that is sparse and ill defined (or mainly absent) (5). This absence is not due to degenerative changes, but rather to mechanical damage of the fragile cytoplasm during smear preparation. The pattern of exfoliation of these cells, with the nuclei lying in rows, pairs, or dense clumps, is highly characteristic. The cells can be found in less than 0.5% of smears derived from sexually mature females, most often at the time of ovulation.

Subcolumnar reserve cells are seen in the vicinity of columnar cells and show the same morphologic pattern of exfoliation as ectocervical reserve cells. The nuclei of subcolumnar reserve cells may be somewhat rounder than that of ectocervical reserve cells in an atrophic smear pattern. Occasionally, there may be a small amount of poorly defined, sparse cytoplasm, but the nuclei are mostly stripped of cytoplasm or "naked".

We hypothesized that the atypical variant of reserve cell hyperplasia displays the same characteristics as those of reserve cells in smears; thus, they have stripped nuclei, but these nuclei are atypical and larger, with irregularities in shape and chromatin pattern. Indeed, we found such stripped nuclei in great abundance in smears that also contained dysplastic and malignant cells. Similar to benign reserve cells, these atypical nuclei lie in rows, pairs, and clumps, and, in the latter, nuclear molding is evident. The naked nuclei, when very large, often appear to be collapsed on themselves, with the nuclear membrane forming folds, much like the folds of an almost completely deflated balloon. Another commonly observed phenomenon is the folding of part of the large bare nucleus over itself, in the manner of a pancake edge rolling over toward the center. Recently, we observed that the bare atypical nuclei are easily damaged in the smear process, resulting in smudged, fragmented, or disrupted nuclei (Figure 2). In the deformation of the nuclei, one can reconstruct the direction in which the material was smeared on the glass slide. The nuclear shapes can be deformed by the smear process; in addition, other features can be observed, including small irregularities in nuclear contour, indentations, and protrusions. The bare nuclei are more easily dehydrated when compared with the other cells in the smear, such as dysplastic cells. Accordingly, one can find air-dried bare nuclei of the atypical reserve cells (with still well-visible nuclear protrusions) in an otherwise well-fixed smear.

The chromatin pattern of atypical reserve cells is abnormal. The chromatin distribution is always uneven, but this might be the only sign of abnormality. The chromatin may be slightly coarse and some hyperchromasia may occur, although not as marked as in malignant or in dysplastic cells, and many nuclei even appear to be normochromatic or slightly hypochromatic. In some cases, anisokaryosis is quite marked, with extremely large hypochromatic nuclei admixed with very small ones. In both of these nuclei, the chromatin is granular alternating with clear areas, and one or more nucleoli are often present.

In the early 1980s, we published the above description of what we consider to be the cytologic presentation of atypical reserve cells (22a). Until now, we remain the only group attempting to identify atypical reserve cells in smears. We recommend that atyp-

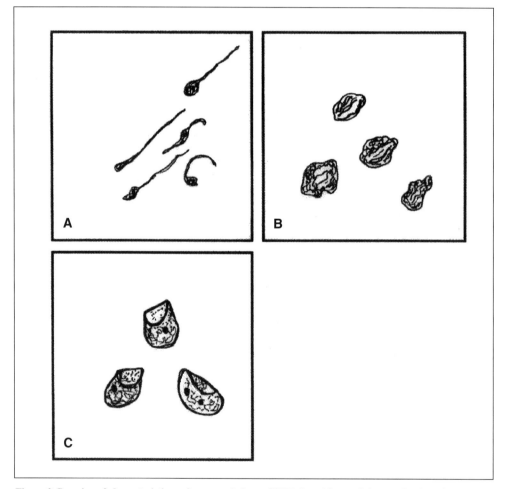

Figure 2. Drawing of characteristic nuclear morphology of MIB-1-positive nuclei occurring bare in cytologic smears. Several nuclear morphologies are shown, including: (A) disrupted, elongated nuclear smudges indicating the increased fragility of bare reserve cell nuclei; (B) deflated balloon nuclei showing folds of the nuclear membrane; and (C) pancake nuclei showing folding of one side of the flattened nucleus toward the center.

ical reserve cells be identified on the *absence* of a feature (absence of cytoplasm), not on the presence of something. This is an unusual thinking process for the diagnostician.

The MIB-1 method is well suited for closer examination of both benign and atypical reserve cells, because we anticipate that many of these immature cells proliferate (e.g., stand out in the MIB-1 stain). Indeed, we observed that some benign reserve cells stain positive for MIB-1, but that atypical reserve cells stain even more. When staining a smear that contains atypical reserve cells with MIB-1, we find many more of these cells than were initially noticed in the Papanicolaou-stained smear. Also, the air-dried nuclei stain very well, whereas only a few endocervical cylindrical cells stain MIB-1 positive. The fact that the bare atypical reserve cells stain positive in these above-mentioned procedures illustrates once again that these cells are not a degenerative form of cylindrical endocervical cells, but are a vital, proliferating cell population. The damaged atypical reserve cell nuclei in particular stain positive; thus, we can find many more deformed, fragmented, and smudged nuclei than were originally observed in the Papanicolaou-stained specimen (Figure 2). In addition, the other phenomena such as the deflated balloon and the pancake effect, often observed in very large atypical reserve cell nuclei, are highlighted by the MIB-1 stain (Figure 2). The contrast between positive and negative staining nuclei is so good that it is possible to detect the positive nuclei even when they are beneath several others. From our observations, it is clear that MIB-1 staining of cervical smears is a powerful technique to obtain insight in this, until now, neglected cell population in cervical smears.

For instance, we learned that when we base our cytologic diagnosis mainly on the degree of abnormality of the MIB-1-positive bare nuclei and less on the (mainly dead) dysplastic cells, the correlation between the histologic and the cytologic diagnosis improves (5). In other words, the MIB-1 method can be used to fine-tune the diagnosis of abnormal smears. Last but not least, it is important to mention that the reserve cells are selected by the PAPNET system and, as a consequence, are highlighted in the diagnostic process when PAPNET is applied for primary screening.

VISUALIZING NORMAL AND ABNORMAL PROLIFERATING ENDOCERVICAL CELLS

In the last two decades, we have seen a relative increase of glandular malignant lesions (ACs) of the endocervix. Without doubt, this is partly attributable to the difficulties involved in recognizing the premalignant cells (those derived from AIS). MIB-1 staining might be of help here. For histology, it is reported that the labeling index for AIS varied in one series between 57% and 96% and was over 60% in a second series (15,24). Labeling indices of benign endocervical epithelium were always below 30%. In our diagnostic laboratory, we tested the MIB-1 method on five (false-negative) smears preceding the diagnosis of AIS. In these cases, we searched for glandular epithelial fragments and established the percentage of MIB-1-positive nuclei, or the proliferation index (PI). All contained epithelial fragments with PI values exceeding 70%. In contrast, truly negative smears contained epithelial glandular fragments with PI values not exceeding 20% and were mostly unlabeled. With great success, we have employed the MIB-1 method in the last two years to analyze abnormal glandular cells in cervical smears and, accordingly, have fine-tuned the diagnosis of AIS and AC. The additional advantage of the MIB-1 stain is that the abnormal glandular cells are highlighted because they become brown (when diaminobenzidine is used) and thus are easily detected in the smear.

SOLVING THE PROBLEM OF UNSATISFACTORY SMEARS WITH THE MIB-1 METHOD

Smears containing blood and/or thick inflammatory infiltrate covering the epithelial cells are graded in our laboratory as unsatisfactory. Smears with dense epithelial fragments in which no details could be observed are also classified as unsatisfactory. In all of these cases, part of the smear could not be evaluated by light microscopy because all details were lost. In the past, a repeat smear was required. However, "doing more of the same" was clearly not the answer. Often the repeat smear was hardly better than the original. Thus, we had to look for another solution, that is, to upgrade the original unsatisfactory smear itself. An option here is to stain the diagnostic cells and to leave the overlying nondiagnostic material (blood and granulocytes) unstained, thus rendering the important cells in the smear diagnosable. This is possible by MIB-1 staining. This way, the blood and granulocytes are left virtually unstained, and the MIB-1-positive nuclei stand out clearly and are visualized in every small detail.

GRADING THE MIB-1-POSITIVE UNSATISFACTORY AND SATISFACTORY SMEARS

When staining positive for MIB-1, the smear can be graded based on the MIB-1 staining of the epithelial fragments. Note that single positive cells cannot be used for grading. This proved to not be a problem because, in all cases studied, epithelial fragments with MIB-1-positive cells were also found. The positive- and negative-staining nuclei were counted in these epithelial fragments, these numbers were summed, and the percentage of positive-staining nuclei for each fragment was calculated. The smear was graded according to the epithelial fragment with the highest MIB-1 percentage. The MIB-1 grading corresponds roughly with cytologic diagnoses.

Borderline MIB-1 grading corresponds with the cytologic diagnosis of atypical cells of unknown significance/atypical glandular cells of unknown significance (ASCUS/AGUS). In such smears, epithelial fragments are found with 1% to 20% MIB-1-positive nuclei (Figure 3).

MIB-1 grade I corresponds with the cytologic diagnosis CIN I. In grade I smears, epithelial fragments with 21% to 35% MIB-1-positive nuclei are found (Figure 3). MIB-1 grade II corresponds to between 36% and 50% MIB-1-positive nuclei, and MIB-1 grade III has 51% or more MIB-1-positive nuclei (Figure 3).

Of the 84 817 smears screened in 18 months (beween 1994 and 1995), 82 749 were satisfactory, and 2068 (2.4%) were unsatisfactory. The MIB-1 classification of the unsatisfactory smears and the cytologic classification of the satisfactory smears are given in Table 3. To test the difference between the scores in corresponding classes found in satisfactory versus unsatisfactory smears, the Z test was applied; for $\alpha = 0.005$, values greater than +1.96 or lower than -1.96 indicate that the scores in the two groups differ significantly. In the unsatisfactory group, more than twice as many cases were graded as borderline than as ASCUS. These differences were statistically significant. Approximately the same ratio was seen for grade II versus CIN II, and grade III versus CIN III or higher. The differences between unsatisfactory and satisfactory scores for these groups were also significant. The grade I score was higher than the CIN I score, but here the difference was not statistically significant.

Of the 2068 women with unsatisfactory smears, there were 74 with a MIB-1 grad-

Table 3. MIB-1 Grading of Unsatisfactory Smears and Cytologic Classification of Satisfactory Smears

MIB-1 grading	Unsatisfactory smears		Cytologic classification	Satisfactory smears	
	No.	%		No.	%
Negative	1701	82.25	Negative	75 185	90.86
Borderline	293	14.17	ASCUS	5543	6.70
Grade I	40	1.93	CIN I	1253	1.51
Grade II	19	0.92	CIN II	389	0.47
Grade III	15	0.73	≥CIN III	379	0.46
Total	2068	100.00		82 749	100.00

ASCUS, atypical cells of unknown significance; CIN, cervical intraepithelial neoplasia.

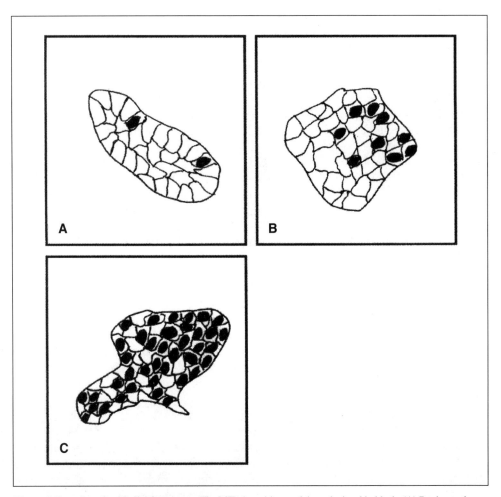

Figure 3. Drawing of epithelial fragments. The MIB-1-positive nuclei are depicted in black. (A) Benign endocervical cells. (B) MIB-1 grade I, 30% MIB-1-positive nuclei. (C) MIB-1 grade III, 75% MIB-1-positive staining nuclei.

Table 4. Histologic Follow-Up of MIB-1-Positive Cases with Upgraded Unsatisfactory Smears

MIB-1	No. of cases ≥ grade I	No histology	Histologic diagnosis		
			CIN I	CIN II	≥ CIN III[a]
Grade I	40	34	5	0	1
Grade II	19	12	1	1	5
Grade III	15	5	2	4	4
Total	74	51	8	5	10

CIN, cervical intraepithelial neoplasia.

[a]This category includes three severe dysplasias, four carcinomas in situ, one invasive squamous carcinoma, and two adenocarcinomas of the endocervix

ing of I or higher, of whom 51 were followed cytologically without a biopsy. Almost all cases (40 all together) with MIB-1 grade I had only this type of follow-up. Of these 40 patients, only one case with CIN I was found. Of the 19 cases with MIB-1 grade II, 8 had only cytology, with 1 diagnosis of CIN I. There was one case in which cylindrical epithelium was characterized as MIB-1 grade II. In that case, an AC of the endocervix was found. In the group of 15 cases with MIB-1 grade III, only four had cytologic follow-up, all with a negative repeat smear.

Finally, 23 women had a histologic follow-up, in some cases following a repeat smear that was classified as CIN III or greater. All of these women proved to have CIN or invasive carcinoma (Table 4). There was a clear relationship between MIB-1 grading and histology: most of the CIN I cases were found in the MIB-1 grade I group, while, of the 15 patients with MIB-1 grade III, four proved to have CIN III or higher. Of the 10 patients within the histology CIN III or higher, 3 had severe dysplasia, 4 had CIS, and 3 had invasive carcinoma, of which 2 were ACs. Thus, the permillage for invasive carcinoma in this group of 2068 women was 1.5.

CLINICAL RELEVANCE OF UPGRADING UNSATISFACTORY SMEARS WITH THE MIB-1 METHOD

When a false-negative smear is reevaluated, it is often found to be unsatisfactory because of a thick inflammatory infiltrate hiding the cancer cells, or because of blood influencing the staining characteristics of the diagnostic cells. In retrospect, it would have been better to be critical toward the quality of such smears and to use directly adjunctive procedures such as the MIB-1 method described here. Accordingly, unsatisfactory smears can be upgraded by the MIB-1 method because the hidden diagnostic cells can then be visualized, as is shown in the present paper. In this group of otherwise discarded smears, a remarkably high number of cases graded as MIB-1 grade I or higher were found, indicating that there might be an underlying (pre)neoplasia. Indeed, no less than three dysplasias, four carcinomas in situ, and three invasive carcinomas were detected in the histologic sections of those women in which the diagnosis could not be made on the Papanicolaou-stained smear. The permillage for invasive cervical carcinoma was 10 times larger in the unsatisfactory group than in the satisfactory group. Thus, the MIB-1 method has further enhanced our diagnostic acumen for these difficult types of smears.

PAPNET SCANNING OF MIB-1-STAINED SMEARS

In our laboratory, we have acquired extensive experience with the PAPNET system for prescreening cervical smears (4,20). The system uses neural network programming for the detection of abnormal cells in cervical smears (16). The selected microscopic fields are displayed on a high-definition videoscreen (64 on page 1 for single cells, and 64 on page 2 for epithelial fragments). The PAPNET system is also able to collect epithelial fragments with dark brown nuclei (positive immunostaining) from the smear. Therefore, we decided to perform an analysis of MIB-1-stained cervical smears and histologic sections using PAPNET.

Out of extensive clinical material, the following smears were chosen for this study:

1. *Moderate dysplasias*: One hundred cases of moderate dysplasia were stained for MIB-1. Of these, only 27 contained MIB-1-positive cells. Five of these could not be used for PAPNET because the slides were broken; the remaining 22 could be used for quantitation.

2. *Repair cells*: Five smears with many epithelial fragments consisting of repair cells were stained for MIB-1. Repair cells are defined as cells with large nuclei containing large nucleoli but lacking chromatin changes. Often, these epithelial fragments contain a mitotic figure. Of these five smears with repair cells, all contained MIB-1-positive nuclei and could be used for quantitation.

3. *Carcinoma in situ*: Fourteen smears with a cytologic diagnosis of CIS were taken from the files. All contained MIB-1-positive cells and could be used for quantitation.

4. *False positives*: Three smears with positive cytology (CIS) and negative histology were chosen from the files. All contained MIB-1-positive cells and could be used for quantitation.

5. *False negatives*: Two cases were selected with positive histology (CIS) and negative cytology. These smears were devoid of diagnostic cells (true false negatives). Both smears did not contain MIB-1-positive cells and could not be used for quantitation.

PAPNET Procedure

The MIB-1-stained slides were scanned with the PAPNET system. In the PAPNET procedure, all 300 000 or more cells were first scanned using a low-power objective to find areas of cellularity to which the medium-powered lens was directed (4). Then some 3000 or 30 000 potentially interesting objects, selected by the algorithmic computer, were sent to the neural network computer. The images were stored on a CD Rom, and review of the images was performed in the laboratory.

In all cases selected for quantitation, epithelial fragments with MIB-1-positive nuclei were present in the 64 video tiles of page 2. In addition, these tiles contained some fragments with hyperchromatic nuclei lacking positive MIB-1 staining, or mucus staining intensely blue (or dark blue) with hematoxylin. From the 64 tiles of page 2, a maximum of 16 tiles with epithelial fragments containing brown (MIB-1-positive) nuclei was collected by the operator on a summary screen. Of these 16 tiles, the one with the largest number of brown nuclei was chosen for quantitation.

Quantitation of MIB-1-Positive PAPNET Images

For quantitation, the selected PAPNET images were transferred with FASTTILE™

Table 5. MIB-1 Quantitative Parameters: Definitions with Area in μm^2

PPN (proportion-positive nuclei; %)	$\dfrac{\text{summed area of positive nuclei}}{\text{summed area of cytoplasm}} \times 100$
PAN (proportion-all nuclei; %)	$\dfrac{\text{summed area of all nuclei}}{\text{summed area of cytoplasm}} \times 100$
NDPos (nuclear density-positive; per 10^6 μm^2)	$\dfrac{\text{number of positive nuclei}}{\text{summed area of cytoplasm}}$
PI (proliferation index; %)	$\dfrac{\text{number of positive nuclei}}{\text{number of all nuclei}} \times 100$

Table 6. MIB-1 Quantitative Parameters: Values for Moderate Dysplasia and Carcinoma In Situ

Parameter	Smear (moderate dysplasia) (n = 22)	Smear (CIS) (n = 14)
PPN (in %)	15 ± 6	59 ± 11
PAN (in %)	42 ± 12	78 ± 12
NDPos (per 10^6 μm^2)	21 ± 10	56 ± 18
PI (in %)	35 ± 17	71 ± 21

CIS, carcinoma in situ. For other abbreviations, see Table 5.

(NSI, Suffern, NJ, USA) to be loaded into Mocha (Jandel Scientific, San Rafael, CA, USA). The PAPNET images thus appeared in the image window of Mocha in color, allowing the operator to see the brown (MIB-1-positive) nuclei, the blue (MIB-1-negative) nuclei, and the cytoplasmic area of the epithelial fragment. Mocha offers a highly flexible and comprehensive set of measurement capabilities using manual, flood fill, and automatic measurements. The manual measurements served our purpose best, i.e., the measurement of the nuclear area of a brown nucleus and a blue nucleus, and the complete cytoplasmic area of the epithelial fragment (thus of the summed cells). With manual measurement, the chosen object (one of the three defined above) was delineated by the operator using the computer mouse. Particularly in the CIS smears, many fragments had overlapping nuclei; here, the operator completed (with the cursor) the part of the measured nucleus hidden under its neighbor. The measured areas were tabulated, and from each measured epithelial fragment, the parameters defined in Table 5 were calculated. The parameter proportion-positive nuclei (PPN) depended on both the size and the number of the brown nuclei in the fragment. Note that the parameter proportion-all nuclei (PAN) depends on both the size and the number of all nuclei. In the parameters NDPos (nuclear density-positive) and PI, only the number of nuclei is taken into account.

Table 6 gives values of the quantitative parameters for the cytologic smears with moderate dysplasia and CIS. For the distinction between moderate dysplasia and CIS, PPN proved to be superior, but also for PAN, NDPos, and PI, the values for dysplasia were significantly lower than those for CIS.

Table 7 shows values of the five cases with repair cells. Values for all four parameters fall in the range of those of moderate dysplasias (compare with Table 6). The

Table 7. Values of Quantitative Parameters in Five Smears with Repair Cells

Case no.	PPN (%)	PAN (%)	NDPos (per 10^6 μm^2)	PI (%)
1	18	38	21	40
2	23	58	27	44
3	21	46	23	40
4	12	39	18	43
5	24	41	31	43

For abbreviations, see Table 5.

Table 8. Values of Quantitative Parameters of False Positives

Case no.	PPN (%)	PAN (%)	NDPos (per 10^6 μm^2)	PI (%)
1	48	58	51	76
2	67	78	59	80
3	48	72	49	79

For abbreviations, see Table 5.

values for PI are higher than the mean value for the moderate dysplasias. In Table 8, values for the three false-positive smears are presented. For all three cases, values fall in the range of the CIS smears (compare with Table 6).

With this quantitation method, we cannot distinguish repair cells from moderate dysplasia. However, we can separate these two entities on the basis of staining pattern of the nuclei, with repair cells showing mainly a nucleolar MIB-1 staining and moderate dysplasia showing a nuclear one. In this context, it is important to mention that only one-quarter of the smears with moderate dysplasia contained MIB-1-positive cells. In a recent study, we showed that the presence of MIB-1-positive cells has prognostic significance (5).

Quantitation of MIB-1 staining of epithelial fragments has proved to be highly efficient for the distinction between moderate dysplasia and CIS. Here the parameter PPN, in which the area and the number of positive nuclei are taken into account, was a more effective classifier than the PI. We warn readers that the values for cytology cannot be used for histology because, in histology, the distance between the nuclei is larger than in cytology (5).

In summing up PAPNET and MIB-1, MIB-1-positive PAPNET images have provided us with insight into the biologic characteristics of various cervical lesions, and their quantification has provided an added numerical value to our visual observations. In addition, MIB-1 staining is valuable in the evaluation of false-negative and false-positive smears; thus, even without quantitation, MIB-1 staining can be used to fine-tune the cytologic diagnosis when PAPNET is used for the primary screening.

REFERENCES

1. **Al-Saleh, W., P. Delvenne, R. Greimers, V. Fridman, J. Doyen, and J. Boniver.** 1995. Assessment of Ki-67 antigen immunostaining in squamous intraepithelial lesions of the uterine cervix. Correlation with the histologic grade

and human papillomavirus type. Am. J. Clin. Pathol. *104*:154-160.

2. **Al-Saleh, W., P. Delvenne, F.A. van den Brule, S. Menard, J. Boniver, and V. Castronovo.** 1997. Expression of the 67 KD laminin receptor in human cervical preneoplastic and neoplastic squamous epithelial lesions: an immuno-histochemical study. J. Pathol. *181*:287-293.

3. **Avall-Lundqvist, E.H., C. Silfversward, U. Aspenblad, B.R. Nilsson, and G.U. Auer.** 1997. The impact of tumour angiogenesis, p53 overexpression and proliferative activity (MIB-1) on survival in squamous cervical car-cinoma. Eur. J. Cancer *33*:1799-1804.

4. **Boon, M.E. and L.P. Kok.** 1993. Neural network processing can provide means to catch errors that slip through human screening of Pap smears. Diagn. Cytopathol. *9*:411-416.

5. **Boon, M.E., F.M.F. van Dunné, and N.J. Vardaxis.** 1995. Recognition of atypical reserve cell hyperplasia in cer-vical smears and its diagnostic significance. Mod. Pathol. *8*:786-794.

6. **Cattoretti, G., M.H.G. Becker, G. Key, M. Duchrow, C. Schlüter, J. Galle, and J. Gerdes.** 1992. Monoclonal antibodies against recombinant parts of the Ki-67 antigen (MIB 1 and MIB 3) detect proliferating cells in microwave-processed formalin-fixed paraffin sections. J. Pathol. *168*:357-363.

7. **Cina, S.J., M.S. Richardson, R.M. Austin, and R.J. Kurman.** 1997. Immunohistochemical staining for Ki-67 antigen, carcinoembryonic antigen, and p53 in the differential diagnosis of glandular lesions of the cervix. Mod. Pathol. *10*:176-180.

8. **Dunton, C.J., K.H. van Hoeven, A.J. Kovatich, R.E. Oliver, R.Q. Scacheri, J.R. Cater, and J.A. Carlson.** 1997. Ki-67 antigen staining as an adjunct to identifying cervical intraepithelial neoplasia. Gynecol. Oncol. *64*:451-455.

9. **Garzetti, G.G., A. Ciavattini, G. Lucarini, G. Goteri, M. de Nictolis, M. Muzzioli, N. Fabris, C. Romanini, and G. Biagini.** 1995. MIB-1 immunostaining in stage I squamous cervical carcinoma: relationship with natural killer cell activity. Gynecol. Oncol. *58*:28-33.

10. **Garzetti, G.G., A. Ciavattini, G. Lucarini, G. Goteri, M. de Nictolis, C. Romanini, and G. Biagini.** 1995. Mod-ulation of expression of p53 and cell proliferation in locally advanced cervical carcinoma after neoadjuvant combi-nation chemotherapy. Eur. J. Obstet. Gynecol. Reprod. Biol. *63*:31-36.

11. **Garzetti, G.G., A. Ciavattini, M. de Nictolis, G. Lucarini, G. Goteri, C. Romanini, and G. Biagini.** 1996. MIB-1 immunostaining in cervical intraepithelial neoplasia: prognostic significance in mild and moderate lesions. Gynecol. Obstet. Invest. *42*:261-266.

12. **Garzetti, G.G., A. Ciavattini, G. Lucarini, G. Goteri, M. de Nictolis, and G. Biagini.** 1997. MIB-1 immunos-taining in cervical carcinoma of young patients. Gynecol. Oncol. *67*:184-187.

13. **Gibbons, D., F. Fogt, J. Kasznica, J. Holden, and S. Nikulasson.** 1997. Comparison of topoisomerase II alpha and MIB-1 expression in uterine cervical squamous lesions. Mod. Pathol. *10*:409-413.

14. **Hietala, K.A., V.M. Kosma, K.J. Syrjanen, S.M. Syrjanen, and J.K. Kellokoski.** 1997. Correlation of MIB-1 antigen expression with transcription factors Skn-1, Oct-1, AP-2, and HPV type in cervical intraepithelial neoplasia. J. Pathol. *183*:305-310.

15. **Leteurtre, E., F. Boman, M.O. Farine, J.L. Leroy, and B. Gosselin.** 1998. Importance of the study of the expres-sion of MIB-1 (Ki-67) for the diagnosis of endocervical glandular lesions. Ann. Pathol. *18*:172-177 (in French).

16. **Mango, L.J.** 1994. Computer-assisted cervical screening using neural networks. Cancer Lett. *77*:155-162.

17. **McCluggage, W.G., P. Maxwell, and H. Bharucha.** 1998. Immunohistochemical detection of metallothionein and MIB-1 in uterine cervical squamous lesions. Int. J. Gynecol. Pathol. *17*:29-35.

18. **Mittal, K. and J. Palazzo.** 1998. Cervical condylomas show higher proliferation than do inflamed or metaplastic cervical squamous epithelium. Mod. Pathol. *11*:780-783.

19. **Oka, K., T. Nakano, and T. Hoshi.** 1996. Analysis of response to radiation therapy of patients with cervical ade-nocarcinoma compared with squamous cell carcinoma. MIB-1 and PC10 labeling indices. Cancer *77*:2280-2285.

20. **Ouwerkerk-Noordam, E., M.E. Boon, and S. Beck.** 1994. Computer-assisted primary screening of cervical smears using the PAPNET method: comparison with conventional screening and evaluation of the role of the cytol-ogist. Cytopathology *5*:211-218.

21. **Payne, S., N.M. Kernohan, and F. Walker.** 1996. Proliferation in the normal cervix and in preinvasive cervical lesions. J. Clin. Pathol. *49*:667-671.

22. **Resnick, M., S. Lester, J.E. Tate, E.E. Sheets, C. Sparks, and C.P. Crum.** 1996. Viral and histopathologic cor-relates of MN and MIB-1 expression in cervical intraepithelial neoplasia. Hum. Pathol. *27*:234-239.

22a. **Ruiter, D.J. and M.E. Boon.** 1982. Atypical indifferent (reserve) cells in the cervical epithelium and their exfo-liative pattern. Acta Cytol. *25*:292-298.

23. **Van Hoeven, K.H., A.J. Kovatich, R.E. Oliver, M. Nobel, and C.J. Dunton.** 1996. Protocol for immunocyto-chemical detection of SIL in cervical smears using MIB-1 antibody to Ki-67. Mod. Pathol. *9*:407-412 [published erratum appears in Mod. Pathol. 1996. *9*:790].

24. **Van Hoeven, K.H., L. Ramondetta, A.J. Kovatich, M. Bibbo, and C.J. Dunton.** 1997. Quantitative image analy-sis of MIB-1 reactivity in inflammatory, hyperplastic, and neoplastic endocervical lesions. Int. J. Gynecol. Pathol. *16*:15-21.

25. **Ziol, M., C. Di Tomaso, A. Biaggi, M. Tepper, P. Piquet, L. Carbillon, M. Uzan, and C. Guettier.** 1998. Viro-logical and biological characteristics of cervical intraepithelial neoplasia grade I with marked koilocytotic atypia. Hum. Pathol. *29*:1068-1073.

Microwave-Enhanced In Situ End-Labeling of Apoptotic Cells in Tissue Sections: Pitfalls and Possibilities

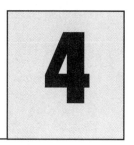

4

Paul J. Lucassen[1,2], Françoise Labat-Moleur[3], Adrien Negoescu[3], and Menno Van Lookeren Campagne[4]

[1]Division of Medical Pharmacology, LACDR, Leiden University, Leiden, [2]Institute Neurobiology, Faculty of Science, University of Amsterdam, Amsterdam, The Netherlands, [3]Laboratoire de Pathologie Cellulaire CHRU, Grenoble, France, and [4]Department of Immunology, Genentech, South San Francisco, CA, USA

INTRODUCTION

Apoptosis, a form of cell death, is characterized by specific morphological and biochemical changes in the cell (29,86). In the absence of an unequivocal, specific biochemical marker for apoptosis, the associated DNA fragmentation detected by in situ end-labeling (ISEL) and terminal deoxynucleotidyl transferase (TdT)-mediated dUTP-biotin nick end-labeling (TUNEL) has been widely applied in developmental studies, oncology, immunology, aging, and neurodegenerative research to identify apoptotic cells in tissue sections (2,8,17,18,24,27,28,35,45,49,64,75,81,83). ISEL is a common denominator for two enzyme-based techniques, in situ nick translation (ISNT), using DNA polymerase I or its Klenow fragment, and TUNEL. TdT covalently adds labeled nucleotides to the 3′ OH ends of DNA fragments, and TUNEL is considered more sensitive and specific for the detection of double-stranded DNA breaks than ISNT and is now widely used (2,15,16,19–21,33,55,85).

Due to the nature of its target, TUNEL suffers from two types of limitations:

1. **Limitations in specificity.** Because of the unavoidable presence of low numbers of 3′ OH DNA ends in virtually all healthy cells and the high amounts of 3′ OH ends in necrotic cells, TUNEL is not always specific for apoptosis. Furthermore, (TUNEL-detectable) DNA breaks can, in theory, occur artifactually

Antigen Retrieval Techniques
Edited by Shan-Rong Shi, Jiang Gu, and Clive R. Taylor
©2000 Eaton Publishing, Natick, MA

following ischemia, DNA repair processes, mitosis, and endonuclease activation or autolysis during the postmortem period (PMD) (12,36,50,52), possibly leading to false-positive labeling.

2. **Limitations in sensitivity.** Because of the combined effects of DNA hypercondensation during stages of the apoptotic process and chemical cross-linking of DNA and histone proteins by (formalin) fixation, accessibility of the DNA for the TdT enzyme is hampered and may lead to false-negative results.

Furthermore, apoptosis is a rapid process that is completed in several hours, which makes identification in thin sections obtained from tissues with a prolonged disease duration very difficult (3,26,41,56,57). In addition, TUNEL positivity alone is insufficient to identify apoptosis because morphological criteria, such as membrane blebbing, apoptotic bodies, and chromatin condensation, are required as established hallmarks of apoptosis (7,8,29,86). Nuances in this morphological definition have increased as different intermediate forms between apoptosis and necrosis have been described, exemplified by changes in the early phase of apoptosis (namely, nuclear enlargement rather than condensation) that are accompanied by DNA fragmentation (6,7,9,11,54,72,86).

Consequently, several recent reports have raised doubts about the specificity, suitability, and reproducibility of TUNEL for archival tissue or (postmortem) brain tissue (4,22,31,51,56,58,63,87), whereas others have reported specific adaptations for TUNEL to overcome these limitations (10,34,39,53,58,63,74,78,84). One of the adaptations recommended for overfixed tissue is the microwave antigen retrieval (MW-AR) technique that has already proved to be so valuable to unmask antigens in immunocytochemistry (14,39,40,65,69,74,80). Perfusion-fixed tissue samples benefit from a rapid, homogeneous, and well-controlled fixation, whereas tissues fixed by immersion, which is the case in most routine pathological specimens, are subject to heterogeneity in fixative penetration that depends on temperature, duration, tissue density, lipid content, form, size, and thickness of the sample. All these variables may contribute to variation in TUNEL results.

In this chapter, we summarize current literature and joint experimental data on the application of MW-AR to optimize TUNEL in four conditions associated with apoptotic or necrotic cell death in differently fixed tissues: *(i)* autopsy brain tissue of Alzheimer's disease patients and control subjects; *(ii)* perfusion-fixed rat brains following unilateral excitatory amino acid-induced brain injury; *(iii)* immersion-fixed thyroid tissue in Graves' disease; and *(iv)* rat prostate tissue, immersion-fixed three days after castration.

MATERIALS AND METHODS

Tissues

Postmortem Human Brain

Human brain material was obtained from the Netherlands Brain Bank (coordinator Dr. R. Ravid) and consisted of occipital cortex and hippocampal tissue of two control subjects (PMDs of 4 h, 30 min and 12 h, 5 min) and two Alzheimer's disease patients (PMDs of 4 h and 11 h). The hippocampus in Alzheimer's disease patients frequently shows considerable numbers of TUNEL-positive glial and neuronal cells, whereas the occipital cortex is generally not affected.

NMDA-Treated Rat Brain

As a model system for apoptotic and necrotic neuronal death, 7-day-old neonatal rats were unilaterally injected with *N*-methyl-D-aspartate (NMDA) intrastriatally. Because rats of this age are particularly vulnerable to NMDA, large amounts of apoptotic and necrotic cells occur unilaterally in the hippocampus, the cerebral cortex, and, more ventrally, the mammillary nucleus (MN) (43,82). The contralateral side of the brain served as an internal control because it was not affected by the NMDA injection.

Intrastriatal injections of NMDA or vehicle were performed in postnatal day 7 pups as previously described (43). Briefly, injections were performed in ether-anesthetized rat pups with a 5-μL Hamilton syringe that was positioned in the left striatum 2.5-mm lateral of the bregma at a depth of 4 mm. Control animals received 0.5 μL of 50 mol/L Tris-HCl buffer (pH 7.4). Experimental animals were injected with 0.5 μL Tris-HCl containing 20 nmol of NMDA. Twenty-four hours later, animals were perfused with 0.9% NaCl followed by 4% paraformaldehyde in phosphate-buffered saline (PBS), decapitated, and the heads were left in the same fixative overnight at 4°C, after which the brain was removed and postfixed for either 3 or 10 days in fixative that was refreshed daily, prior to paraffin embedding (Histowax). Sections (7 μm) were mounted on aminoalkylsilane (AAS)-coated slides (25).

Graves' Disease

Graves' disease is caused by the binding of IgGs that mimic the action of thyrotropin on the thyrotropin receptor, whose activation induces hyperfunction and hyperplasia of the follicular epithelium. The disease evolves following IgG variations; low IgGs have the same effect as withdrawal of throphic hormonal signal on the target organ. Consequent involution of the goiter is completed through Bax/Bcl-2-regulated apoptosis of thyrocytes. There is no interference with necrosis in this condition (Reference 34 and unpublished observations).

Two types of samples were submitted to TUNEL:
1. Controlled-fixed tissue fragments measuring 5 to 8 mm and 3 mm thick (volume about 0.5 cm^3), were fixed by immersion for 20 hours in aldehyde (cross-linking) or Bouin's liquid (cross-linking and precipitating) fixatives. With regard to the strength of fixation, it may be considered medium. Tissue fragments had been obtained from the surgeon without delay.
2. Noncontrolled-fixed larger samples measuring 1 to 5 cm^2 and 1.5 to 3 mm thick were taken from a thyroid lobe with one-half fixed in 4% neutral formalin and the other half in Bouin's liquid. Fixation lasting 20 hours to 4 days is always nonhomogeneous from one sample to another, and tissues may be mostly considered overfixed, but variably so.

Rat Prostate

We used rat prostate as a convenient model for apoptosis because it yielded large numbers of apoptotic cells in the luminal wall of the follicles that were induced by steroid hormone withdrawal following castration (13,61,85). The prostate of a young adult rat was removed three days after castration and fixed for 5 days in neutral buffered formalin.

The different tissue treatments are summarized in Table 1.

Table 1. Tissue Conditions

	Human Brain	Rat Brain	Human Thyroid	Rat Prostate
Tissue parameters				
Approximate sample volume (cm^3)	2.25–8	2–3	0.5[a] 6–80[b]	0.2
Postsurgical or post-mortem delay to fixation (h)	4–12	0	0–24	0
Fixation				
Fixative	4% NBF	4% PFA	4% NBF or Bouin's liquid	4% NBF
Mode	Immersion	Perfusion + Immersion	Immersion	Immersion
Duration	6 weeks	3–10 days	20 h to 4 days	5 days
Temperature	RT	RT	RT	RT
Histological preparation				
Embedding medium	Paraffin	Paraffin	Paraffin	Paraffin
Section thickness (μm)	10	7	4	4
Slide coating	Aminoalkylsilane (AAS) or aminopropyltriethoxylsilane (APES)			
Slide drying	24–48 h, 37°C	24–48 h 37°C	24–48 h 37°C	24–48 h 37°C

NBF, neutral-buffered formalin; PFA, paraformaldehyde; RT, room temperature.
[a]Controlled fixation parameters.
[b]Uncontrolled fixation parameters.

Materials and Reagents

- PBS 0.05 mol/L, pH 7.4
- Tris-buffered saline (TBS; 0.05 mol/L Tris, 0.9% NaCl, pH 7.6)
- Tris-HCl, pH 7.4
- Ethanol 50%, 70%, 90%, 100% series followed by xylene
- Paraformaldehyde, methanol-free (4% in PBS, pH 7.4; Sigma, St. Louis, MO, USA)
- NMDA 20 nmol in Tris-HCl
- Triton® X-100 (Sigma) 0.1% (vol/vol)
- 0.1% sodium citrate (Merck, West Point, PA, USA) in distilled water (DW)
- 20% normal sheep serum (Jackson Immuno Research Laboratories, West Grove, PA, USA) in 0.1 mol/L TBS
- Proteinase K (PK; stock >600 U/mL) (Roche Molecular Biochemicals, Indianapolis, IN, USA) prepared as 20 mg/mL stocks in PBS or in 10 mmol/L Tris buffer + 2.6 mmol/L CaCl$_2$, final pH 7.5
- TdT (25 U/μL) (Roche Molecular Biochemicals)
- TdT reaction buffer (0.2 mol/L sodium cacodylate, 0.025 mol/L Tris-HCl, and 0.25 mg/mL bovine serum albumin (BSA), pH 6.6

- Biotin-16-2′ deoxyuridine-5′ triphosphate (bio-16-dUTP; 1 nmol/mL) (Roche Molecular Biochemicals)
- Cobalt chloride (25 mmol/L)
- Peroxidase-conjugated avidin (ABC-Elite kit; Vector, Burlingame, CA, USA)
- Diaminobenzidine (DAB; Sigma) reaction mixture (0.05 mg/mL DAB in 0.05 mol/L Tris-HCl, pH 7.5, with 0.02% H_2O_2)
- 0.1 mol/L Sodium citrate buffer (consisting of 102.5 mL 0.2 mol/L acetic acid, 22.5 mL 0.2 mol/L sodium acetate, 125 mL DW, pH 4.0)
- 0.6% Methylgreen in sodium citrate buffer
- Peroxidase-labeled fluorescein sheep FAb antibody with 3% BSA in 1% (wt/vol) blocking reagent (Roche Molecular Biochemicals)
- Plastic Coplin jars (Merck)
- Microwave oven: SMC model E70TFA, 600 W or AEG Micromat, 850 W

Tissue Pretreatments Before TUNEL

Pretreatments generally aim to facilitate access of TdT and labeled nucleotides to DNA breaks in the fixed tissue matrix. The conditions compared, either separately or in combination, included the following:
1. No pretreatment.
2. Addition of detergent, namely, Triton X-100 0.1% (vol/vol) in 0.1% sodium citrate in distilled water for 2 minutes, ice-cooled.
3. Enzymatic digestion by PK at 20 µg/mL in various buffers [PBS, pH 4.4, or PK buffer (10 mmol/L Tris, 2.6 mmol/L $CaCl_2$, pH 7.0, and adjusted to pH 8.0)] after preliminary tests with varying concentrations (2, 10, 20, and 40 µg/mL; not shown) and incubation times (5, 10, and 15 min) at room temperature (RT).
4. Microwave irradiation. According to Shi's classic paper on MW-AR in immuno-histochemistry, MW-AR procedures were adapted from earlier protocols (39,69,74) using 0.1 mol/L citrate and Tris buffers. In view of the importance of the incubation fluid (pH, chemical composition, volume) and of the irradiation conditions (power, temperature, duration), these parameters were explored as summarized in Tables 2 and 3.

In brief, after rehydration to TBS or PBS, slides were washed in DW and placed in plastic jars that were filled with 200 mL of buffer and covered with loose-fitting caps. The jars were placed in the middle of a microwave oven. During MW oven heating, two filled jars, irrespective of the number of sections, were always placed in the oven for standarization puposes. In addition, to prevent variation due to hot and cold spots in the oven, the jars were rotated.

Microwave Irradiation Conditions

For each setting, power values were calculated. Temperatures were measured at the end of one or two cycles of 5 minutes, for 200 mL of buffer for the AEG machine and at the end of 2 cycles of 200 mL for the SMC machine. Between two cycles, it was sometimes necessary to adjust the volume of the jar due to evaporation. With domestic ovens lacking fiberoptic thermometers, minor temperature imprecisions cannot be avoided. The same holds for the time needed to reach boiling, which may differ for different machines and must be assessed empirically.

Because of the sometimes vigorous pretreatments and incubation in boiling carbonate and Tris buffers at extreme pH values, there is a serious risk of detachment and loss of the tissue sections. This necessitated two adjustments; first, for TUNEL, it was essential to use tissue mounted on glass slides coated with a strong adhesive. Good results were obtained with AAS (25), poly-L-lysine, or electrostatically coated slides (SuperFrost® Plus, Fisher Scientific, Pittsburgh, PA, USA). Second, to prevent vigorous boiling, the temperature was set at 95°C, which allows a rapid rise in temperature but prevents tissue damage or detachment by the formation of air bubbles. Furthermore, a standard 2 cycles of 5 minutes full-power MW incubation and 15 minutes of progressive cooling at RT was compared with a brief 5-minute MW incubation and subsequent rapid cooling on ice or rapid changing with RT buffer.

Pretreatment Combinations

1. Triton X-100 followed by PK (15, 20, and 25 µg/mL).
2. Microwaves followed by Triton X-100.
3. Microwaves followed by PK (15, 20, and 25 µg/mL).
4. Microwaves followed by Triton X-100 and then by PK (15, 20, and 25 µg/mL).
All pretreatments ended in PBS, pH 7.4.

TUNEL

Brain and prostate tissue were labeled with a laboratory protocol, and thyroid tissue was labeled with the Roche Molecular Biochemicals In Situ Cell Death Detection Kit.

Laboratory Protocol

1. Deparaffinize and rehydrate tissue sections in two cycles in xylene for 15 minutes, two cycles in 100% ethanol for 10 minutes, and 96%, 90%, 70%, and 50% in ethanol for 5 minutes each.
2. Wash sections briefly in DW and once in PBS.
3. Pretreat sections according to one of the abovementioned MW protocols.
4. Place sections for preincubation in TdT buffer for 15 minutes at RT.
5. Incubate for 60 minutes at 37°C with a reaction mixture made out of the same TdT buffer, which also contains: 0.1 µL (= 2.5 U) TdT per 100 µL reaction mixture, 0.5 µL (= 0.5 nmol) biotin-16-dUTP per 100 µL reaction mixture, and cobalt chloride (25 mmol/L; 5% of the final volume). To optimize signal in overfixed (human) brain tissue, adaptation of these concentrations of label and enzyme can be considered or titrated with varying pretreatment conditions on adjacent sections.
6. End incorporation of labeled oligonucleotides by rinsing the sections in water and PBS, pH 7.4, for 5 minutes at RT.
7. In the case of immersion-fixed tissue, block endogenous peroxidase activity by incubating in 0.1% H_2O_2 in PBS for 20 minutes at RT.
8. Wash sections for 2×5 minutes in PBS.
9. Preincubate sections in PBS/1% BSA for 15 minutes, during which both components of the ABC kit are joined together (according to the manufacturer's instructions) and left at RT for another 15 minutes for complex formation. Incubate the sections with peroxidase-conjugated avidin (ABC-Elite kit) diluted 1:1000 in PBS/1% BSA, leave at RT for 30 minutes, and place overnight at 4°C.

10. Wash in PBS for 3 × 5 minutes, and wash in 0.05 mol/L Tris-HCl, pH 7.5, for 5 minutes.
11. Check pH of the buffer again, incubate with 0.5 mg/mL DAB in 0.05 M Tris-HCl, pH 7.5, with 0.01% H_2O_2 for 10 minutes and monitor color development in a positive control slide under a microscope; just before massive labeling of intact nuclei becomes detectable in this slide, stop reaction by washing all slides in DW.
12. Wash 2× in PBS.
13. Counterstain slides lightly with methyl green or cresyl violet according to routine protocols before mounting coverslips in Entallan (Merck).

Roche Molecular Biochemicals In Situ Cell Death Detection Kit

The kit was used essentially according to the manufacturer's instructions. We introduced two adaptations: the first was before incubation with the TdT buffer (also called TUNEL mixture) and consisted of preincubation in 3% BSA and 20% normal bovine serum (Jackson) in PBS, pH 7.4, for 30 minutes at RT; the second step was introduced before the peroxidase-labeled fluorescein sheep FAb antibody and consisted of 3% BSA and 20% normal sheep serum (Jackson) in 1% (wt/vol) blocking reagent in 0.1 mol/L TBS for 30 minutes at RT. The sheep FAb antibody 1:3 dilution yielded an optimal signal/background ratio.

Development of the DAB precipitate (same technique in both protocols) was consistently monitored under the microscope slide by slide and lasted from 10 seconds to 1 minute, rarely more, for the Graves' thyroid tissue, whereas longer DAB times were needed for brain tissue (up to 10 min). Negative controls, consisting of omitting TdT, showed no signal at all. Positive controls were provided by buffered 10% formalin-fixed, weaning mammary glands (ApopTag Control Slides; Oncor, Gaithersburg, MD, USA). After counterstaining with Harris' hematoxylin, slides were dehydrated and mounted in Merckoglas (Merck).

RESULTS

TUNEL on Fixed Tissues: Necessity of Pretreatments

For Graves' thyroid tissue, the masking effect of fixation was assessed by comparing the fraction of cells with clear apoptotic features versus all TUNEL-positive cells. If no MW-AR or PK treatment was used, very little (if any) labeling was observed (also in the human brain tissue), and the positive fraction in thyroid sections ranged from 8% to 50%.

A direct correlation between TUNEL sensitivity and the strength of fixation was clearly apparent in two of the tissue models:
1. *NMDA-treated perfusion-fixed rat brain.* In perfusion-fixed tissue, the number of neurons displaying apoptotic and necrotic DNA fragmentation as well as the size of the lesion was clearly influenced by the duration of postfixation; in perfused and 10-day postfixed rat brain, ISEL signal was generally weak, very variable, and less outspoken than in 3-day postfixed, perfusion-fixed tissue. As a consequence, the exact borders of the lesion were difficult to delineate (compare Figure 1A with 1B).

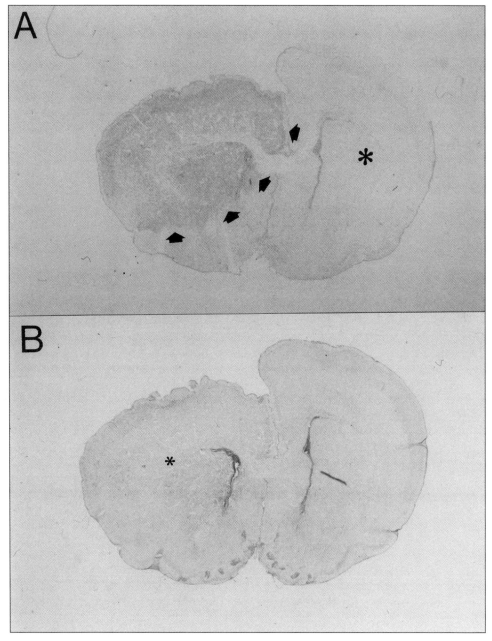

Figure 1. NMDA-injected rat brain. Pattern of TUNEL-detected DNA fragmentation in adjacent frontal paraffin sections of a 7-day-old rat pup brain 24 h after unilateral injection of the neurotoxin NMDA in the striatum. Brain tissue was perfusion-fixed and subsequently postfixed for 10 days in paraformaldehyde (shown in panel B). Weak TUNEL signal of variable intensity is observed in the ipsilateral side (small asterisk) of the brain, whereas the contralateral side is also weakly positive. Panel A shows a section adjacent to the one shown in panel B, but after microwave pretreatment in pH 3.0 citrate buffer. Clear and increased labeling is now observed, allowing the lesion area to be clearly delineated (arrowheads), whereas nonspecific labeling is absent in the contralateral side (large asterisk). Reprinted with permission from Reference 39. **(See color plate A3).**

Table 2. Test Settings for Two Brands of Microwave Oven[a]

	Setting	Power (W)	T (°C)
AEG Micromat 850 W[b]			
	2	188	54
	4	376	86
	8	752	99.6
SMC E70TFA 600 W[c]			
	1	200	40
	3	400	75
	5	600	98

[a]We advise that each lab test its own MW oven to determine optimal conditions.
[b]Boiling T° was 99.6°C for all solutions, reached in 3 min at 752 W for 200 mL.
[c]Boiling T° was reached in 4 min, 30 s at full power (600 W).

Table 3. Microwave Tissue Treatments for TUNEL

	Microwave conditions							
Buffers	188 W 5′ (min)	188 W 5′ × 2	376 W 5′	376 W 5′ × 2	600 W 5′ × 2	752 W 5′	752 W 5′ × 2	Tissues tested
Citrate 0.01 mol/L, pH 3.0	+	+	+	+	nd	+	+	HB, RB, HT, RP
Citrate 0.01 mol/L, pH 6.0	+	+	+	+	nd	+	+	HB, RB, HT, RP
SHC 0.01 mol/L, pH 9.0	nd	nd	nd	nd	nd	+*	nd	HT
Tris 0.05 mol/L, pH 10.6	nd	nd	nd	nd	+	nd	nd	HB, RB, HT, RP
Tris-citrate 1/1 (vol/vol), pH 9.0	nd	nd	nd	nd	nd	+	+	HB, RB, HT, RP

nd, not tested; SHC, sodium hydrogen carbonate; HB, human brain; RB, rat brain; HT, human thyroid; RP, rat prostate.
The temperature of various microwave conditions are: 188 W = 50°–54°C; 376 W = 86°–90°C; 600 W = 98°C; 752 W = 99.6°C. +* = 752 W for 3 min to reach boiling followed by adjustment of the power to 376 W for 2–22 min.

2. *Graves' thyroid.* In small tissue samples subjected to a well-controlled, relatively long fixation (20 h at RT) for this size of fragment, the best pretreatment proved to be proteinase K (20 µg/mL, 15 min at RT) with about 60% (Bouin's) to 70% [4% neutral-buffered formalin (NBF)] of apoptotic cells being labeled. On overfixed larger samples, these scores dropped to 10% and 40%, respectively.

Pretreatment Effects on TUNEL: Single or Combined

1. *Detergent: Triton X-100 0.1%.* On heavily fixed tissues, as presented here, detergent must be considered only as an adjuvant, since it contributed to lower background levels but did not seem to influence signal intensity.
2. *Enzymatic digestion.* Of the PK concentrations tested, the most optimal proved to be 20 µg/mL for 15 minutes at RT, as higher concentrations and longer durations caused extensive nonspecific labeling and often worsened tissue morphology. However, this may be batch dependant and should be tested prior to comparing groups. PK turned out to be essential, as its exclusion resulted in an absence of labeling (e.g., in Bouin's-fixed thyroid perfusion-fixed rat as well as immersion-fixed human brain tissue).
3. *Microwave irradiation: alone or combined with PK.* Our test revealed the importance of different MW parameters: temperature, cycle number, and duration, with buffer pH as one of the strongest effects, as it influenced TUNEL results drastically. However, depending on the MW condition and tissue type, MW-AR for TUNEL could also introduce adverse effects, causing massive nonspecific labeling of almost all nuclei, e.g., in postmortem brain tissue but also in the prostate (see Figures 2D and 3C).

In NMDA-treated perfusion-fixed rat brain that was postfixed for another 10 days, MW pretreatment in citrate buffer, pH 3.0, resulted in a clear labeling of apoptotic nuclei in many ipsilaterally affected brain areas, including the mamillary nucleus, striatum, hippocampus, and cortex, but not in the contralateral side of the same brain (Figure 1A); the same MW pretreatment at pH 6.0 also improved TUNEL signal but was less prominent (Table 3), whereas pH 9.0 and 10.6 often induced tissue detachment or massive nonspecific nuclear labeling.

In perfusion-fixed tissue that was postfixed for 3 days as well as in immersion-fixed adult rat brain tisssue, MW pretreatment in citrate buffer at all four pH values induced extensive nonspecific staining of almost every nucleus in the section. For perfusion-fixed tissue postfixed for 10 days, MW treatments in general had minimal adverse effects and gave more reproducible results.

If no MW-AR pretreatment was used in human brain tissue, hardly any labeling was observed in the human occipital cortex tissue, whereas the hippocampus of Alzheimer's disease patients showed considerable numbers of positive cells using standard label and enzyme concentrations. Typical apoptotic morphology could not be observed in human brain. At higher magnification, labeled neurons often showed positive nuclear staining with sometimes disrupted nuclear membranes, suggestive of necrosis rather than apoptosis. TUNEL-positive cells also often showed glia-like morphology in the Alzheimer's disease hippocampus (see also Reference 38).

Standard MW pretreatment for TUNEL (i.e., 2 × 5 min plus cooling at RT) on occipital cortex and hippocampal tissue, irrespective of the pH of the citrate buffer induced extensive nonspecific labeling with standard enzyme and label concentrations (Figure 3C). However, following reduction of the enzyme and label concentra-

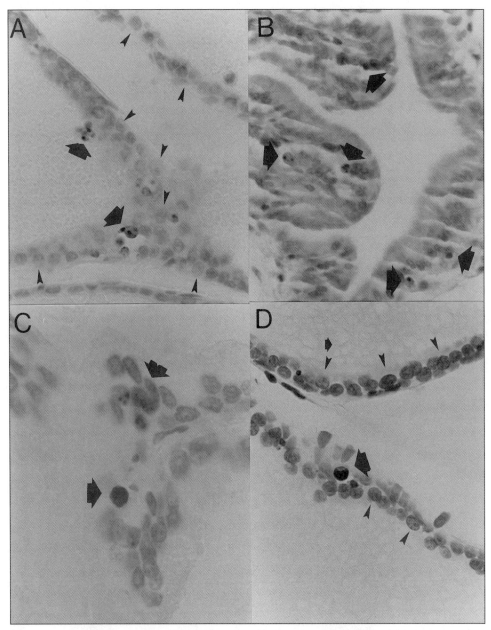

Figure 2. TUNEL-positive, apoptotic cells in the rat prostate 3 days after castration identified after MW pretreatment and a 50% reduction in standard enzyme and label concentrations. (A) MW pretreatment at pH 3.0 resulted in a clear identification of apoptotic cells (arrows), but with some weak background, also seen in nonapoptotic cells (arrowheads). (B) Background staining is absent following incubation at pH 9.0 and shows clear staining of apoptotic cells (arrows). (C) MW pretreatment at pH 9.0 reveals prominent staining of individual apoptotic cells (arrows), whereas no background staining was apparent. (D) Standard enzyme conditions in combination with MW and PK pretreatment caused all nuclei, including intact ones, to be stained (arrowheads), although a possibly apoptotic nucleus (large arrow) can still be recognized. Small arrows indicate prostate vesicle lumen wall. **(See color plate A4).**

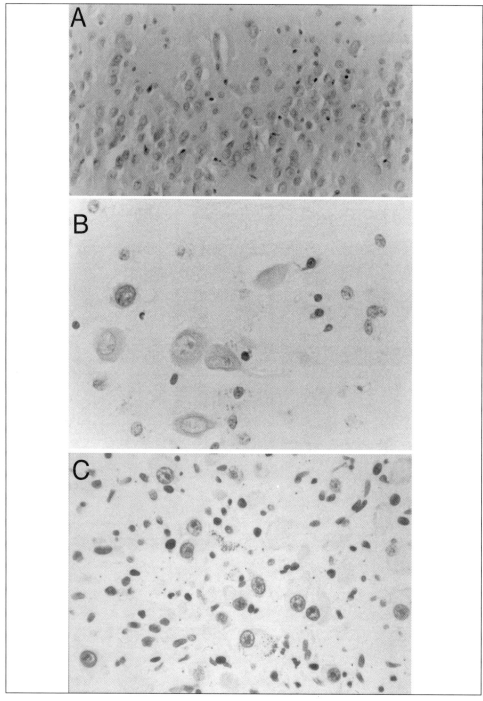

Figure 3. Human hippocampus tissue of an Alzheimer patient (PMD 4h) following TUNEL. (A) No labeling is observed if no MW pretreatment is applied. (B) In adjacent sections, following a short MW protocol at pH 3.0 in combination with rapid cooling (see text for details), an optimal staining pattern was achieved, as revealed by labeling of only some hippocampal neurons and smaller glia cells, in the absence of background labeling. (C) Almost every nucleus (neuron or glia) has become positive following standard (2× 5 minutes full power) microwave pretreatment of human postmortem brain tissue in pH 3.0 or 6.0 buffer including 15 minutes cooling at room temperature and standard enzyme and label concentrations. Local differences in specific signal can no longer be assessed. **(See color plate A5).**

tions by 50% and an adapted short MW-AR protocol at pH 3.0 in combination with a rapid change with cold buffer, some clear and isolated TUNEL-positive cells were observed in the hippocampus without increased background levels (Figure 3B). Isolated glia-like positive cells were also observed. Both cell types were absent in adjacent, non-MW-treated sections (Figure 3A). Other pH values of 6.0 and 9.0 yielded no clear improvement for the short protocol with rapid cooling, as already slightly enhanced background labeling was found.

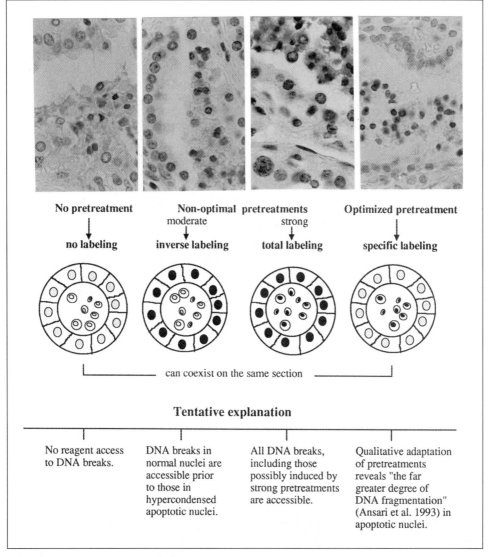

Figure 4. Possible TUNEL patterns in relation to tissue pretreatment. Tissue fixation, i.e., protein and DNA cross-linking, in addition to extensive condensation of the chromatin during apoptosis, will hamper the TUNEL enzyme mixture components from reaching the fragmented 3' OH DNA ends that are present in much larger amounts in apoptotic cells than in intact cells. The adaptation of fixation conditions, pretreatment, and enzyme/label concentrations, in addition to a careful monitoring of color development after TUNEL, will allow specific identification of apoptotic cells, before the lower amounts of DNA breaks in nonapoptotic cells becomes detectable. Reprinted with permission from Reference 34. **(See color plate A6).**

In the thyroid study, MW application was crucial (Figure 4). No gain in TUNEL result was obtained on medium-fixed small fragments by introducing a short MW heating step (1 min at 750 W, 86°C in 50 mL of citrate buffer, pH 6.0, rapidly cooled) followed by classic PK digestion as described previously (74). Conversely, when TUNEL was applied to overfixed samples, combined with PK, only MW treatment allowed us to restore, or even exceed the scores of specific staining achieved on tissues fixed for shorter periods. With regard to buffers, the carbonate solution (pH 9.0 and 10.6) altered histological features and tended to detach sections. Tris-citrate (pH 9.0), although less aggressive, and citrate buffer (pH 6.0) provided no decisive TUNEL improvement than was obtained with extreme pH values in citrate buffer (pH 3.0), twice for 5 minutes at 752 W for formalin-fixed samples, with about 80% apoptotic cells labeled and very low background; the basic Tris solution (pH 10.6) with a comparable energy (3 min at 752 W followed by 7 min at 376 W) combined with classic Triton X-100 and PK steps yielded similar improvement. In Bouin's-fixed samples, the addition of detergent Triton clearly reduced residual background levels.

In prostate tissue, 3 days after castration, many apoptotic cells are present in the wall of the vesicle lumen that were not detected in the absence of MW or PK pretreatment. Combined MW and PK pretreatment, with a reduction in the concentration of the TdT enzyme and labeled UTP by 50%, as has been described previously (45), yielded a similar staining intensity as after higher PK concentrations alone. Furthermore, MW pretreatment in pH 3.0 resulted in a clear identification of apoptotic cells, but with some background in nonapoptotic cells (Figure 2A). Treatment in pH 6.0 yielded similar results for the intensity of specific apoptotic cell staining but with somewhat lower background levels, which was absent following incubation at 9.0 (Figure 2B) and also showed prominent staining of individual cells (Figure 2C), which was judged the best condition for this tissue.

Standard enzyme conditions in combination with MW and PK yielded all nuclei to be stained, although a possibly apoptotic nucleus can still be recognized (Figure 2D).

TUNEL Technique: Brief Comments

1. Two different conditions for TUNEL were used. For brain and prostate staining, incorporated nucleotides were biotinylated and then incubated with avidin-peroxidase and DAB-H_2O_2 solution. This system is well known in immunohistochemistry for its high sensitivity. For thyroid tissue, protocols were used based on nucleotides labeled with fluorescein in the Roche Molecular Biochemicals kit and digoxigenin in a previous laboratory protocol described elsewhere (34,52), which were subsequently detected by specific monoclonal FAb antibodies. The latter approach tends to favor specificity over sensitivity.

2. Specific blocking solutions may be helpful against background, such as: *(i)* serum albumin or normal serum, and *(ii)* serum albumin or normal serum of the animal in which the labeled antibody was raised.

3. Monitoring of DAB development under the microscope is essential to prevent overdeveloping and massive aspecific labeling. In particular, for different tissues and different methods or durations of fixation, nucleotide incorporation may have been variable between patients and can seriously interfere with the variation in TUNEL outcome between patients. For example, development of approximately 10 minutes yielded acceptable signal-to-noise ratios for brain tissue, whereas for the Graves' thyroid tissue, much shorter DAB times (i.e., 1

min) were already sufficient.

4. As for TdT and UTP concentration, the original concentrations described by Wijsman et al. (85) turned out to be necessary for the often overfixed brain tissue that otherwise (i.e., at 50% of the enzyme and label concentration) showed no TUNEL-positive cells. Pretreatment with MW improved considerably the signal for prostate and perfused brain tissue, such that 50% of the original TdT and UTP concentrations could be used, which was beneficial from a financial point of view as well. However, increasing TdT and UTP concentrations can help to enhance TUNEL sensitivity in cases of rare tissue, or for tissue that has already been mounted on glass slides coated with weak adhesives, such as protein-based gelatin coating, for which PK or MW pretreatment cannot be used, as detachment may occur.

DISCUSSION

In the present study, we investigated the influence of MW-AR and other pretreatments on TUNEL results in rat and human brain tissue, prostate, and Graves' thyroid tissue. Heating sections in an MW oven in citrate buffer of pH 3.0 combined with PK treatment of 20 µg/mL for 15 minutes at RT proved to enhance TUNEL in the Graves' thyroid and in 10-day postfixed, NMDA-injected rat pup brain. Slightly enhanced TUNEL was found in similarly treated immersion-fixed postmortem human brain tissue, but only with an adapted, short MW-AR protocol and rapid cooling and clear variations between patients. In addition, MW pretreatment allowed the reduction of enzyme and label concentrations without compromising the labeling of apoptotic nuclei in the perfused rat brain.

The effect on TUNEL for formalin tissue by pretreating with MW-AR heating in citrate buffer at pH 3.0 is in agreement with previous immunocytochemical studies, showing optimal retrieval of mainly nuclear antigens at low pH (66,68,79). It is striking that two aldehyde-fixed glandular tissues yielded opposite results regarding the optimal pH value: a better sensitivity and clear background was found at acidic pH for thyroid, in contrast with basic pH for prostate. Although the only noticeable differences that may explain these results were fixation time (10 days for prostate vs. 20 h for thyroid), size, and/or lipid content, the underlying mechanism remains unclear.

Detection of DNA fragmentation is seriously hampered by prolonged fixation, as became clear by comparing the 3- and 10-day postfixation conditions in the NMDA-treated rat brain model. Unlike the 3-day postfixed tissue, the lesion area was difficult to delineate following 10 days of postfixation, indicating that in (perfused) brain tissue, duration of postfixation (and thus the extent of protein cross-linking) seriously hampers accessibility of DNA. Literature data support this (10,34,39,78).

Beneficial effects of MW-AR for TUNEL have been described in the literature, mentioning similar limitations and cautionary suggestions for tissue-specific adaptations (22,34,39,52,53,62,63,74,87). It was Iseki (27) who suggested that differences in DNA accessibility and chromatin structure, due to overfixation or hypercondensation during various stage of the apoptotic process, might result in varying rates of enzymatic incorporation and thus TUNEL outcome. Others have also studied and discussed this possibility, but with different results; no relation could be established between duration of formalin fixation and TUNEL signal in age-matched human brain tissue (1,10,35,38,39,59,71), whereas such a link was indeed found in brain lymphoma and rat testis (10), or rat spleen and thymus tissue (10,78). For instance, for colon and thymus tissue with much shorter fixation times than presently used for brain tissue, only very brief MW-AR pretreatments were necessary (74), which is in agreement with the results on perfused rat brain tissue that was fixed in a stronger fashion and required relatively strong MW-AR conditions.

Immersion fixation obviously induces a gradient from the periphery to more central areas of the tissue and apparently can induce clear variations in TUNEL outcome depending on tissue size. Different gradations can be recognized in fixation strength or cross-linking intensity, starting with perfusion fixation followed by prolonged post-fixation; these gradations require stronger or more extreme MW-AR or combined PK pretreatments, than, for example, briefly immersion-fixed, small tissue samples such as rat prostate tissue. Immersion-fixed postmortem brain or larger thyroid tissue samples apparently represent a different situation, as duration of fixation did not seem to influence TUNEL much (34,39,53). Sample size of the tissue is thus a parameter that may be critical in the influence of fixation.

PMD may also influence TUNEL outcome (31,60), which is particularly relevant for human brain tissue and has been studied extensively, but without a clear relation noticeable up to 24 (1,63), 42 (38,39), or even 72 hours (58) for rat and human brain or rat intestine. Although fixation may be interrelated here, clusters of TUNEL-labeled cells began to appear following PMDs of 48 and 72 hours in mouse and rat brain (39,63) or after 2 or 4 hours at 4°C in rat spleen and thymus (78). Obviously, depending on tissue size and surface/content ratio, differences in cooling rate will occur. This would support earlier data showing the rapid induction of many DNA breaks in rat cortex when tissue is kept at 37°C for 3 hours postmortem, while almost no breaks were induced in the same tissue kept at 0°C. This was interpreted as an effect of temperature-dependent activity of endonucleases during the postmortem period (50,63).

Various other factors have been tested in relation to improvement of TUNEL sensitivity. For instance, blocked DNA termini caused by phosphorylation of the 3' OH ends, during postmortem or apoptotic processes (5,42), have been suggested to hamper enzyme accessibility. However, dephosphorylation prior to MW-AR and TUNEL, as commonly used for immunohistochemistry for e.g., tau-related antigens (23,76), did not result in any beneficial effect (39). Also, hydrochloric or formic acid pretreatments, frequently used in in situ hybridization or immunocytochemical studies, will induce acid hydrolysis and could enhance signal-to-background ratios (32,39). For TUNEL, depending on prior proteolytic digestion, mild acid treatment was reported to induce increased TUNEL signal in both apoptotic and normal-appearing nuclei, which is in agreement with these predictions. Also, pretreating immersion-fixed rat brain sections with formic acid (pH 0.0) for 30 minutes or HCl (pH 2.0) for 60 minutes at RT yielded extensive nonspecific labeling (39).

In addition, pH of the cerebrospinal fluid (CSF), which may influence the activation of endonucleases and thus DNA fragmentation patterns may influence TUNEL outcome (38,39), although a recent paper suggests otherwise. Similar to conservation of RNA integrity during the postmortem period, the pH of the CSF or tissue affected the outcome of TUNEL staining (30,31). To what extent these findings apply to human brain tissue with many other post- and antemortem variables cannot be answered at present (60), but matching for this parameter when studying patient groups seems necessary. As far as PK is concerned, although others (19) have described beneficial effects of increasing PK concentrations, the current consensus is that 20 µg/mL is sufficient and higher concentrations may result in tissue detachment, worsened tissue morphology, and increased background staining. As PK batches may differ considerably, every new batch should be validated again and, in view of the enzyme's optimum, pH of the PK buffer should be controlled accurately, as pH 8.0 (in contrast to the commonly used pH 7.0 of the PK buffer) may cause clear increases in TUNEL signal. Finally, calcium chelation, which was recently shown to interfere with MW-AR results in immunocytochemistry (47,48) could also, in theory, be of importance for effects of MW-AR on TUNEL as well.

In addition to these methodological aspects, it is important to realize that apoptosis is a very rapid process, which is completed within hours in the rodent brain (7,9, 17,26) and requires frequent sampling in space and time. As discussed and calculated before (37,38,56,57,72), identification in thin sections is hence very difficult in chronic disorders. Assuming a gradual decay approximately 1 in 4000 cells should be undergoing apoptosis at any given time in a chronic disorder with a duration of several decades, which comes down to one or two positive cells per tissue section, that may be very difficult to find. Furthermore, although TUNEL positivity alone is insufficient evidence to identify the presence of apoptosis, as this requires additional morphological criteria, like apoptotic bodies, and nuclear and chromatin condensation, the criteria discriminating apoptosis from necrosis have become more complex now that intermediate and overlapping phenotypes have been described (7,59,77).

CONCLUSION

TUNEL detects DNA fragmentation associated with cell death in tissue sections or cell preparations. It is now widely applied to identify apoptosis on archival, biopsy, or autopsy material fixed for prolonged periods of time. As TUNEL in fact does not detect apoptosis, but rather the associated increase in DNA breaks, conservation of DNA integrity that can be compromised by e.g., postmortem delay, as well as accessibility of DNA, which is hampered by fixation and chromatin hypercondensation, is very important.

Prolonged formalin postfixation following perfusion fixation can mask the enzyme's substrate but can be counteracted by MW pretreatment, with best results with citrate buffer at pH 3.0 in case of formalin-fixed tissue. For Graves' thyroid tissue, pH 3.0 yielded optimal results for formalin fixation and pH 10.6 for Bouin's-fixed tissue. Standard MW pretreatment proved to be not beneficial for every tissue, because it can induce extensive nonspecific labeling in immersion-fixed rat and human brain tissue at standard label and enzyme concentrations. Brief MW pretreatment for 5 minutes and rapid cooling, or adaptation of the enzyme and label concentrations to 50% can improve signal-to-background ratios in brain. The influence of fixation on TUNEL appears to depend also on tissue sample size. Small-sized prostate tissue and small fragments of thyroid parenchyma showed a different result as compared to larger samples of brain tissue.

In conclusion, MW pretreatments are beneficial for TUNEL on small-sized samples of immersion-fixed prostate, thyroid tissue, and perfused brain tissue. Brief MW pretreatments and mild TUNEL conditions are advisable for human postmortem and immersion-fixed rat brain tissue only. Individual factors, like postmortem delay and pH of the CSF may further influence TUNEL results as well. Thus, TUNEL detection of apoptosis is a powerful and useful technique that requires careful matching and pilot optimization for every tissue condition before comparing different experimental groups or conditions. Importantly, as TUNEL labels fragmented DNA, which can also be associated with necrosis, autolysis, or phagocytosed DNA fragments inside macrophages, specific morphological criteria, in addition to TUNEL positivity, are essential for the convincing identification of apoptosis.

The main problems with TUNEL can be summarized as follows:

1. For archival tissue such as brain or Graves' thyroid, pretreatments with either PK or MW are needed for specific labeling. Tissue pretreatments are used in an attempt to overcome the masking of the DNA by a matrix of fixed tissue. The effectiveness of the pretreatment also optimizes detection of infrequent DNA breaks present in nonapoptotic cells.

2. Fixation type and duration of fixation, and thus tissue sample size, are crucial for a reproducible TUNEL outcome, but these may differ in archival tissue.

Also, other variables such as pH of the CSF, tissue sample size, and PMD will have to be taken into account and matched for future studies (30,34,52,53).

3. On tissues fixed for prolonged periods of time, TUNEL needs to be facilitated by pretreatments or by adapting enzyme and label concentrations: the longer the fixation, the stronger (and more aggressive) the pretreatment needed.

4. PK appears to be indispensable for fixed tissue for 15 minutes at RT, with an optimal concentration of 20 µg/mL (0.3 µg/mL on frozen sections) in our hands.

5. Detergent (0.1% Triton X-100) only acts as an adjuvant is not essential and appears mostly to reduce background staining.

6. MW irradiation plays a key role, as it strongly improves TUNEL outcome in overfixed tissues. Although variation can be induced by differences in fluid volume, MW oven power, and incubation pH and duration, a standard protocol that tests (combinations of) Tris and citrate buffers at pH 3.0, 6.0, and 9.0 allows one to judge optimal pretreatment conditions for a given tissue while sparing morphological detail (e.g., see References 66 and 67).

7. The type of detection system used in TUNEL protocols may influence sensitivity and specificity. For each tissue type, an optimal detection system must be empirically determined.

Once adapted, TUNEL remains an excellent technique to identify apoptotic cells in a variety of tissues and conditions.

ACKNOWLEDGMENTS

P.J.L. is supported by NWO and the Internationale Stichting Alzheimer Onderzoek (ISAO).

REFERENCES

1. **Anderson, A.J., J.H. Su, and C.W. Cotman.** 1996. DNA damage and apoptosis in Alzheimer's disease: colocalization with c-jun immunoreactivity, relationship to brain area, and effect of postmortem delay. J. Neurosci. *16*:1710-1719.

2. **Ansari, B., B.D. Coates, B.D. Greenstein, and P.A. Hall.** 1993. In situ end labeling detects DNA strand breaks in apoptosis and other physiological and pathological states. J. Pathol. *170*:1-8.

3. **Bursch, W., S. Paffe, B. Putz, G. Barthel, and R. Schulte-Hermann.** 1990. Determination of the length of the histological stages of apoptosis in normal liver and in altered hepatic foci of rats. Carcinogenesis *11*:847-853.

4. **Cervos-Navarro, J. and T.E. Schubert.** 1996. Pitfalls in the evaluation of apoptosis using TUNEL. Brain Pathol. *6*:347-348.

5. **Chaudun, E., C. Arutti, Y. Courtois, F. Ferrag, J.C. Jeanny, B.N. Patel, C. Skidmore, A. Torriglia, and M.F.**

Counis. 1994. DNA strand breakage during physiological apoptosis of the embryonic chick lens: free 3′ OH end single strand breaks do not accumulate even in the presence of a cation-independent deoxyribonuclease. J. Cell Physiol. *158*:354-364.

6. **Clarke, P.G.** 1990. Developmental cell death: morphological diversity and multiple mechanisms. Anat. Embryol. *181*:195-213.

7. **Clarke, P.G.H.** 1999. Apoptosis versus necrosis: how valid a dichotomy for neurons? p. 3-28. *In* V.E. Koliatsos and R.R. Ratan (Eds.), Cell Death and Diseases of the Nervous System. Humana Press, Totowa, NJ.

8. **Cohen, J.J.** 1993. Apoptosis. Immunol. Today *14*:126-130.

9. **Conti, A.C., R. Raghupathi, J.Q. Trojanowski, and T.K. McIntosh.** 1998. Experimental brain injury induces regionally distinct apoptosis during the acute and delayed post-traumatic period. J. Neurosci. *18*:5663-5672.

10. **Davison, F.D., M. Groves, and F. Scaravilli.** 1995. The effects of formalin fixation on the detection of apoptosis in human brain by in situ end labeling of DNA. Histochem. J. *27*:983-988.

11. **Desjardins, L.M. and J.P. MacManus.** 1995. An adherent cell model to study different stages of apoptosis. Exp. Cell Res. *216*:380-387.

12. **Eastman, A. and M.A. Barry.** 1992. The origins of DNA breaks: a consequence of DNA damage, DNA repair, or apoptosis. Cancer Invest. *10*:229-240.

13. **English, H.F., N. Kyprianou, and J.T. Isaacs.** 1989. Relationship between DNA fragmentation and apoptosis in the programmed cell death in the rat prostate following castration. Prostate *15*:233-250.

14. **Evers, P. and H.B.M. Uylings.** 1994. Microwave stimulated antigen retrieval is pH and temperature dependent. J. Histochem. Cytochem. *42*:1555-1563.

15. **Fehsel, K., V. Kolb-Bachofen, and H. Kolb.** 1991. Analysis of TNF α-induced DNA strand breaks at the single cell level. Am. J. Pathol. *139*:251-254.

16. **Fehsel, K., K.D. Krönck, H. Kolb, and V. Kolb-Bachoven.** 1994. In situ nick-translation detects focal apoptosis in thymuses of glucocorticoid- and lipopolysaccharide-treated mice. J. Histochem. Cytochem. *42*:613-619.

17. **Ferrer, I., A. Tortosa, R. Blanco, F. Martin, T. Serrano, A. Planas, and A. Macaya.** 1994. Naturally occurring cell death in the developing cerebral cortex of the rat. Evidence of apoptosis-associated internucleosomal DNA fragmentation. Neurosci. Lett. *182*:77-79.

18. **Gavrieli, Y., Y. Sherman, and S.A. Ben-Sasson.** 1992. Identification of programmed cell death in situ via specific labeling of nuclear DNA fragmentation. J. Cell. Biol. *119*:493-501.

19. **Gold, R., M. Schmied, G. Giegerich, H. Breitschopf, H.P. Hartung, K.V. Tokyka, and H. Lassmann.** 1994. Differentiation between cellular apoptosis and necrosis by combined use of in situ tailing and nick translation techniques. Lab. Invest. *71*:219-225.

20. **Gold, R., M. Schmied, G. Rothe, H. Zischler, H. Breitschopf, H. Wekerle, and H. Lassmann.** 1993. Detection of DNA fragmentation in apoptosis: application of in situ nick translation to cell culture systems and tissue sections. J. Histochem. Cytochem. *41*:1023-1030.

21. **Gorczyca, W., J. Gong, and Z. Darzynkiewicz.** 1993. Detection of DNA strand breaks in individual apototic cells by the in situ TdT and nick translation assays. Cancer Res. *53*:1945-1951.

22. **Grasl-Kraupp, B., B. Ruttkay-Nedecky, H. Koudelka, K. Bukowska, W. Bursch, and R. Schulte-Hermann.** 1995. In situ detection of fragmented DNA (TUNEL assay) fails to discriminate among apoptosis, necrosis and autolytic cell death: a cautionary note. Hepatology *21*:1465-1468.

23. **Grundke-Iqbal, I., K. Iqbal, Y.-C. Tung, M. Quinlan, H.M. Wisniewski, and L. Binder.** 1986. Abnormal phosphorylation of the microtubule-associated protein τ (tau) in Alzheimer cytoskeletal pathology. Proc. Natl. Acad. Sci. USA *83*:4913-4917.

24. **Hammond, L.J., M.W. Lowdell, P.G. Cerrano, A.W. Goode, G.F. Bottazzo, and R. Mirakian.** 1997. Analysis of apoptosis in relation to tissue destruction associated with Hashimoto's autoimmune thyroiditis. J. Pathol. *182*:138-144.

25. **Henderson, C.** 1989. Aminoalkylsilane: an inexpensive, simple preparation for slide adhesion. J. Histotechnol. *12*:123-124.

26. **Hu, Z., K. Yuri, H. Ozawa, H. Lu, and M. Kawata.** 1997. The in vivo time course for elimination of adrenalectomy-induced apoptotic profiles from the granule cell layer of the rat hippocampus. J. Neurosci. *17*:3981-3989.

27. **Iseki, S.** 1986. DNA strand breaks in rat tissues as detected by in situ nick translation. Exp. Cell Res. *167*:311-326.

28. **Kasagi, N., Y. Gomyo, H. Shirai, S. Tsujitani, and H. Ito.** 1994. Apoptotic cell death in human gastric carcinoma: analysis by terminal deoxynucleotidyl transferase-mediated dUTP-biotin nick end labeling. Jpn. J. Cancer Res. *85*:939-945.

29. **Kerr, J.F.R., A.H. Wyllie, and A.R. Currie.** 1972. Apoptosis: a basic biological phenomenon with wide-ranging implications in tissue kinetics. Br. J. Cancer *26*:239-257.

30. **Kingsbury, A.E., O.J. Foster, A.P. Nisbet, N. Cairns, L. Bray, D.J. Eve, A.J. Lees, and C.D. Marsden.** 1995. Tissue pH as an indicator of mRNA preservation in human post-mortem brain. Brain Res. Mol. Brain Res. *28*:311-318.

31. **Kingsbury, A.E., C.D. Mardsen, and O.J. Foster.** 1998. DNA fragmentation in human substantia nigra: apoptosis or perimortem effect? Mov. Disord. *13*:877-884.

32. **Kitamoto, T., K. Ogomori, J. Tateishi, and S.B. Prusiner.** 1987. Formic acid pretreatment enhances immunostaining of cerebral and systemic amyloids. Lab. Invest. *57*:230-236.

33. **Kressel, M. and P. Groscurth.** 1995. Distinction of apoptotic and necrotic cell death by in situ labelling of fragmented DNA. Cell Tissue Res. *278*:549-556.

34. **Labat-Moleur, F., C. Guillermet, P. Lorimier, C. Robert, S. Lantuejoul, E. Brambilla, and A. Negoescu.** 1998. TUNEL apoptotic cell detection in tissue sections: critical evaluation and improvement. J. Histochem. Cytochem. *46*: 327-334.

35. **Lassmann, H., C. Bancher, H. Breitschopf, J. Wegiel, M. Bobinski, K. Jellinger, and H.M. Wisniewski.** 1995. Cell death in Alzheimer's disease evaluated by DNA fragmentation in situ. Acta. Neuropathol. *89*:35-41.

36. **Li, Y., M. Chopp, N. Jiang, F. Yao, and C. Zaloga.** 1995. Temporal profile of in situ DNA fragmentation after transient middle cerebral artery occlusion in the rat. J. Cereb. Blood Flow Metab. *15*:389-397.

37. **Lucassen, P.J.** 2000. Presenilins and DNA damage; a link through amyloid? J. Alzheimers Dis. *2*:61-67.

38. **Lucassen, P.J., W.C.J. Chung, W. Kamphorst, and D.F. Swaab.** 1997. DNA damage distribution in the human brain as shown by in situ end labeling; area specific differences in aging and Alzheimer's disease in the absence of apoptotic morphology. J. Neuropathol. Exp. Neurol. *56*:887-900.

39. **Lucassen, P.J., W.C.J. Chung, J.P. Vermeulen, M. Van Lookeren Campagne, J.H. Van Dierendonck, and D.F. Swaab.** 1995. Microwave-enhanced in situ end-labeling of fragmented DNA: parametric studies in relation to postmortem delay and fixation of rat and human brain. J. Histochem. Cytochem. *43*:1163-1171.

40. **Lucassen, P.J., R. Ravid, N.K. Gonatas, and D.F. Swaab.** 1993. Activation of human supraoptic and paraventricular nucleus neurons with aging and in Alzheimer's disease as judged from increasing size of the Golgi apparatus. Brain Res. *632*:105-113.

41. **Majno, G. and I. Joris.** 1995. Apoptosis, oncosis, and necrosis. An overview of cell death. Am. J. Pathol. *146*:3-15.

42. **Matsuo, E.S., R.-W. Shin, M.L. Billingsley, A. Van deVoorde, M. O'Connor, J.Q. Trojanowski, and V.M. Lee.** 1994. Biopsy-derived adult human brain tau is phosphorylated at many of the same sites as Alzheimer's disease paired helical filament tau. Neuron *13*:989-1002.

43. **McDonald, J.W., F.S. Silverstein, and M.V. Johnston.** 1988. Neurotoxicity of N-methyl-D-aspartate is markedly enhanced in developing rat central nervous system. Brain Res. *459*:200-203.

44. **Migheli, A., A. Attanasio, and D. Schiffer.** 1995. Ultrastructural detection of DNA strand breaks in apoptotic neural cells by in situ end-labelling techniques. J. Pathol. *176*:27-35.

45. **Migheli, A., P. Cavalla, S. Marino, and D. Schiffer.** 1994. A study of apoptosis in normal and pathologic nervous tissue after in situ end labeling of DNA strand breaks. J. Neuropathol. Exp. Neurol. *53*:606-616.

46. **Monti, D., L. Troiano, F. Tropea, E. Grassilli, A. Cossarizza, D. Barozzi, M.C. Pelloni, M.G. Tamassia, G. Bellomo, and C. Franceschi.** 1992. Apoptosis-programmed cell death: a role in the aging process? Am. J. Clin. Nutr. *55*:1208S-1214S.

47. **Morgan, J.M., H. Navabi, and B. Jasani.** 1997. Role of calcium chelation in high-temperature antigen retrieval at different pH values. J. Pathol. *182*:233-237.

48. **Morgan, J.M., H. Navabi, K.W. Schmid, and B. Jasani.** 1994. Possible role of tissue-bound calcium ions in citrate-mediated high-temperature antigen retrieval. J. Pathol. *174*:301-307.

49. **Mori, C., N. Nakamura, Y. Okamoto, M. Osawa, and K. Shiota.** 1994. Cytochemical identification of programmed cell death in the fusing fetal mouse plate by specific labeling of DNA fragmentation. Anat. Embryol. *190*:21-28.

50. **Mullaart, E., M.E. Boerrigter, R. Ravid, D.F. Swaab, and J. Vijg.** 1990. Increased levels of DNA breaks in cerebral cortex of Alzheimer's disease patients. Neurobiol. Aging *11*:169-173.

51. **Mundle, S.D. and A. Raz.** 1995. The two in situ techniques do not differentiate between apoptosis and necrosis but rather reveal distinct patterns of DNA fragmentation in apoptosis. Lab. Invest. *72*:611-613.

52. **Negoescu, A., C. Guillermet, P. Lorimier, E. Brambilla, and F. Labat-Moleur.** 1998. Importance of DNA fragmentation in apoptosis with regard to TUNEL specificity. Biomed. Pharmacother. *52*:252-258.

53. **Negoescu, A., P. Lorimier, F. Labat-Moleur, C. Drouet, C. Robert, C. Guillermet, C. Brambilla, and E. Brambilla.** 1996. In situ apoptotic cell labeling by the TUNEL method: improvement and evaluation on cell preparations. J. Histochem. Cytochem. *44*:959-968.

54. **Pang, Z. and J.W. Geddes.** 1997. Mechanisms of cell death induced by the mitochondrial toxin 3-nitropropionic acid: acute excitotoxic necrosis and delayed apoptosis. J. Neurosci. *17*:3064-3073.

55. **Peitsch, M.C., C. Müller, and J. Tschopp.** 1993. DNA fragmentation during apoptosis is caused by frequent single-strand cuts. Nucleic Acids Res. *21*:4206-4209.

56. **Perry, G., A. Nunomura, P. Lucassen, H. Lassmann, and M.A. Smith.** 1998. Apoptosis and Alzheimer's disease. Science *282*:1268-1269.

57. **Perry, G., A. Nunomura, and M.A. Smith.** 1998. A suicide note from Alzheimer disease neurons? Nature Med. *4*:897-898.

58. **Petito, C.K. and B. Roberts.** 1995. Effect of postmortem interval on in situ end-labeling of DNA oligosomes. J. Neuropathol. Exp. Neurol. *54*:761-763.

59. **Portera Cailliau, C., J.C. Hedreen, D.L. Price, and V.E. Koliatsos.** 1995. Evidence for apoptotic cell death in Huntington's disease and excitotoxic animal models. J. Neurosci. *15*:3775-3787.

60. **Ravid, R., E.J. Van Zwieten, and D.F. Swaab.** 1992. Brain banking and the human hypothalamus—factors to match for, pitfalls and potentials. Progr. Brain Res. *93*:83-90.

61. **Sandford, N.L., J.W. Searle, and J.F.R. Kerr.** 1984. Successive waves of apoptosis in the rat prostate after repeat-

ed withdrawal of testosterone stimulation. Pathology *16*:406-410.

62. **Sasano, H.** 1995. In situ end labeling and its applications to the study of endocrine disease: how can we study programmed cell death in surgical pathology materials? Endocr. Pathol. 2:87-89.

63. **Schallock, K., W.J. Schulz-Schaeffer, A. Giese, and H.A. Kretzschmar.** 1997. Postmortem delay and temperature conditions affect the in situ end-labeling (ISEL) assay in brain tissue of mice. Clin. Neuropathol. 16:133-136.

64. **Schwartzman, R.A. and J.A. Cidlowski.** 1993 Apoptosis: the biochemistry and molecular biology of programmed cell death. Endocr. Rev. *14*:133-151.

65. **Shi, S.R., B. Chaiwun, L. Young, R.J. Cote, and C.R. Taylor.** 1993. Antigen retrieval technique utilizing citrate buffer or urea solution for immunohistochemical demonstration of androgen receptor in formalin-fixed paraffin sections. J. Histochem. Cytochem. *41*:1599-1604.

66. **Shi, S.R., R.J. Cote, and C.R. Taylor.** 1997. Antigen retrieval immunohistochemistry: past, present, and future. J. Histochem. Cytochem. *45*:327-343.

67. **Shi, S.R., R.J. Cote, C. Yang, C. Chen, H.J. Xu, W.F Benedict, and C.R. Taylor.** 1996. Development of an optimal protocol for antigen retrieval: a "test battery" approach exemplified with reference to the staining of retinoblastoma protein (pRB) in formalin-fixed paraffin sections. J. Pathol. *179*:347-352.

68. **Shi, S.R., S.A. Imam, L. Young, R.J. Cote, and C.R. Taylor.** 1995. Antigen retrieval immunohistochemistry under the influence of pH using monoclonal antibodies. J. Histochem. Cytochem. *43*:193-201.

69. **Shi, S.R., M.E. Key, and K.L. Kalra.** 1991. Antigen retrieval in formalin-fixed, paraffin-embedded tissues: an enhancement method for immunohistochemical staining based on microwave oven heating of tissue sections. J. Histochem. Cytochem. *39*:741-748.

70. **Simic, G., D. Seso-Simic, P.J. Lucassen, A. Islam, A. Cviko, Z. Krsnik, M. Gnjidic, N. Barisic, B. Winblad, I. Kostovic, and B. Kruslin.** Ultrastructural and immunocytochemical evidence for motor neuron apoptosis in Werdnig-Hoffmann's disease. J. Neuropathol. Exp. Neurol. (In Press).

71. **Smale, G., N.R. Nichols, D.R. Brady, C.E. Finch, and W.E. Horton.** 1995. Evidence for apoptotic cell death in Alzheimer's disease. Exp. Neurol. *133*:225-230.

72. **Stadelmann, C., W. Bruck, C. Bancher, K. Jellinger, and H. Lassmann.** 1998. Alzheimer disease: DNA fragmentation indicates increased neuronal vulnerability, but not apoptosis. J. Neuropathol. Exp. Neurol. 57:456-464.

73. **Staunton, M.J. and E.F. Gaffney.** 1998. Apoptosis: basic concepts and potential significance in human cancer. Arch. Pathol. Lab. Med. *122*:310-319.

74. **Sträter, J., A.R. Günthert, S. Brüderlein, and P. Möller.** 1995. Microwave irradiation of paraffin-embedded tissue sensitizes the TUNEL method for in situ detection of apoptotic cells. Histochem. Cell Biol. *103*:157-160.

75. **Sugaya, K., M. Reeves, and M. McKinney.** 1997. Topographic associations between DNA fragmentation and Alzheimer's disease neuropathology in the hippocampus. Neurochem. Int. *31*:275-281.

76. **Swaab, D.F., I. Grundke-Iqbal, K. Iqbal, H.P.H. Kremer, R. Ravid, and J.A.P. Van de Nes.** 1992. τ and ubiquitin in the human hypothalamus in aging and Alzheimer's disease. Brain Res. *590*:239-245.

77. **Tan, S., M. Wood, and P. Maher.** 1998. Oxidative stress induces a form of programmed celldeath with characteristics of both apoptosis and necrosis in normal cells. J. Neurochem. *71*:95-105.

78. **Tateyama, H., T. Tada, H. Hattori, T. Murase, W.X. Li, and T. Eimoto.** 1998. Effects of prefixation and fixation times on apoptosis detection by in situ end-labeling of fragmented DNA. Arch. Pathol. Lab. Med. *122*:252-255.

79. **Taylor, C.R., S.R. Shi, B. Chaiwun, L. Young, S.A. Imam, and R.J. Cote.** 1994. Strategies for improving the immunohistochemical staining of various intranuclear prognostic markers in formalin-paraffin sections: androgen receptor, estrogen receptor, progesterone receptor, p53 protein, proliferating cell nuclear antigen, and Ki-67 antigen revealed by antigen retrieval techniques. Hum. Pathol. 25:263-270.

80. **Taylor, C.R., S.R. Shi, C. Chen, L. Young, C. Yang, and R.J. Cote.** 1996. Comparative study of antigen retrieval heating methods: microwave, microwave and pressure cooker, autoclave, and steamer. Biotech. Histochem. *71*:263-270.

81. **Thiry, M.** 1992. Highly sensitive immunodetection of DNA on sections with exogenous terminal deoxynucleotidyl transferase and non-isotopic nucleotide analogues. J. Histochem. Cytochem. *40*:411-419.

82. **Van Lookeren Campagne, M., P.J. Lucassen, J.P. Vermeulen, and R. Balázs.** 1995. NMDA and Kainate induce internucleosomal DNA fragmentation and apoptotic cell death in the neonatal rat brain. Eur. J. Neurosci. 7:1627-1640.

83. **Vincent, V.A.M., C.J.A. DeGroot, P.J. Lucassen, P. Portegies, D. Troost, F.J.H. Tilders, and A.M.W. van Dam** 1999. Nitric oxide synthase expression and apoptotic cell death in brains of AIDS and AIDS dementia patients. AIDS *13*:317-326.

81. **Whiteside, G., N. Cougnon, S.P. Hunt, and R. Munglani.** 1998. An improved method for detection of apoptosis in tissue sections and cell culture, using the TUNEL technique combined with Hoechst stain. Brain Res. Protoc. 2:160-164.

85. **Wijsman, J.H., R.R. Jonker, R. Keijzer, C.J.H. van de Velde, C.J. Cornelisse, and J.H. van Dierendonck.** 1993. A new method to detect apoptosis in paraffin sections: ISEL of fragmented DNA. J. Histochem. Cytochem. *41*:7-12.

86. **Wyllie, A.H., J.F.R. Kerr, and A.R. Currie.** 1980. Cell death: the significance of apoptosis. Int. Rev. Cytol. *68*:251-306.

87. **Yasuda, M., S. Unemura, Y. Osamura, T. Kenjo, and Y. Tsutsumi.** 1995. Apoptotic cells in the human endometrium and placental villi: pitfalls in applying the TUNEL method. Arch. Histol. Cytol. *58*:185-190.

Antigen Retrieval and Unmasking for Immunoelectron Microscopy

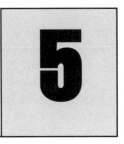

John W. Stirling

Department of Anatomical Pathology, SouthPath, Flinders Medical Centre, Bedford Park, Australia

INTRODUCTION

The use of colloidal gold probes to visualize antibodies bound to epitopes in thin sections (postembedding immunogold labeling) for electron microscopy (EM) was introduced by Faulk and Taylor in 1971 (22). Immunogold labeling for EM (IEM) is a versatile and sensitive affinity probe system with wide-ranging applications in biomedical research and diagnostics. By facilitating the high-resolution localization of epitopes, IEM allows the qualitative and semiquantitative analysis of cell and tissue components. IEM also facilitates the investigation of dynamic biologic processes. The critical aspect of IEM protocols, as in all immunocytochemical procedures, is the optimization of immunolabeling. Achieving maximum sensitivity in IEM studies is a more complex issue than for light microscopy (LM), and many epitopes cannot be labeled successfully because of the effects of fixation, processing, and embedding. Therefore, techniques that facilitate labeling, or improve sensitivity, are mandatory for some studies. Of the strategies available, heat-induced antigen retrieval, introduced by Shi et al. (60) is a simple, rapid, and cost-effective method that facilitates the labeling of many difficult epitopes.

OPTIMIZING IMMUNOREACTIVITY BEFORE RETRIEVAL

Unfortunately, it is often difficult to predict whether an epitope will label after EM

Antigen Retrieval Techniques
Edited by Shan-Rong Shi, Jiang Gu, and Clive R. Taylor
©2000 Eaton Publishing, Natick, MA

fixation and processing. The joint aims of preserving immunoreactivity and ultrastructural detail may be difficult to achieve and, in fact, mutually exclusive. In particular, fixation for EM is more complete than for LM; this is essential for retaining high-quality ultrastructural detail. Of particular concern are the effects of the complex chemistry associated with glutaraldehyde fixation and the cross-linking of tissue and resin components (24,47). Specifically, the cross-linking of tissue components by fixation (24,47), the cross-linking of proteins with resin components (19), and the extent of cross-linking between the resin components themselves can all influence immunoreactivity (24,47). In addition, resin embedding results in the physical masking of epitopes. Particulate gold probes do not penetrate resin sections and, unlike paraffin wax sections, the embedding media used for EM cannot be removed easily prior to labeling.

Before proceeding to antigen retrieval (AR), the initial step in any IEM study (unless only archival material is available) must be to optimize fixation and processing to maximize immunoreactivity and thus labeling. After taking into account the labeling dynamics of the antigen from LM studies, the effects of each processing step should be considered. The principal criteria are as follows: how will the antigen be affected by fixatives, dehydrants, resin components, heat (including polymerization exotherm) and resin masking? The range of strategies available to optimize labeling is briefly summarized here. For full details of the overall factors that influence immunogold labeling, the variety of labeling strategies available, and their underlying rationales, see general texts and reviews (4,5,24,28,29,47,54,65,68).

Modified Fixation

- Reduce the glutaraldehyde concentration to approximately 0.5% and decrease the fixation time (24,47).
- Substitute formaldehyde for glutaraldehyde wholly, or partly, (24,47). When glutaraldehyde is unsuitable for fixation, 4% formaldehyde in phosphate or cacodylate buffer (pH 7.0 to 7.4) is an excellent alternative that gives acceptable preservation at the ultrastructural level. The fixative should be made from paraformaldehyde (avoid commercial solutions containing methanol) and used within 48 hours to maximize immunoreactivity (68). Tissue prepared for LM and reprocessed for EM from wax blocks may also be acceptable.
- Reduce, or omit, osmium postfixation or substitute tannic acid or uranyl acetate for the osmium (68).
- Substitute microwave fixation for chemical fixation (33,38).
- Use cryofixation and cryosectioning (24).
- Eliminate chemical fixation and replace it with inert dehydration using ethanediol combined with direct embedding in low-acid glycol methacrylate (66,69).

Modified Embedding

- Embed the tissue in an immunocompatible resin such as low-acid glycol methacrylate or the LR, or Lowicryl, resin types (7,24,47,66,69).
- Use an immunocompatible resin with a modified, or low temperature, embedding protocol (47).
- Increase the accelerator concentration in the epoxy resin mixture (11,12) or, during processing, add *para*-phenylendramine to the dehydration and resin infiltration steps to reduce antigen–resin cross-linking (14).

EPITOPES THAT ARE NONREACTIVE DUE TO THEIR MOLECULAR OR STRUCTURAL CONFIGURATION

Epitopes may not be immunoreactive for reasons other than the effects of processing. In particular, the epitope may be hidden due to the molecular configuration of the native molecule or because of its orientation in respect to related structures. Typical examples are amyloid (1) and the unique epitopes hidden within the NC1 globular domains of collagen IV, which define the collagen IV subtypes (α1–α6) (79). In addition to enzymatic digestion, such epitopes may be exposed by chemical denaturation (in some cases before embedding) using urea (27,79), guanidine hydrochloride (51), acid, alkali (1,30,34,44,51), or sodium methoxide treatment (35,57). The labeling of oligosaccharide-associated sugar moieties can also be improved using enzyme treatment. In this case, the removal of the oligosaccharides probably reduces steric hinderance (25).

SIGNAL AMPLIFICATION TECHNIQUES FOR ELECTRON MICROSCOPY

Signal amplification techniques are used in immunocytochemical procedures to improve probe visibility. In immunogold studies, this may be done by increasing probe size or density (probe density being the number of probe particles bound per unit area). The size of the immunogold probes is enhanced using silver or gold (29,43). Additional probe particles are applied using an antibody-gold probe sandwich technique (6) or by labeling both sides of the section. Immunoenzyme techniques can also be utilized (either before or after embedding) to enhance the amount of label deposited. Methods include protocols based on diaminobenzidine (DAB) and the dinitrophenol (DNP) hapten sandwich staining procedure (21,24,31,47–49). The biotinyl-tyramide protocol for LM immunocytochemistry has also been modified for EM (39). The biotin-tyramide polymer can be labeled on-section using immunogold probes (31).

ANTIGEN RETRIEVAL VERSUS SIGNAL AMPLIFICATION FOR IMMUNOGOLD ELECTRON MICROSCOPY

AR techniques are fundamentally different from signal amplification protocols. AR techniques unmask tissue epitopes and revive their immunoreactivity. As a result, the amount of epitope detected is increased, and the detection threshold of the epitope is lowered. Thus, AR improves sensitivity where sensitivity is defined as the minimum amount of antigen detected by the technique (5). Lowering the detection threshold reduces the possibility of a false-negative result or, equally as important, a misleading false-negative result in the presence of positive labeling. In contrast, signal amplification protocols enhance label visibility. However, amplification does not necessarily increase the amount of epitope detected (even when both sides of the section are labeled), and the detection threshold may be unaltered.

The aim of immunocytochemical studies at the ultrastructural level is to localize epitopes at high resolution. To achieve this, immunogold localization combined with heat induced AR (where increased sensitivity is required) is the method of choice. In general, signal amplification, especially immunoenzyme techniques that produce a diffusible reaction product and antibody-gold probe sandwich methods, will reduce spatial resolution. In addition, immunoenzyme labels are not easily quantified and, in contrast to discrete gold probe particles with high electron density, are not easily distinguished from biologic structures at the ultrastructural level.

DEOSMICATION AND PHYSICAL UNMASKING (RESIN ETCHING)

For material processed using routine techniques (glutaraldehyde/osmium fixation and embedding in epoxy resin), the principal unmasking method utilized in IEM studies has been to deosmicate the tissue. The standard protocol is to incubate thin sections with a saturated aqueous solution of sodium metaperiodate for 1 hour (8). The treatment appears to deosmicate the tissue at the section surface, without significant resin etching or loss, and with no effect on heavy metal staining. Thus, localization is improved without reducing section, or image, quality (8). LR and Lowicryl sections may also be treated with metaperiodate (46,64). Prolonged exposure of Lowicryl sections to metaperiodate can increase background labeling, and brief incubation (5–15 min) is recommended (46). Metaperiodate treatment may cause false-positive labeling, and adequate controls are essential (64,67,68). The physical masking of epitopes in epoxy sections is reduced by etching the resin with hydrogen peroxide or sodium ethoxide. However, unlike metaperiodate, these compounds may damage the sections structurally and cause bleaching and loss of ultrastructural detail (8). The hydrophilicity of epoxy resin sections may be increased by oxidation with potassium permanganate or periodic acid (19). Acrylic resins can be etched with organic solvents, thereby increasing the surface area of the material exposed on the surface of the section. However, the tissue may also be damaged, and this strategy is not recommended (47).

UNMASKING USING ENZYMES

Proteolytic enzymes are extremely effective for exposing epitopes and improving immunolabeling for LM, although, in most cases, heat-induced antigen retrieval is superior (23). Enzyme digestion, although not used widely in IEM studies, has been applied to resin sections (e.g., acrylics and low-acid glycol methacrylate) (15,32,47,76). The immunoreactivity of some epitopes deteriorates slowly after embedding in methyl methacrylate. Thus, although trypsinization alone is effective for sections of freshly embedded tissue, epitopes in sections cut from old blocks may require a combination of trypsinization and heat-induced AR for succesful labeling (26). Heating during enzyme incubation may also improve labeling (10). Enzyme treatment of epoxy sections is likely to be less effective because the resin is hydrophobic. However, etching with hydrogen peroxide followed by trypsinization has been used in an IEM study of amyloid (1). Treatment of cryosections with N-glycanase F and exposure to acidic conditions (pH 5.5) has been found to improve the labeling of carbohydrate and protein antigens (25).

HEAT-INDUCED ANTIGEN RETRIEVAL: PROTOCOLS FOR IMMUNOGOLD ELECTRON MICROSCOPY

The application of heat-induced AR to IEM has been relatively restricted. In contrast, a large number of protocols have been developed for LM, and the mechanisms underlying the retrieval process have been investigated (17,18,23,52,57,59). Despite the added complications resulting from EM processing, the principles and techniques established for LM (including retrieval media, heating methods, etc.) can, in general, be extrapolated to IEM. Published studies (Table 1) indicate that heat-induced retrieval is effective for some epitopes in glutaraldehyde- as well as formaldehyde-fixed tissue. When planning a study, of particular relevance are LM protocols utilizing plastic-embedded tissue (Table 2); epitopes that can be demonstrated by LM in resin sections should be amenable to IEM using similar retrieval strategies.

Heating Methods

Initial protocols for LM involved boiling tissue sections in retrieval medium using a microwave oven (10,17,18,60). It is now recognized that microwave boiling per se is not necessarily essential and that high-temperature heating is the critical factor influencing retrieval (57,60). The effectiveness of the technique is temperature and time dependent so that, as temperature increases, the length of incubation decreases (57). The degree of retrieval is also reported to be proportional to the number of cycles of heating and cooling. For microwave heating, up to four periods of heating, followed by 15 to 20 minutes of cooling (to room temperature), are recommended (18,74). In some cases, the cooling period is essential for retrieval to occur (23). Overfixed tissue may require heating for a longer period to achieve the maximum retrieval effect (45). A drawback of microwave retrieval is that heating may be uneven due to the presence of high-intensity hot spots; these can cause uneven labeling (10,50,74). As an alternative to microwave heating, retrieval can be achieved by incubating in a water bath or steamer, or superheating in a pressure cooker or autoclave (57,60,74). Superheating in a plastic pressure cooker by microwave heating is also effective (74). Using these methods, heating may be more even and easier to control (74); additional benefits include speed and improved reproducibility (50). Finally, it should be noted that the overall labeling pattern of individual epitopes may be influenced by the retrieval protocol used (41).

In IEM studies, heat has been applied using a hot plate (70), a hot plate with a water bath (55), a standard bench-top oven (62), simple boiling (78), a microwave oven (77,78), an autoclave, a pressure cooker (78), and a polymerase chain reaction machine (12,13) (Table 1). In a study comparing simple boiling, microwaving, pressure cooking, and autoclaving (Table 1), all treatments gave similar retrieval levels. However, pressurized boiling produced ultrastructural damage that increased with time (78). For practical reasons it may be best to avoid actual boiling, because bubble formation disrupts the sections and reduces contact with the retrieval medium (70). In addition, when boiling in a microwave using small volumes or drops, the grids may be dislodged or lost from the surface of the retrieval medium (77). Thus, if a microwave is used for heating, the grids should be immersed in a reasonable volume of fluid, and, when boiling is essential, gentle boiling (simmering) using a low energy setting is recommended.

Recent reviews suggest that, overall, no single heating method is superior (57,74). The ultimate choice of a heating method for IEM will therefore depend on practical issues such as retention of section integrity and the type of equipment available.

Low-Temperature Heating

A small number of LM studies have been performed by incubating sections for a long period at a relatively low temperature (60°–80°C) (52). When sections of human breast tissue were incubated overnight at 60°C in boric acid (0.2 mol/L, pH 7.0) the

Table 1. Examples of IEM Protocols Utilizing Heat-Induced Antigen Retrieval

Reference	Tissue and fixation	Resin-section pretreatment	Retrieval protocol	Epitope	Comments
Stirling & Graff, 1995 (70)	Human cornea (IgG crystalloids) 4% buffered formalin + 1% osmium tetroxide and 2% aqueous uranyl acetate (en bloc) postfixation	Epoxy resin: Araldite Pretreatment: Yes/no, two media used 1. 10% sodium ethoxide for 2 min 2. saturated aqueous sodium metaperiodate for 60 min at room temperature	Single heating protocol using three media *Retrieval media:* 1. 0.01 mol/L citrate buffer, pH 6.0 2. Water 3. 50% aqueous sodium metaperiodate *Heating:* Hot plate • Heat at 95°–100°C for 10 min • Cool on retrieval medium for 15 min	IgG	Comparative study testing pretreatment protocols and AR, alone and combined. Metaperiodate pretreatment followed by retrieval with citrate buffer gave the highest probe density (186 particles/μm^2). Metaperiodate pretreatment alone gave 20 particles/μm^2 Retrieval alone (using various media) gave: citrate, 64 particles/μm^2; water, 84 particles per/μm^2; metaperiodate, 65 particles/μm^2
Brorson, 1998 (12)	Kidney (human and pig) 4% paraformaldehyde, 1% glutaraldehyde mixture	Epoxy resin: LX-112 Acrylic resin: LR White No pretreatment	*Retrieval medium:* • 0.01 mol/L citrate buffer pH 6.0 *Heating:* PCR machine • Heat at 95°C for 15 min	Fibrin IgG	Labeling of both epitopes improved by retrieval (epoxy and LR White resin). Labeling on retrieved high-accelerator epoxy sections was greater than that on nonretrieved LR White sections.
Brorson, 1999 (13)	Kidney (pig) 4% paraformaldehyde, 1% glutaraldehyde mixture Tissue in epoxy resin postfixed: 1% osmium tetroxide	Epoxy resin: LX-112 Acrylic resin: LR White Pretreatment Yes/no Sections of osmicated tissue in epoxy resin	*Retrieval medium:* • 0.01 mol/L citrate buffer, pH 6.0 *Heating:* PCR machine • Heat at 95°C for 15 min	IgG	Untreated LR White sections had highest label density. Using epoxy resin, label density on retrieved sections of nonosmicated tissue increased with accelerator concentration (highest density was 70% of LRW sections). Label density on sections of retrieved nonosmicated tissue in epoxy resin was greater than

Table 1. Examples of IEM Protocols Utilizing Heat-Induced Antigen Retrieval (continued)

Reference	Tissue and fixation	Resin-section pretreatment	Retrieval protocol	Epitope	Comments
		treated with saturated aqueous sodium ometaperiodate for 6 min at room temperature			that on sections of retrieved osmicated tissue treated with metaperiodate. Recommendation is to use unosmicated tissue embedded in epoxy resin with moderately increased accelerator concentration, combined with citrate retrieval.
Wilson et al., 1996 (77)	Rat tissue Human oral mucosa LR White tissue: 0.25% glutaraldehyde, 0.15% picric acid mixture Epoxy resin tissue: 2.5% glutaraldehyde, 2% osmium tetroxide	Epoxy resin: TAAB Acrylic resin: LR White No pretreatment	*Retrieval medium:* • 0.01 mol/L citrate buffer, pH 6.0 *Heating:* Microwave (700 W) • Heat for 5 min to reach 70°–80°C at end of incubation	Human and rat: Pan cytokeratin Collagen type I Collagen type III Collagen type IV Collagen type VI Laminin	In LR White sections: Labeling of human pan cytokeratin collagen types III, IV, and VI all significantly improved over nonretrieved sections. In TAAB resin sections: Labeling of human collagen type IV significantly improved over non-retrieved sections.
Leong and Sormunen, 1998 (37)	Breast carcinoma Fixation not stated	Acrylic resin: LR White No pretreatment	*Retrieval medium:* • 0.01 mol/L citrate buffer, pH 6.0 *Heating:* Microwave • Heat as 85°–90°C for 5 min • Cool on retrieval medium for 20 min	Vimentin Cytokeratin Type IV collagen β-catenin IgA IgG	Conjoint LM study Labeling of all epitopes reported as enhanced by retrieval.

Table 1. Examples of IEM Protocols Utilizing Heat-Induced Antigen Retrieval (continued)

Reference	Tissue and fixation	Resin-section pretreatment	Retrieval protocol	Epitope	Comments
Sormunen and Leong, 1998 (63)	Breast carcinoma Kidney 4% paraformaldehyde, 0.05% glutaraldehyde mixture	Acrylic resin: LR White No pretreatment	*Retrieval medium:* • 0.01 mol/L citrate buffer, pH 6.0 *Heating:* Two heating protocols Microwave 1. Heat at 90°C for 5 min • Cool on retrieval medium for 20 min 2. Heat retrieval medium until boiling, then simmer for 2 min • Cool on retrieval medium for 20 min	Vimentin Cytokeratin Type IV collagen β-catenin IgA IgG	Conjoint LM study Vimentin, cytokeratin, type IV collagen, and β-catenin labeling all enhanced by retrieval. Labeling of IgA and IgG similar to non-retrieved sections.
Xiao et al., 1996 (78)	Normal Human liver Hepatocellular carcinoma Hepatoblastoma: 3% paraformaldehyde, 0.1% glutaraldehyde mixture	Resin: Lowicryl K4M (low temperature embedding) No pretreatment	Four heating protocols with each of four media *Retrieval media:* 1. 0.01 mol/L citrate buffer, pH6.0 2. 0.01 mol/L citrate buffer, pH 8.0 3. 0.01 mol/L EDTA, pH 8.0 4. 0.001 mol/L EDTA, pH 8.0 *Heating:* 1. Microwave (700 W) • 3 cycles of heating at 100°C, each of 5 min 2. Autoclave • Heat at 120°C for 10 min 3. Pressure cooker	Cytokeratin 18 (CK 18)	Study comparing various retrieval protocols and enzyme treatment. No difference found in efficiency of heating methods. 0.01 mol/L EDTA, pH 8.0, and 0.01 mol/L citrate buffer, pH 6.0 gave best results. Enzyme treatment (pronase) ineffective. Pressurized boiling produced ultrastructural damage with increasing time.

Table 1. Examples of IEM Protocols Utilizing Heat-Induced Antigen Retrieval (continued)

Reference	Tissue and fixation	Resin-section pretreatment	Retrieval protocol	Epitope	Comments
			• Heat at 120°C for 1, 2, or 5 min 4. Simple boiling • Heat at 100°C for 15 min All treatments: After heating, grids allowed to cool at room temperature for 20–30 min		
Chicoine and Webster, 1998 (20)	Pancreas Cultured J774 Cells	Cryosections (sucrose-infiltrated tissue)	*Retrieval medium:* None (dry heat)	Amylase Ia MHC class II	Only amylase labeling in pancreas improved by retrieval.
	4% formaldehyde, ± 0.5% glutaraldehyde postfixation	No pretreatment	*Heating:* Microwave Heat at 25°C for 0, 2, 4, 6, and 10 min	Dinitrophenol (DNP)	Optimal incubation times were 2 min and 10 min for formalin-fixed tissue, 6 min for glutaraldehyde-postfixed tissue.
Röecken and Roessner, 1999 (55)	Various tissues containing amyloid	Epoxy resin: Epon	Single heating protocol using three media *Retrieval media:* 1. water	AA amyloid ATTR amyloid Aκ amyloid	Comparative study testing pretreatment protocols and antigen retrieval, alone and combined. The best methods were: AA amyloid: Retrieval with EDTA alone; metaperiodate pretreatment followed by retrieval with EDTA. ATTR amyloid: Retrieval with EDTA alone; H_2O_2 or metaperiodate pretreatment followed by retrieval with EDTA. Pretreated specimens had high background. Aκ amyloid: Retrieval with EDTA alone; metaperiodate pretreatment followed by retrieval with EDTA.
	Combinations of formalin and glutaraldehyde +2% osmium tetroxide with 3% aqueous- and 1% ethanolic uranyl acetate (en-bloc) post-fixation	Pretreatment: Yes/no, two media used 1. 3% H_2O_2 for 10 min 2. saturate aqueous sodium metaperiodate for 60 min at room temperature	2. 0.01 mol/L citrate buffer, pH 6.0 3. 0.001 mol/L EDTA, pH 8.0 *Heating:* Hot plate with hot water bath • Heat at 91°C for 30 min		

Table 2. Examples of LM Protocols Utilizing Plastic-Embedded Tissue

Reference	Tissue and fixation	Resin-section pretreatment	Retrieval protocol	Epitope	Comments
Blythe et al., 1998 (9)	Bone marrow trephine biopsies (undecalcified) 10% formalin	Methyl methacrylate Pretreatment: Xylene at 37°C for 20 min	*Retrieval medium:* 0.01 mol/L citrate buffer pH 6.0 *Heating:* Microwave (800 W) • Heat for 8 min • Cool for 5 min • Heat for 3 min • Cold wash	Panel of 47 epitopes to screen for hematologic malignancies	Trypsinization followed by retrieval best for some epitopes. Tissues fixed in other formalin-based fixatives gave similar results and were compatible with retrieval (see Hand et al., 1996 below).
Hand et al., 1996 (26)	Normal and pathologic human tissue, including skin, kidney, lymph node, uterus, breast, and bone marrow 10% formalin 10% formal saline 10% formal calcium	Methyl methacrylate Pretreatment: Xylene at 37°C, two changes, each of 10 min	*Retrieval medium:* 0.01 mol/L citrate buffer, pH 6.0 *Heating:* Microwave Two heating protocols 1. Microwave (700 and 800 W) • Heat for 8 min • Cool for 5 min • Heat for 5 min • Cool for 20 min • Wash in cold water 2. Microwave (450, 650, and 700 W) • Heat for 20 min • Wash in cold water	Panel of 27 epitopes	Retrieval improved labeling of all epitopes. Results depend on time elapsed since tissue embedded (retrieval required for older blocks rather than trypsinzation alone). Results comparable using all fixatives and either heating protocol. Trypinzation followed by retrieval best for some epitopes.

Table 2. Examples of LM Protocols Utilizing Plastic-Embedded Tissue (Continued)

Reference	Tissue and fixation	Resin-section pretreatment	Retrieval protocol	Epitope	Comments
Suurmeijer and Boon, 1993 (71) Boon and Kok, 1994 (10)	Specific tissue not stated Formalin Kryofix	Glycol methacrylate No pretreatment	*Retrieval medium:* 0.01 mol/L citrate buffer, pH 6.0 *Heating:* Microwave • 3 cycles of boiling, each of 10 min	Vimentin MIB-1 Keratin	Retrieved sections were positive, but alternative trypsin treatment gave negative results. Diluting antibodies in Triton® X-100 improved MIB-1 labeling
Leong and Sormunen, 1998 (37)	Breast carcinoma Fixation not stated	Acrylic resin: LR White No pretreatment	*Retrieval medium:* • 0.01 mol/L citrate buffer, pH 6.0 *Heating:* Microwave (750 W) • Bring to boil, then simmer for 10 min • Cool in buffer for 20 min	Vimentin Cytokeratin Smooth muscle actin Type IV collagen Laminin β-catenin IgA IgG	Labeling of all epitopes improved by retrieval.
Sormunen and Leong, 1998 (63)	Breast carcinoma Kidney 4% paraformaldehyde, 0.05% glutaraldehyde mixture	Acrylic resin: LR White No pretreatment	*Retrieval medium:* • 0.01 mol/L citrate buffer, pH 6.0 *Heating:* Microwave • Heat for 5 min	Vimentin Cytokeratin Type IV collagen β-catenin IgA IgG	Immunogold labeling with silver enhancement. Labeling of all epitopes improved by retrieval except IgA and IgG, which showed no improvement.

Table 2. Examples of LM Protocols Utilizing Plastic-Embedded Tissue (Continued)

Reference	Tissue and fixation	Resin-section pretreatment	Retrieval protocol	Epitope	Comments
Krenács and Rosendaal, 1998 (36)	Bone marrow 4% paraformaldehyde	Epoxy resin: Araldite Durcupan Pretreatment: Sodium ethoxide for 8–12 min	*Retrieval medium:* 0.01 mol/L citrate buffer, pH 6.0 *Heating:* Microwave (850 W) • Heat for 20 min	Connexin43 Collagen III CD34	Retrieval gave good results. Connexin43 labeled using combined trypsinization and retrieval. Some sections also double-labeled after combined treatment.
McCluggage . et al., 1995 (40)	Bone marrow trephine biopsies 10% neutral buffered formalin	Epoxy resin: Polarbed 812 Pretreatment: Sodium ethoxide for 25 min	*Retrieval medium:* 0.01 mol/L citrate buffer, pH 6.0 *Heating:* Microwave (850 W) • Heat for 30 min • Allow to cool at room temperature	Panel of 22 epitopes to screen for bone marrow disorders.	Good-quality labeling with all epitopes except CD61 and neutrophil elastase. Morphology better than wax sections.
Barou et al., 1997 (2)	Trabecular bone 70% ethanol	Epoxy resin: Embed 812 Pretreatment: Sodium ethoxide (various concentrations and incubation times)	*Retrieval medium:* 0.1 mol/L citrate buffer, pH 6.0 *Heating:* Microwave (700 W) • Heat for 5 min	BrdU	Retrieval caused shrinkage and damage to sections. No improvement over BrdU labeling

localization of estrogen and progesterone receptors was comparable to pressure cooking for 90 seconds in citric acid (0.1 mol/L, pH 6.0). Furthermore, tissue morphology was improved (52). This approach has not been utilized for IEM but may be appropriate for some specimens.

Retrieval Media

A wide variety of retrieval media (including commercial products) have been utilized or tested in LM studies, and their effectiveness is frequently epitope dependent. A range of buffers have been tested in comparative trials, and a number are in common use (Table 3) (3,17,18,23,57,59). Original media based on lead compounds are no longer recommended for safety reasons (57,60).

Media utilized in IEM studies include the following: water (55,70), citrate buffer (12,13,37,55,63,70,78), sodium metaperiodate (70), and EDTA (53,55,78) (Table 1). Dry microwave heating has also been utilized with variable results (Table 1) (20). In an IEM study of IgG crystalloids in formalin-fixed, post-osmicated tissue embedded in epoxy resin, heating with water was slightly more effective than using citrate retrieval medium. Heating with either citrate or water was considerably better than deosmication using metaperiodate alone. However, the highest probe densities were obtained when thin sections were pretreated with sodium metaperiodate followed by heat-induced AR using citrate (Table 1) (70). In a study using paraformaldehyde–glutaraldehyde-fixed tissue (no osmication) embedded in Lowicryl K4M, there was no difference between citrate buffer and EDTA retrieval medium (Table 1) (78). In contrast, EDTA was superior to citrate when applied to amyloid deposits (55).

In summary, citrate buffer (0.01 mol/L, pH 6.0; see protocol described below) is consistently reliable and a popular retrieval medium for all applications (LM, resin sections, and IEM; Tables 1 and 2). However, no single universal medium has been found, and media other than citrate should be considered (Table 3), particularly EDTA, which is superior to citrate for some epitopes (55). Commercial media may also be applicable. The conditions required to maximize retrieval can be established using a test battery, as recommended for LM (57–59,74). The test battery is used to select an appropriate retrieval medium and define the variables of heating method, temperature, time, pH, and molarity. High-temperature heating is the most important factor, and the pH value of the medium is also critical. Three levels of heating time and pH (pH 1.0 to 2.0, pH 7.0 to 8.0, and pH 10.0 to 11.0) are recommended (57,58). Retrieval media containing metal salts are not recommended if the gold probe is subsequently silver enhanced because of the danger of causing nonspecific silver deposition (75). Urea may not be suitable for high-temperature heating because it breaks down if heated above 100°C (74).

PROTOCOLS

Basic Unmasking and Retrieval Methods

The following methods are basic protocols for unmasking (deosmication and etching) and heat-induced AR (70). The protocols may be modified as required. Unmasking and retrieval can be used singly or combined, the choice depending on the relative probe densities achieved. Unmasking using sodium metaperiodate is recommended for osmi-

Table 3. Media in Common Use for High-Temperature Antigen Retrieval

Retrieval medium	Summary information and citations
Citrate buffer	• An aqueous solution of sodium citrate, 0.01 mol/L adjusted to pH 6.0 with HCl. Used widely (16–18,70) • 0.01 mol/L sodium citrate (pH 6.0) gave equal, or better, results when compared with enzyme treatment (23) • Also effective at 0.1 mol/L (pH 6.0) (3,56,73)
Sodium acetate	• Evaluated using test battery. Recommended as suitable for most antigens using 0.01 mol/L solution at pH 8.0–9.0 (59) • Evaluated using test battery. Recommended as best medium for retinoblastoma protein (pRB) using 0.01 mol/L solution at pH 1.0–2.0 (58)
Sodium bicarbonate buffer	• 0.01 mol/L (pH 6.0) solution superior to citrate when applied to tissue fixed in acidic fixatives (Bouin's, etc.) (18) • 0.01 mol/L (pH 6.0) solution one of best media tested (17) • Background increased when 0.01 mol/L solution used at pH 7.8 (23)
Sodium carbonate buffer	• 0.01 mol/L (pH 6.0) solution one of best media tested (17) • 0.0015 mol/L solution effective at pH 8.0 (42)
Tris base, pH 10.0	• 0.5 mol/L (pH 10.0) solution one of best with difficult epitopes. More effective with more antigens than 3 mol/L urea or 0.1 mol/L citrate (pH 6.0) (3)
Tris-HCl	• 0.05 mol/L Tris buffer (pH 7.49 and pH 7.2) not as effective as citrate (3,23) • Evaluated using test battery. Better results at high pH than other media. Recommended as suitable for most antigens using 0.01 mol/L solution at pH 8.0–9.0 (59)
Tris-HCl with urea	• Make 0.1 mol/L Tris-HCl buffer (pH 10.0), add 5% urea, and adjust to pH 9.5 (74) • Effective for a wide range of epitopes (74) • Urea unstable above 100°C (74)
Urea	• Comparable to citrate and $AlCl_4$ when used at 0.01 mol/L and 0.8 mol/L (18) • Unmasks additional epitopes when used at 4–6 mol/L (17,18) • At 0.01 mol/L and 6 mol/L, one of best media tested (17) • 3 mol/L solution one of best media tested. Leaves white deposit on any surface where it dries (3) • 5% solution not as good as 0.1 mol/L citrate or glycine-HCl (73) • 5% solution similar to 0.1 M citrate (61)
EDTA-NaOH	• EDTA- and EGTA-NaOH (0.01–0.001 mol/L, pH 8.0) better than citrate (0.01 mol/L, pH 6.0 and 8.0) (42,53,55)
Aluminium chloride	• Comparable to citrate when used at 0.3 mol/L (18) • Reveals additional epitopes to citrate (18) • Some antigens detected best with 0.01 mol/L $AlCl_4$ and three boiling cycles (18) • 0.01 mol/L solution almost as effective as citrate (17) • 4% (0.3 mol/L) solution similar to 6 mol/L urea in selected cases (17) • 4% solution recommended for vimentin (72) • Possibly not suitable if retrieval used in conjunction with silver enhancement (75)

cated tissues. In some cases, sodium metaperiodate treatment alone may be sufficiently effective, but it is possible that subsequent heat-induced retrieval may increase probe levels considerably (70). Resin unmasking using an etching treatment may reduce physical masking on epoxy sections but is also liable to cause section damage. Combining sodium metaperiodate treatment with etching is not generally recommended.

Section Collection and Incubation Technique

Collect sections on coated (e.g., Formvar or Butvar) nickel grids or, alternatively, on uncoated grids, if both sides of the section are to be labeled (double-sided labeling). The compatibility of grid coating agents and embedding resins with solvents and other reagents (e.g., alcoholic stains and sodium ethoxide) should be established prior to use. Sections must be robust and should be cut slightly thicker than for routine ultrastructural studies (straw to gold interference color: 80–100 nm). Sections are incubated by floating the grids face-down on the relevant solution (i.e., the sections in full contact with the fluid). For double-sided labeling, sections must be fully immersed. All drops of reagent for incubation must be placed on a clean surface.

Protocol for Sodium Metaperiodate Unmasking: Deosmication

Materials and Reagents

- A saturated aqueous solution of sodium metaperiodate (sodium periodate; sodium m-periodate, $NaIO_4$).
- A humid incubation chamber. Use a closed container (such as a 9-cm Petri dish) with a large drop of water to reduce the evaporation of the sodium metaperiodate solution.
- Distilled or deionized water.

Procedure

1. Incubate the grids for 1 hour (at room temperature) in a humid chamber on large drops of a saturated aqueous solution of sodium metaperiodate.
2. Wash the grids thoroughly in distilled or deionized water.
3. Proceed to heat-induced AR or immunolabeling.

Protocol for Sodium Ethoxide Etching to Reduce Physical Masking by Epoxy Resin

Materials and Reagents

- A solution of approximately 10% sodium ethoxide. The sodium ethoxide stock reagent is a saturated solution of sodium hydroxide in anhydrous ethanol. The solution is usually allowed to mature for a day (or more) before use and becomes more effective with time. The stock reagent is diluted to the concentration required with anhydrous ethanol. Sodium methoxide can be substituted for sodium ethoxide and is made similarly using sodium hydroxide and anhydrous methanol. *CARE*: These solutions are flammable and caustic. Avoid skin contact. Store in polyethylene or polypropylene containers; avoid glass.

• An incubation chamber. Use a closed container (such as a 9-cm plastic Petri dish—avoid glass) with a large drop of alcohol to reduce the evaporation of the sodium ethoxide solution.
• Distilled or deionized water.

Procedure

1. Incubate the grids for approximately 2 minutes (at room temperature) on large drops of approximately 10% sodium ethoxide.
2. Wash grids carefully and thoroughly in distilled or deionized water.
3. Proceed to heat-induced AR or immunolabeling.

Note:

• Use coated grids to maintain section integrity and reduce damage.
• The incubation period is determined empirically; adjust the incubation time or reagent concentration to give the desired effect. Excess etching will produce holes, and the sections will contaminate easily during staining and labeling steps.

Protocol for Heat-Induced Antigen Retrieval Using a Hot Plate

Materials and Reagents

• 0.01 mol/L citrate buffer retrieval medium. Dissolve 2.94 g of tri-sodium citrate dihydrate (0.01 mol/L) in water and adjust to pH 6.0 with 0.1 mol/L HCl. Make the volume up to 1.0 L (64). Alternative formulations can be used, and buffer (pH 6.0) based on (A) 0.2 mol/L disodium hydrogen orthophosphate and (B) 0.1 mol/L citric acid (add 63.1 mL of A to 36.9 mL of B) is also effective (62). See Table 3 for additional retrieval media.
• A hot plate set at 95° to 100°C.
• A 50-mL beaker.
• Distilled or deionized water.

Procedure

1. Float the grids on retrieval medium in a 50-mL beaker and incubate at 95° to 100°C on a hot plate for 10 minutes.
2. Remove the beaker from the hot plate and allow the beaker and the grids to cool by leaving them to stand for 15 minutes.
3. Wash the grids thoroughly in distilled or deionized water.
4. Proceed to immunolabeling.

Note:

• Do not allow the retrieval medium to boil vigorously or bubbles to form on the grids during heating. Vigorous boiling may damage the sections, and bubbles will reduce contact with the retrieval medium.
• To avoid excessive evaporation, the beaker of retrieval medium can be preheated to boiling point in a microwave oven before placing it on the hot plate.

• As an alternative to using a hot plate, grids may be incubated on (or in) a beaker of preheated retrieval medium in an oven at 95°C. Microwaving and other heating methods may also be effective—refer to heating methods above.

Immunogold Labeling

After antigen retrieval, sections are labeled using a standard immunogold procedure (24,28,47,68,70). Antibody solutions may require titration to optimize labeling and minimize background. Appropriate antibody and gold probe concentrations can be established using a range of dilutions combined as follows:

1. Incubate grids with the primary antibody. Use a range of dilutions, e.g., 1:10, 1:50, 1:100, 1:200, 1:500, 1:750, 1:1000. Select a range of antibody dilutions to cover the known or expected level of antibody activity. Incubate multiple grids (e.g., four) per dilution. Thus, in this example, seven antibody dilutions requires a total of 28 grids.
2. Incubate grids with the gold probe. Use a range of gold probe dilutions for each antibody dilution. In this example (four grids available at each antibody dilution), gold probe could be used at 1:10, 1:50, 1:75, and 1:100.

The antibody-gold probe concentrations of choice are the lowest dilutions that give the maximum probe density (probe per unit area) with the minimum background. Controls can be omitted during initial trials but must be included when final dilutions are established. Trials can be carried out in stages, as handling large numbers of grids may be difficult.

Controls

It is essential to use adequate controls in conjunction with unmasking and retrieval procedures to ensure that the epitope distribution revealed is genuine (67,68). A serious concern is the creation of nonspecific binding with a restricted distribution that mimics a genuine labeling pattern (false positive labeling). To avoid this situation, and in addition to procedural checks and tests for the presence of contaminating antibodies (e.g., absorption of the antibody with purified antigen), the following controls must be included: (67,68)

1. Omit the primary antibody and incubate with antibody diluent only, followed by gold probe. This control identifies nonspecific binding by the gold probe. If a link antibody is used, this must also be omitted.
2. Substitute the primary antibody with another directed against a different epitope, or with pooled normal, or preimmune, serum. The substituting antibody must be at the same concentration, be derived from the same species, and be the same immunoglobulin class and subclass as the primary antibody. This control identifies nonspecific binding by the primary antibody.

If a multistep procedure with a link antibody is used and control 2 (above) is positive, nonspecific binding by the link antibody can be identified by omitting the primary antibody (incubate with antibody diluent only) and then incubating with the link antibody (or antibodies), followed by the gold probe.

LABELING NEW EPITOPES: EXPERIMENTAL STRATEGY

First, it must be re-emphasized that, to label an epitope with optimal sensitivity, consideration must be given to specimen preparation. Second, it may be difficult to choose a retrieval strategy, because no single ideal method has been established, and published results are often variable. Presumably, this variability is a reflection of how appropriate the technique was for the epitope in question and whether the retrieval conditions were fully optimized.

The basic heat-induced AR protocol described above may produce a positive result. However, the optimal method that maximizes immunoreactivity (thus reducing the possibility of a false negative) should be established using the experimental test battery concept. Ultimately, provided that heating has been optimized in relation to time and temperature, the method of heating will, in most cases, be a matter of practicality and convenience. Finally, additional strategies to consider include combining heat-induced AR with other methods such as the unmasking of hidden epitopes prior to embedding, enzyme treatment of sections, deosmication, and resin unmasking.

The application of immunogold labeling at the ultrastructural level has greatly expanded our understanding of cell structure and function. Currently, few IEM studies have utilized AR. However, as the technique evolves and the benefits are realized, AR, and heat-induced retrieval in particular, will allow us to push the frontier of our knowledge forward.

REFERENCES

1. **Arbustini, E., P. Morbini, L. Verga, M. Concardi, E. Porcu, A. Pilotto, I. Zorzoli, P. Garini, E. Anesi, and G. Merlini.** 1997. Light and electron microscopy immunohistochemical characterisation of amyloid deposits. Int. J. Exp. Clin. Invest. *4*:157-170.

2. **Barou, O., N. Laroche, S. Palle, C. Alexandre, and M.-H. Lafage-Proust.** 1997. Pre-osteoblastic proliferation assessed with BrdU in undecalcified, epon-embedded adult rat trabecular bone. J. Histochem. Cytochem. *45*:1189-1195.

3. **Beckstead, J.H.** 1994. Improved AR in formalin-fixed, paraffin-embedded tissues. Appl. Immunocytochem. *2*:274-281.

4. **Beesley, J.E.** 1989. Colloidal Gold: A New Perspective for Cytochemical Marking. Royal Microscopical Society Microscopy Handbook 17. Oxford University Press, The Royal Microscopical Society, Oxford.

5. **Bendayan, M.** 1995. Colloidal gold post-embedding immunocytochemistry. Prog. Histochem. Cytochem. *29*:1-159.

6. **Bendayan, M. and M.-A. Duhr.** 1986. Modification of the protein-A gold immunocytochemical technique for the enhancement of its efficiency. J. Histochem. Cytochem. *34*:569-575.

7. **Bendayan, M., A. Nanci, and F.W.K. Kan.** 1987. Effect of tissue processing on colloidal gold cytochemistry. J. Histochem. Cytochem. *35*:983-996.

8. **Bendayan, M. and M. Zollinger.** 1983. Ultrastructural localization of antigenic sites on osmium-fixed tissues applying the protein A-gold technique. J. Histochem. Cytochem. *31*:101-109.

9. **Blythe, D., N.M. Hand, P. Jackson, R.D. Bradbury, and A.S. Jack.** 1997. Use of methyl methacrylate resin for embedding bone marrow trephine biopsy specimens. J. Clin. Pathol. *50*:45-49.

10. **Boon, M.E. and L.P. Kok.** 1994. Microwaves for Immunohistochemistry. Micron *25*:151-170.

11. **Brorson, S.-H.** 1998. Antigen detection on resin sections and methods for improving the immunogold labeling by manipulating the resin. Histol. Histopathol. *13*:275-281.

12. **Brorson, S.-H.** 1998. The combination of high-accelerator epoxy resin and AR to obtain more intense immunogold labeling on epoxy sections than on LR-white sections for large proteins. Micron *29*:89-95.

13. **Brorson, S.-H.** 1999. AR on epoxy sections based on tissue infiltration with moderately increased amount of accelerator to detect immune complex deposits in glomerular tissue. Histol. Histopathol. *14*:151-155.

14. **Brorson, S.-H., I. Halvorsen, L.-C. Lønning, G. Slaattun, M. Sletten, and S. Rashid.** 1999. Increased yield of immunogold labeling of epoxy sections by adding *para*-phenylendiamine in the tissue processing. Micron *30*:561-566.

15. **Casanova, S., U. Donini, N. Zini, R. Morelli, and P. Zuchelli.** 1983. Immunohistochemical staining on hydroxyethyl-methacrylate-embedded tissues. J. Histochem. Cytochem. *31*:1000-1004.

16. **Cattoretti, G., M.H.G. Becker, G. Key, M. Duchrow, C. Schlüter, J. Galle, and J. Gerdes.** 1992. Monoclonal antibodies against recombinant parts of the Ki-67 antigen (MIB 1 and MIB 3) detect proliferating cells in microwave-processed formalin-fixed paraffin sections. J. Pathol. *168*:357-363.

17. **Cattoretti, G., S. Pileri, C. Parravicini, M.H.G. Becker, S. Poggi, C. Bifulco, G. Key, L. D'Amato, E. Sabat-**

tini, E. Feudale, et al. 1993. Antigen unmasking on formalin-fixed, paraffin-embedded tissue sections. J. Pathol. *171*:83-98.

18.**Cattoretti, G. and A.J.H. Suurmeijer.** 1995. Antigen unmasking on formalin-fixed paraffin-embedded tissues using microwaves: a review. Adv. Anat. Pathol. 2:2-9.

19.**Causton, B.E.** 1984. The choice of resins for electron immunocytochemistry, p. 29-36. *In* J.M. Polak and I.M. Varndell (Eds.), Immunolabelling for Electron Microscopy, Ch. 3. Elsevier Science Publishers, Amsterdam.

20.**Chicoine, L. and P. Webster.** 1998. Effect of microwave irradiation on antibody labeling efficiency when applied to ultrathin cryosections through fixed biological material. Microsc. Res. Tech. *42*:24-32.

21.**Doerr-Schott, J.** 1989. Colloidal gold for multiple staining, p. 145-190. *In* M.A. Hayat (Ed.), Colloidal Gold. Principles, Methods, and Applications, Vol. 1. Academic Press, San Diego.

22.**Faulk, W.P. and G.M. Taylor.** 1971. An immunocolloid method for the electron microscope. Immunochemistry 8:1081-1083.

23.**Gown, A.M., N. de Wever, and H. Battifora.** 1993. Microwave-based antigenic unmasking: a revolutionary new technique for routine immunohistochemistry. Appl. Immunohistochem. *1*:256-266.

24.**Griffiths, G.** 1993. Fine Structure Immunocytochemistry. Springer-Verlag, Berlin.

25.**Guhl, B., M. Ziak, and J. Roth.** 1998. Unconventional antigen retrieval for carbohydrate and protein antigens. Histochem. Cell Biol. *110*:603-611.

26.**Hand, N.M., D. Blythe, and P. Jackson.** 1996. Antigen unmasking using microwave heating on formalin-fixed tissue embedded in methyl methacrylate. J. Cell. Pathol. *1*:31-37.

27.**Hausen, P. and C. Dreyer.** 1982. Urea reactivates antigens in paraffin sections for immunofluorescent staining. Stain Technol. *57*:321-324.

28.**Hayat, M.A. (Ed.).** 1989-1991. Colloidal Gold: Principles, Methods, and Applications. Vols. 1-3. Academic Press, San Diego.

29.**Hayat, M.A. (Ed.).** 1995. Immunogold-Silver Staining: Principles, Methods, and Applications. CRC Press, Boca Raton.

30.**Hulette, C.M., B.T. Downey, and P.C. Burger.** 1992. Macrophage markers in diagnostic neuropathology. Am. J. Surg. Pathol. *16*:493-499.

31.**Humbel, B.M., M.D.M. De Jong, W.H. Müller, and A.J. Verkleij.** 1998. Pre-embedding immunolabeling for electron microscopy: an evaluation of permeabilisation methods and markers. Microsc. Res. Tech. *42*:43-58.

32.**Ishida-Yamamoto, A., H. Tanaka, H. Nakane, H. Takahashi, and H. Iizuka.** 1999. Antigen retrieval of loricrin epitopes at desmosomal areas of cornified cell envelopes: an immunoelectron microscopic analysis. Exp. Dermatol. *8*:402-406.

33.**Jamur, M.C., C.D. Faraco, L.O. Lunardi, R.P. Siraganian, and C. Oliver.** 1995. Microwave fixation improves antigenicity of glutaraldehyde-sensitive antigens while preserving ultrastructural detail. J. Histochem. Cytochem. *43*:307-311.

34.**Kitamoto, T., K. Ogomori, J. Tateishi, and S.B. Prusiner.** 1987. Formic acid pretreatment enhances immunostaining of cerebral and systemic amyloidosis. Lab. Invest. *57*:230-236.

35.**Krenács, L., L. Tiszalvicz, T. Krenács, and L. Boumsell.** 1993. Immunohistochemical detection of CD1A antigen in formalin-fixed and paraffin-embedded tissue sections with monoclonal antibody 010. J. Pathol. *171*:99-104.

36.**Krenács, T. and M. Rosendaal.** 1998. Connexin43 gap junctions in normal, regenerating, and cultured mouse bone marrow and in human leukemias: their possible involvement in blood formation. Amer. J. Pathol. *152*:993-1004.

37.**Leong, A.S.-Y. and R.T. Sormunen.** 1998. Microwave procedures for electron microscopy and resin-embedded sections. Micron *29*:397-409.

38.**Login, G.R., T.-C. Ku, and A.M. Dvorak.** 1995. Rapid primary microwave-aldehyde and microwave-osmium fixation: improved detection of rat parotid acinar cell secretory granule α-amylase using a postembedding immunogold ultrastructural morphometric analysis. J. Histochem. Cytochem. *43*:515-523.

39.**Mayer, G. and M. Bendayan.** 1997. Biotinyl-tyramide: a novel approach for electron microscopic immunocytochemistry. J. Histochem. Cytochem. *45*:1449-1454.

40.**McCluggage, W.G., S. Roddy, C. Whiteside, J. Burton, H. McBride, P. Maxwell, and H. Bharucha.** 1995. Immunohistochemical staining of plastic-embedded bone marrow trephine biopsy specimens after microwave heating. J. Clin. Pathol. *48*:840-844.

41.**Mighell, A.J., P.A. Robinson, and W.J. Hume.** 1995. Patterns of immunoreactivity to an anti-fibronectin polyclonal antibody in formalin-fixed, paraffin-embedded oral tissues are dependant on methods of antigen retrieval. J. Histochem. Cytochem. *43*:1107-1114.

42.**Morgan, J.M., H. Navabi, K.W. Schmid, and B. Jasani.** 1994. Possible role of tissue-bound calcium ions in citrate-mediated high-temperature antigen retrieval. J. Pathol. *174*:301-307.

43.**Morris, R.E., G.M. Ciraolo, and C.B. Saelinger.** 1991. Gold enhancement of gold-labeled probes: gold-intensified staining technique (GIST). J. Histochem. Cytochem. *39*:1585-1591.

44.**Mukai, M., C. Torikata, H. Iri, J. Hata, M. Naito, and T. Shimoda.** 1992. Immunohistochemical identification of aggregated actin filaments in formalin-fixed, paraffin-embedded sections. I. A study of infantile digital fibromatosis by a new pretreatment. Am. J. Surg. Pathol. *16*:110-115.

111

45.**Munakata, S. and J.B. Hendricks.** 1993. Effect of fixation time and microwave oven heating time on retrieval of the Ki-67 antigen from paraffin-embedded tissue. J. Histochem. Cytochem. *41*:1241-1246.

46.**Nanci, A., M. Mazariegos, and M. Fortin.** 1992. The use of osmicated tissues for lowicryl K4M embedding. J. Histochem. Cytochem. *40*:869-874.

47.**Newman, G.R. and J.A. Hobot.** 1993. Resin Microscopy and On-Section Immunocytochemistry. Springer-Verlag, Berlin.

48.**Newman, G.R. and B. Jasani.** 1984. Post-embedding immunoenzyme techniques, p. 53-70. *In* J.M. Polak and I.M. Varndell (Eds.), Immunolabelling for Electron Microscopy, Ch. 5. Elsevier Science Publishers, Amsterdam.

49.**Newman, G.R., B. Jasani, and E.D. Williams.** 1983. Metal compound intensification of the electron-density of diaminobenzidine. J. Histochem. Cytochem. *31*:1430-1434.

50.**Norton, A.J., S. Jordan, and P. Yeomans.** 1994. Brief, high temperature heat denaturation (pressure cooking): a simple and effective method of antigen retrieval for routinely processed tissues. J. Pathol. *173*:371-379.

51.**Peränen, J., M. Rikkonen, and L. Kääriäinen.** 1993. A method for exposing hidden antigenic sites in paraformaldehyde-fixed cultured cells, applied to initially unreactive antibodies. J. Histochem. Cytochem. *41*:447-454.

52.**Peston, D. and S. Shousha.** 1998. Low temperature heat mediated antigen retrieval for demonstration of oestrogen and progesterone receptors in formalin-fixed paraffin sections. J. Cell Pathol. *3*:91-97.

53.**Pileri, S.A., G. Roncador, C. Ceccarelli, M. Piccioli, A. Briskonatis, E. Sabattini, S. Ascani, D. Santini, P.P. Piccaluga, O. Leone, et al.** 1997. Antigen retrieval techniques in immunohistochemistry: comparison of different methods. J. Pathol. *183*:116-123.

54.**Polak, J.M. and I.M. Varndell (Eds.).** 1984. Immunolabelling for Electron Microscopy. Elsevier Science Publishers, Amsterdam.

55.**Röcken, C. and A. Roessner.** 1999. An evaluation of antigen retrieval procedures for immunoelectron microscopic classification of amyloid deposits. J. Histochem. Cytochem. *47*:1385-1394.

56.**Shi, S.-R., B. Chaiwun, L. Young, R.J. Cote, and C.R. Taylor.** 1993. Antigen retrieval technique utilizing citrate buffer or urea solution for immunohistochemical demonstration of androgen receptor in formalin-fixed paraffin sections. J. Histochem. Cytochem. *41*:1599-1604.

57.**Shi, S.-R., R.J. Cote, and C.R. Taylor.** 1997. Antigen retrieval for immunohistochemistry: past, present, and future. J. Histochem. Cytochem. *45*:327-343.

58.**Shi, S.-R., R.J. Cote, C. Yang, C. Chen, H.-J. Xu, W.F. Benedict, and C.R. Taylor.** 1996. Development of an optimal protocol for antigen retrieval: a 'test battery' approach exemplified with reference to the staining of retinoblastoma protein (pRB) in formalin-fixed paraffin sections. J. Pathol. *179*:347-352.

59.**Shi, S.-R., S.A. Imam, L. Young, R.J. Cote, and C.R. Taylor.** 1995. Antigen retrieval immunocytochemistry under the influence of pH using monoclonal antibodies. J. Histochem. Cytochem. *43*:193-201.

60.**Shi, S.-R., M.E. Key, and K.L. Kalra.** 1991. Antigen retrieval in formalin-fixed, paraffin-embedded tissues: an enhancement method for immunohistological staining based on microwave oven heating of tissue sections. J. Histochem. Cytochem. *39*:741-748.

61.**Shi, S.-R. and Q. Tian.** 1993. Development of an antigen retrieval technique for immunohistochemistry on archival celloidin-embedded sections. J. Histochem. Cytochem. *41*:1121.

62.**Skehel, P.A., R. Fabian-Fine, and E.R. Kandel.** 2000. Mouse VAP33 is associated with the endoplasmic reticulum and microtubules. Proc. Natl. Acad. Sci. USA *97*:1101-1106.

63.**Sormunen, R. and A. S.-Y. Leong.** 1998. Microwave-stimulated antigen retrieval for immunohistology and immunoelectron microscopy of resin-embedded sections. Appl. Immunohistochem. *6*:234-237.

64.**Stirling, J.W.** 1989. Ultrastructural localization of lysozyme in human colon eosinophils using the protein-A gold technique: effects of processing on probe distribution. J. Histochem. Cytochem. *37*:709-714.

65.**Stirling, J.W.** 1990. Immuno- and affinity probes for electron microscopy: a review of labeling and preparation techniques. J. Histochem. Cytochem. *38*:145-157.

66.**Stirling, J.W.** 1992. Unfixed tissue for electron immunocytochemistry: a simple preparation method for colloidal gold localization of sensitive epitopes using ethanediol dehydration. Histochem. J. *24*:190-206.

67.**Stirling, J.W.** 1993. Controls for immunogold labeling. J. Histochem. Cytochem. *41*:1869-1870.

68.**Stirling, J.W.** 1995. Immunogold labelling: resin sections, p. 9.3-1–9.3-21. *In* A.E.Woods and R.C. Ellis (Eds.), Laboratory Histopathology: A Complete Reference. Electron Microscopy (Section 9), Chapter 3. Churchill Livingstone, Edinburgh.

69.**Stirling, J.W., M. Coleman, and J. Brennan.** 1990. The use of inert dehydration and glycol methacrylate embedding for immunogold localization of glomerular basement membrane components. Lab. Invest. *62*:655-663.

70.**Stirling, J.W. and P. Graff.** 1995. Antigen unmasking for immuno-electron microscopy: labeling is improved by treating with sodium ethoxide or sodium metaperiodate then heating on retrieval medium. J. Histochem. Cytochem. *43*:115-123.

71.**Suurmeijer, A.J.H. and M.E. Boon.** 1993. Notes on the application of microwaves for antigen retrieval in paraffin and plastic tissue sections. Eur. J. Morphol. *31*:144-150.

72.**Suurmeijer, A.J.H. and M.E. Boon.** 1993. Optimising keratin and vimentin retrieval in formalin-fixed, paraffin-embedded tissue with the use of heat and metal salts. Appl. Immunohistochem. *1*:143-148.

73.**Taylor, C.R., S.-R. Shi, B. Chaiwun, L. Young, S.A. Imam, and R.J Cote.** 1994. Strategies for improving the immunohistochemical staining of various intranuclear prognostic markers in formalin-paraffin sections: androgen receptor, estrogen receptor, progesterone receptor, p53 protein, proliferating cell nuclear antigen, and Ki-67 antigen revealed by antigen retrieval techniques. Hum. Pathol. 25:263-270.

74. Taylor, C.R., S.R. Shi, C. Chen, L. Young, C. Yang, and R.J. Cote. 1996. Comparative study of antigen retrieval heating methods: microwave, microwave and pressure cooker, autoclave, and steamer. Biotech. Histochem. 71:263-270.

75. Van de Kant, H.J.G., M.E. Boon, and D.G. de Rooij. 1993. Microwave applications before and during immunogold-silver staining. J. Histotechnol. 16:209-215.

76. Van Goor, H., G. Harms, P.O. Gerrits, F.G.M. Kroese, S. Poppema, and J. Grond. 1988. Immunhistochemical antigen demonstration in plastic-embedded lymphoid tissue. J. Histochem. Cytochem. 36:115-120.

77. Wilson, D.F., D.-J. Jiang, A.M. Pierce, and O.W. Wiebkin. 1996. Antigen retrieval for electron microscopy using a microwave technique for epithelial and basal lamina antigens. Appl. Immunocytochem. 4:66-71.

78. Xiao, J.-C., A. Adam, P. Ruck, and E. Kaiserling. 1996. A comparison of methods for heat-mediated antigen retrieval for immunoelectron microscopy: demonstration of cytokeratin no. 18 in normal and neoplastic hepatocytes. Biotech. Histochem. 71:278-285.

79. Yoshioka, K., A.F. Michael, J. Velosa, and A.J. Fish. 1985. Detection of hidden nephritogenic antigen determinants in human renal and non-renal basement membranes. Am. J. Pathol. 121:156-165.

Target Retrieval for In Situ Hybridization

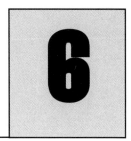

Jiang Gu[1], Reagin Farley[1], Shan-Rong Shi[2], and Clive R. Taylor[2]

[1]Department of Biomedical Sciences, University of South Alabama, Mobile, AL, and [2]Department of Pathology, University of Southern California Keck School of Medicine, Los Angeles, CA, USA

INTRODUCTION

Commonly used formalin fixation frequently masks antigenic epitopes and renders them inaccessible to immunohistochemical detection. Restoration of immunoreactivity can be achieved by pretreatment of the tissue sections. Similar problems exist for DNA or RNA detection during in situ hybridization. A tissue fixation with formalin causes proteins to cross-link and block binding sites not only to antigens for immunohistochemistry, but also to nucleotide sequences for in situ hybridization. Pretreatments must be performed to reveal those target sites. However, for in situ hybridization, the range of targets and probes varies to a greater extent (2), and therefore the optimal pretreatment for each procedure differs. In immunohistochemistry, the most widely accepted antigen retrieval step has been to treat tissue sections in a boiling water or buffer bath, heated either by a microwave oven or by other means. For in situ hybridization, however, the popular pretreatment has been enzyme digestion.

Recent studies tested novel approaches, including a microwave heating pretreatment following the success of heating-assisted antigen retrieval first reported by Shi et al. (27). Several groups reported that microwave pretreatment improves the results of in situ hybridization. An interesting observation is that microwave pretreatment combined with a short enzyme digestion resulted in the strongest signal. The findings did vary with the method and duration of fixation, embedding material, pretreatment

Antigen Retrieval Techniques
Edited by Shan-Rong Shi, Jiang Gu, and Clive R. Taylor
©2000 Eaton Publishing, Natick, MA

buffers, type of tissue, and other variables. The literature includes studies with plastic embedding media and cryostat sections, but most studies utilized the conventional, formalin-fixed, paraffin-embedded tissue sections. Also reported were observations of experiments with varying pretreatment durations, solution times, enzyme varieties and concentrations, and so forth.

In situ hybridization is a method by which a particular sequence of a cell's DNA or its transcript messages are identified in their original locations. The DNA in the nucleus and the RNA in the cytoplasm can be identified on tissue sections with intact morphology. This procedure allows the location of the sequences in the tissue structures to be pinpointed; it was first employed in 1969 and has been gradually popularized. Many variables in the protocols have become more generalized and streamlined.

Compared with immunohistochemistry, in situ hybridization is a more challenging and laborious procedure. Apart from probe preparation and optimization of incubation and washing conditions, tissue pretreatment is a complicating factor. In formalin-fixed tissue sections, DNA and RNA targets are generally not detectable without proper pretreatment of tissue sections. This pretreatment usually entails digestion of the sections with one of a number of enzymes at various concentrations for different durations at a range of temperatures. Enzyme digestion can be a delicate and sometimes tricky step that often calls for individual optimization with each probe and tissue type. There has long been a need for simplified and standardized protocols for tissue pretreatment, which would contribute to an easier and more reproducible procedure for this important technique. This chapter reviews the current literature in this regard and recommends protocols for future applications. The main contributors in this field and their major observations are summarized in Table 1.

PRETREATMENT PROTOCOL FACTORS

Microwave and Enzyme Digestion Combinations

More than half of the literature on pretreatment for in situ hybridization reported that microwave irradiation in combination with a short enzyme digestion was the simplest and most effective step for producing strong, clear, uniform results with low background and good morphology for formalin-fixed, paraffin-embedded tissue sections (1,3,6,12,14,16,17,19–21,29,31). The use of these two different means of exposing nucleotide sequences and aiding probe diffusion was found to be better than prolonged treatment with either one. The postulated effects of microwaving tissue, in combination with the proteolytic action of the protease, seem to produce a cumulative effect on tissue and target sequences that results in a significantly improved in situ hybridization signal detection (24).

Morphology

Enzyme digestion disintegrates proteins, which inevitably compromises the morphology of the tissue section. Because the microwave irradiation does not act to destroy integral cell components, morphology is preserved when it is utilized. Indeed, even when the microwave pretreatment is accompanied by a shortened period of enzyme digestion, the morphology is drastically better than that obtained using enzyme digestion alone for durations sufficient to produce acceptable staining intensity. In their experiments, McMahon and McQuaid (24) observed that, unlike tissue sections that have been overdigested by proteolytic enzymes, there was no evidence of poor morphology in any of the combination-treated sections.

Signal Intensity

Wilkins et al. (31) compared the effects of microwave pretreatment with those of conventional enzymatic digestion on the detection of κ/λ light chain mRNA and obtained the best results when microwave irradiation was followed by a short proteinase K digestion. With the optimized protocol [microwave irradiation (30 min at a power of 900 W) followed by a short proteinase K digestion (10 mg/mL for 2 min)], signal intensity was markedly increased in those cases with duration of fixation longer than 24 hours (31). Sperry et al. (29) investigated the effects of microwave treatment, enzyme digestion, and simple heating in standard saline citrate (SSC) on the detection of RNA and DNA in formalin-fixed, paraffin-embedded tissue sections in an attempt to improve the detecting sensitivity of in situ hybridization. They found that, in contrast to the antigen retrieval methods for immunohistochemistry, in which either microwave treatment or protease digestion may be adequate for optimum results, a combination of microwave treatment with a shortened protease digestion produced the best results. Use of the microwave in conjunction with enzyme digestion increased the number of positive cases detected, strengthened the positive signal, and allowed the detection of nucleotide sequences in cases using a probe concentration low enough to be undetectable when other methods were employed. Sperry et al. (29) found a 10-fold difference in the minimum concentration of albumin probe for which a positive signal could be detected by microwave treatment compared with treating in 2× SSC at 70°C for 30 minutes. Similar results were obtained with CgA and CgB probe cocktail and with the JC probe (29). At the highest probe concentrations, the hybridization signal was stronger in the microwaved specimen compared with the 2 × SSC-treated samples (29). Both signal intensity and number of positive cases among the tumors studied were increased (29).

The order of the elements of the combination does not seem to be important. McMahon and McQuaid (24), also investigating the effectiveness of microwave pretreatment versus enzyme digestion, found that combination pretreatments resulted in the strongest hybridization signals, irrespective of the order in which they were carried out. A marked increase in hybridization signal was observed when protease and microwaving were used in combination compared with the use of either alone (24). Lan et al. (19–21) compared microwave heating during the hybridization step with incubation in a conventional oven and found that a stronger signal was obtained when incubation with the probe was performed in the microwave oven at a power level of 90 W.

Microwave pretreatment has given positive results even in cases for which in situ hybridization without the microwave pretreatment was not successful. Haas et al. (12) used microwave pretreatment in conjunction with enzyme digestion for all tissues on which in situ hybridization did not work with enzyme digestion alone. They found that the procedure was made possible by the microwave pretreatment, although the results were not uniform for all tissues. In addition to investigation of the possible improvements with microwave pretreatment, Haas et al. (12) experimented with various buffer solutions used during microwaving, enzyme digestion, and heating durations. They recommend that the optimal procedure should be determined individually for each tissue even with the use of a microwave oven. It seems that so many vari-

Gu et al.

Table 1. Tissue Pretreatment: Review of the Literature

Reference	Fixative	Tissue		Embedding media	Thickness of sections (µm)	Probe type
		Time before fixation (h)	Fixation duration (h)			
Sibony et al. (28)	4% paraformaldehyde in PBS; Formalin		24 h	Paraffin		cRNA
Church et al. (5)	4% paraformaldehyde in PBS, pH 7.3	6 days	24	Plastic (MMA)	2 4	RNA
Oliver et al. (25)		Immediate fixation	72	Paraffin	6	DNA (oligoprobe)
Tornóczky et al. (30)	Formalin					DNA (oligoprobe)
Lan et al. (19–21)	2% paraformaldehyde-lysine-periodate (PLP)	Immediate or	4	Tissue-Tek OCT compound (cryosections)	6	DNA
Wilkens et al. (31)	10% formalin	Immediate 2, 4, or 6 or unknown	6, 12, 24, 48, or 72 or 7 days or unknown	Paraffin	4	RNA (oligoprobe)
Haas et al. (12)				Paraffin	6	DNA
Sperry et al. (29)	Formalin			Paraffin	5	DNA (oligoprobe)
McMahon and McQuaid (24)	Formalin	Immediate	24	Paraffin	4 6	RNA DNA

ables were involved that a particular buffer/duration/power combination might be preferable for a particular tissue. The authors suggested that their results may facilitate combined in situ hybridization and immunohistochemistry on the same slide. Additionally, in situ hybridization may be used for otherwise unsuitable tissue samples.

Background

Although background reactions were slightly greater in sections subjected to combination pretreatments, this did not reduce signal-to-noise ratio nor cause problems with interpretation in the study conducted by McMahon and McQuaid (24). Lan et al. (19–21), using cryostat sections, found that a single microwave pretreatment of 10 to 20 minutes allowed detection of a strong hybridization signal with very low background in all six tissues examined using a number of different probes. Intensity of the background stain was a factor in evaluating the pretreatments for each study. Microwave usage generally decreased the amount of background staining simply through the reduction of enzyme digestion duration. A prolonged enzyme digestion period disrupts the architecture of the cells, allowing target molecules to migrate away from centers of greater density, thereby increasing the background staining while decreasing signal specificity.

118

Table 1. Tissue Pretreatment: Review of the Literature (Continued)

Reference	Enzyme digestion	Microwave heating	Conventional heating	Other	Buffer	Optimum method
Sibony et al. (28)	Proteinase K 20 µg/mL 20 min	650–700 W 12 min				Microwave pretreatment
Church et al. (5)	Proteinase K 10 mg/mL 37°C 15 min	450 W 20 min		Pressure cooker: 121°C 103 kPa 3 min	Sodium citrate, pH 6.0	Pressure cooker
Oliver et al. (25)	Proteinase K 8 µg/mL 37°C 20, 40, 90 min	800 W 15 min	DEPC-treated H_2O 120 min 90°C	Autoclaving: 130°C 2 bar 40 min	10 mM citrate, pH 6.0	Microwave pretreatment
Tornóczky et al. (30)	Proteinase K 15 µg/mL 20 min	700 W 20 min			0.01 M citrate, pH 6.0	Microwave pretreatment
Lan et al. (19–21)	Proteinase K 5 µg/mL Various durations	900 W Various durations			0.01 M sodium citrate, pH 6.0	MP: 900 W, 2 × 5 min
Wilkens et al. (31)	Proteinase K 10 mg/mL 10–120 min	900 W 5, 30, 60 min		Combination MP + ED: MP: 5, 30, 60 min ED: 1, 2, 5, 10 min	0.01 M citrate, pH 6.0	MP + ED MP: 900 W 30 min ED: 10 mg/mL 2 min
Haas et al. (12)				Combination MP + ED: MP: 700 W 10, 15, 20 min ED: 0.2% protease E 37°C 5–20 min	10 mM citrate, pH 6.0 Enhancer TRS AR-10 Receptor Enhancer Glyca TUF 0.4 M urea in PBS	MP + ED buffer: TRS or Enhancer MP: 700 W 2 × 6.5 min ED: protease E 0.2% 37°C 10 min
Sperry et al. (29)	Proteinase K 25 µg/mL 20 min 37°C	800 W 20 min		Convection heating 2× SSC 30 min 70°C	10 mM citric acid solution, pH 6.0 H_2O SSC PBS TUF	MP + ED, buffer: 10 mM citric acid, pH 6.0 ED: pH 7.2 5 min MP: 800 W 20 Mn
McMahon and McQuaid (24)	Protease VIII 0.5 or 0.1 mg/mL 10 min room temperature	Various power levels 4, 6, 8, 16 min		Combinations	0.01 M urea, pH 6.0, 6 M urea, pH 6.0 0.01 M NaCl, pH 6.0 Distilled H_2O 0.01 M Na^+ citrate, pH 8.2 0.01 M Na^+ citrate, pH 6.0 0.01 M Na_2CO_3, pH 6.0 0.01 M glycine, pH 6.0 0.01 M $MgCl_2$, pH 6.0	MP + ED, buffer: $MgCl_2$ MP: 450 W 2 × 4 min ED: 10 min room temp.

MMA, methylmethacrylate; DEPC, diethyl pyrocarbonate; MP, microwave pretreatment; ED, enzyme digestion; SSC, standard saline citrate; TRS, Target Retrieval Solution; TUF, Target Unmasking Fluid; PBS, phosphate-buffered saline.

Microwaving Alone

Of all the single treatments, microwave heating was generally found to give the best results; it was often found that microwaving alone significantly improved hybridization signals (19–21,25,30,31). Oliver et al. (25) compared microwave pretreatment, enzyme digestion, autoclaving, and simple heating (using a hot plate) in diethyl pyrocarbonate (DEPC)-treated water and found that the most intense signals were produced by the microwave pretreatment for 15 minutes in 10 mmol/L citrate buffer, pH 6.0. Additionally, sections pretreated with microwaving had negligible damage to cell morphology. Tornóczky et al. (30) compared microwave pretreatment with enzyme digestion and found that in the microwave-treated cases the structure of the tissues and the microscopic details were well-preserved, clear cellular outlines could be seen, and strong signal intensity was registered. Microwave pretreatment resulted in better cellular and nuclear details. The signal intensity in the individual cases was moderately stronger or as strong as those treated with proteinase K digestion. Based on these results, the authors recommended microwave pretreatment over enzyme digestion (30). Lan et al. (19–21) using cryostat sections, found that microwave pretreatment produced superior staining. A 10-minute microwave pretreatment step produced no noticeable damage to the fine cell structure or tissue morphology in any tissues examined compared with serial sections without any treatment (19–21) Furthermore, the microwave treatment reduced the minimum incubation time required for the hybridization step; the normal 3-hour period necessary when enzyme digestion is employed was reduced to 20 minutes (19–21). Wilkens et al. (31) reported that microwave pretreatment instead of enzyme digestion significantly enhanced the results of in situ hybridization, particularly with specimens that had been fixed under suboptimal conditions.

Enzyme Digestion Alone

Many studies found the customary enzyme digestion less effective than microwave heating when the two were compared as single pretreatments (19–21,25,30,31). Oliver et al. (25) found that enzyme digestion with proteinase K at 8 µg/mL for 20 minutes was second to microwaving in citrate buffer for 15 minutes as the most effective method in terms of staining intensity, although there was little difference between the two methods in terms of morphology. With the other methods attempted by Oliver et al. (25), autoclaving and heating in DEPC-treated water at 90°C for 120 minutes, the weakest signals were obtained. Although very poor preservation of cell morphology was observed in sections pretreated by autoclaving, when sections were pretreated with heating at 90°C, negligible effects on morphology were seen (25). Tornóczky et al. (30) found that although microwave pretreatment produced strong signal intensity and good preservation of structure and microscopic details, only three of the nine proteinase K digestion-treated cases showed good cellular and nuclear details and were free of overdigestion. In five of the nine cases studied, the cells gave a strong intranuclear signal; in the other four the signal intensity was moderate. Again, although Lan et al. (19–21) used cryostat sections in their studies, their findings agreed. In contrast to the uniform results obtained using the microwave, proteinase K tissue digestion gave variable results in the different tissues and was unable to match the signal strength obtained with microwave pretreatment. The use of prolonged chromagen development times to increase signal strength merely increased background (19–21). Lan et al. also noted the time required for a pretreatment to produce any signal: 1

minute of microwave treatment permitted detection of a very weak signal; however, a minimum of 5 minutes of digestion with proteinase K was required before any hybridization signal could be detected.

Buffers

Several studies examined the effect of different buffers on the outcome of in situ hybridization. These included some new commercial products that have been introduced for use in immunohistochemical procedures. These new buffer solutions were compared with some of the more traditional buffer systems (e.g., 10 mmol/L sodium citrate, pH 6.0) (12,24,29).

There are samples for which adequate hybridization cannot be obtained even with the use of microwave pretreatment. It is thought that the citrate buffer commonly used in these procedures might be partly responsible for the poor quality of results with these tissues (12,13,24,29). To address this concern, Haas et al. (12) tested several recently available buffer systems that have been used for immunohistochemistry with the intention of combining in situ hybridization with immunohistochemistry on the same slides. These authors reported that certain buffers worked in tandem with and actually enhanced the effects of the microwave pretreatment. Of the many buffers tested in this study, Target Retrieval Solution (TRS; DAKO, Carpinteria, CA, USA) and Enhancer (CAMON, Weisbaden, Germany) gave the most promising results. Citrate (10 mmol/L, pH 6.0) and Antigen Retrieval AR-10 Solution (AR-10; Biogenex, San Ramon, CA, USA) were not as good, while all the others examined, including Target Unmasking Fluid (TUF; Dianova, Hamburg, Germany) and 0.4 mol/L urea in phosphate-buffered saline (PBS), gave unacceptable results under the experimental conditions (12). Given a fixed-power output of the microwave oven and a fixed quantity of solutions, the microwave treatment time of 7.5 minutes was optimal for TRS and citrate, whereas treatments of 5 minutes were optimal for Enhancer and AR-10. The use of TRS, Enhancer, and AR-10 combined with a subsequent mild digestion with protease E (0.2% protease E at 37°C for 5–15 min) resulted in high intensity and low background with adequate preservation of morphology even in critical samples (12). Even with the improved technique of combining two pretreatments with an optimal buffer, the best procedure had to be determined individually for each tissue investigated.

Sperry et al. (29) also investigated several buffer solutions. The only commercial product used in this study was TUF. They tested solutions with various pH levels and found that mmol/L citrate buffer, pH 6.0, and water yielded the strongest hybridization signals, while TUF resulted in the weakest signal. SSC and PBS yielded acceptable but not the best results. Regarding the optimal pH level, the use of mmol/L citrate buffer at pH 6.0 resulted in stronger signals compared with pH 1.0 and 10.0 to detect albumin mRNA.

McMahon and McQuaid (24) conducted an additional study in the pursuit of an ideal buffer, comparing nine different solutions, only one of which was a commercial product. They determined that sections of both of their investigated tissue types, microwaved in magnesium chloride contained the highest number of positive cells with moderate staining intensity. Although there were differences in the resulting hybridization signal when using different buffers, it appears that several solutions may be suitable as microwave buffers. Magnesium chloride (0.01 mol/L $MgCl_2$, pH 6.0), urea (0.01 mol/L urea, pH 6.0, and 6 mol/L urea, pH 6.0) and sodium carbonate (0.01 mol/L Na_2CO_3, pH 6.0) all gave similar results in both tissue and probe systems in terms of sensitivity and staining intensity (24).

The studies that examined buffers did not agree on the effectiveness of citrate solution. Haas et al. (12) found several commercial products that were more effective than citrate, but the citrate was not the weakest solution. TUF gave the weakest signals. Sperry et al. (29) found that citrate (and water) gave some of the strongest signals in their study, although they did not examine the same commercial products as Haas et al. (12). They did examine TUF and agreed that it gave weak signals. Had they also used some of the other products, they might have found them superior to citrate. McMahon and McQuaid (24) also examined many noncommercial solutions but found that citrate (at pH 8.2 and pH 6.0) produced very weak signals when compared with other solutions. A magnesium chloride solution was very effective. No other study evaluated magnesium chloride. All studies evaluated citrate at pH 6.0, and Sperry et al. (29) evaluated it at additional pH values as well, only to find that 6.0 was most effective. McMahon and McQuaid (24) and Haas et al. (12) both examined urea. [McMahon and McQuaid used 0.01 mol/L and 6 mol/L urea, both at pH 6.0; Haas et al. (12) used 0.4 mol/L urea in PBS with pH not mentioned.] Haas et al. (12) found that urea gave unacceptable results, while McMahon and McQuaid found it to be suitable at both concentrations.

Other studies (5,19–21,25,30,31) used 10 mmol/L citrate buffer at pH 6.0. Although some buffers used by Haas et al. (12) and McMahon and McQuaid (24) produced better results than citrate, it did prove to be suitable enough for most studies, to the extent that differences could not be observed for the various pretreatments under analysis.

The mode of action of microwave buffer has not been fully elucidated. Although Cattoretti et al. (4a) suggested that salts could modify the hydrophobicity of polypeptide chains and hence affect the protein conformation, this effect has been observed at molarities higher than those used by McMahon and McQuaid (24). Nevertheless, it appears that high temperature is probably the key factor, as a relatively good hybridization signal was obtained using distilled water as a microwave medium (24). In immunohistochemistry, the unveiling of antigenic epitopes by microwave heating was attributed to the breaking of protein cross-links at high temperature. The exact mechanism of the beneficial effects of microwave treatment for in situ hybridization remains to be elucidated, although a similar mechanism seems probable.

Microwave Oven

When discussing microwave treatment, simply stating the duration of irradiation is not adequate. The average energy output of the oven is also determined by the power capacity, the automatic on-and-off cycling time, the humidity, the amount of sample or liquid in the oven, and the position of the samples within the oven (8–11,23). The key factors are the amount of energy received by the tissue section, the duration of heating, and perhaps the speed at which the optimal temperature is reached. For detailed discussion of different types of microwave ovens and the regulation of their power output and energy absorption by tissue samples, please refer to previous publications of the authors (8–11).

Microwave Treatment and Hybridization

Some studies found that use of the microwave during pretreatment (either alone or with enzyme digestion combination) significantly decreased the hybridization duration and probe concentrations necessary to produce a strong signal when compared with those needed when only protease digestion was used (12,19–21,29). Lan et al. (19–21) found that whereas proteinase K digestion required a minimum of 3 hours of hybridization to obtain an optimal signal, sections treated by microwave oven heating gave an optimal signal after as little as 20 minutes of hybridization with a digoxigenin-labeled probe. The comparison was made with incubation in a conventional 42°C convection oven (19–21).

The use of microwave heating at 90 W during the hybridization step further reduced the time required to obtain an optimal signal from tissue already pretreated by microwave heating from 20 to 5 minutes. Haas et al. (12) found that microwave pretreatment with an optimized buffer and adequately fixed samples consumed fewer of the probes and less solution for the detection system. Sperry et al. (29) found that incubation time was decreased significantly when microwave pretreatment was used. The use of microwave treatment reduced the hybridization time for JC virus detection, resulting in a stronger signal after 2 hours of hybridization compared with the usual 20 hours with 2× SSC at 70°C heat treatment (29). The duration of hybridization required for a suitable signal was 10 times shorter when microwave treatment was used, compared with the usual heating with 2× SSC. Sperry et al. (29) also found that while sections that had not undergone microwave pretreatment required 0.01 ng/μL probe concentration, those that had been pretreated in the microwave in 10 mmol/L citrate buffer, pH 6.0, at a power level of 800 W for 20 minutes only required 0.001 ng/μL concentration.

Microwaving also speeds hybridization time by negating the need to calibrate the optimal enzyme concentration and digestion duration needed for each specific tissue (19–21,30,31). Tornóczky et al. (30) pointed out that enzyme digestion requires calibration of enzyme concentrations and time of the digestion. Lan et al. (19–21) found that a simple 10-minute microwave pretreatment proved far more effective than a time-consuming and complicated tissue digestion process involving acid and/or detergent pretreatment, proteinase K digestion, and postfixation. Wilkens et al. (31) stated that the cumbersome testing of single-case adapted proteinase K digestion for in situ hybridization can now be eliminated by microwave pretreatment. Previously, tissue types, length of formalin fixation, and other variables made systematic testing of variable times and/or concentrations of special pretreatment and digestion necessary to obtain optimal results (31).

Formalin Fixation

The mechanism of tissue fixation by formalin is poorly understood but is thought to occur by formation of intermolecular cross-links between protein molecules (14), which allow preservation of morphology. Fixation in formalin produces macromolecular cross-links that immobilize various cell structures. Preservation of RNA and DNA species in tissue embedded in paraffin is usually carried out using cross-linking fixatives, such as formaldehyde (7,19–21,25,26). Cross-linking itself prevents access of probes to the target molecule, and such sections must therefore be treated. Furthermore, formalin does not seem simply to fix the tissue to a particular degree, but rather, the longer a tissue is left in formalin, the greater the degree of fixation. In cases of high degrees of fixation, many more cross-links are formed, and tissue must be treated more aggressively. Additionally, the period of delay prior to fixation seems to have a similar effect of decreasing the sensitivity of a hybridization procedure, probably due to target nucleotide sequence degradation, leakage, and a worsened morphology (18).

The duration of formalin fixation is an important variable that determines the ease of detecting nucleic acids by in situ hybridization. Sperry et al. (29) used microwave treatment to detect JC virus DNA in tissues that had been fixed in formalin for more than 2 years. Whereas these targets were not effectively demonstrated by proteinase K digestion combined with 2× SSC heat treatment at 70°C for 30 minutes, with microwave treatment they obtained positive results.

Wilkens et al. (31) found that a delay of fixation, as well as fixation times exceeding 24 hours, resulted in a considerable decrease in signal intensity when conventional enzymatic pretreatment was performed; after 7 days of formalin fixation, only faint hybridization signals were seen after proteinase K digestion. When an optimized protocol including a combination of microwave irradiation followed by a short proteinase K digestion was performed, signal intensity was dramatically increased. A prolongation of proteinase K digestion for up to 120 minutes also improved signal intensity, but morphology after such extensive enzymatic treatment was seriously impaired. For cases with fixation periods shorter than 24 hours and no delay of fixation, no particular difference was seen between conventional enzymatic pretreatment and microwave pretreatment (31).

In the study conducted by McMahon and McQuaid (24), archival cases of tissue, whose exact fixation history was not known, were subjected to combined protease/microwave pretreatment, and the resulting in situ hybridization signal was compared with sections pretreated with protease alone. The increase in both signal intensity and the number of positive cells following the combined pretreatment was remarkable in all cases (24).

The general finding was that the in situ hybridization signal for tissues that had been fixed for long periods was improved markedly when microwave pretreatment was introduced in addition to traditional enzyme digestion. Although enzyme digestion alone is acceptable for tissues that were fixed under adequate conditions, it proves to be suboptimal when the fixation conditions are not ideal. The addition of microwave heating to the enzyme pretreatment compensates for those conditions. This combination method, in comparison with enzyme digestion alone, significantly increases the signal's intensity, clarity, and specificity without compromising morphology.

Cryostat Sections

Lan et al. (19–21) did not find a comparable additive effect using combinations of microwave oven heating and proteinase K digestion on paraformaldehyde-lysine-periodate (PLP)-fixed cryostat sections. The difference between effective pretreatments when using paraffin-embedded and cryostat sections indicates that the degree of tissue permeability for effective in situ hybridization may depend on the types of fixatives and the methods of tissue processing (19–21). This was the only study to conclude that there was no significant improvement of combinations over one treatment at a time, although the authors recommend that combined pretreatment of tissues with microwave heating and protease digestion be used in examining paraffin-embedded tissues.

Plastic Embedding

Semithin plastic sections are frequently recommended when good tissue morphology and high resolution are required (4). Church et al. (5) used sections embedded in plastic for their experiments, in which three pretreatments were examined: microwave irradiation (slides immersed in 10 mmol/L sodium citrate buffer, pH 6.0, heated for 20 minutes at a power output of 450 W), enzyme digestion (proteinase K at a concentration of 10 mg/mL at 37°C for 15 min), and superheating in a pressure cooker (slides in 1.5 L of 10 mmol/L sodium citrate buffer, pH 6.0, at 121°C and pressure of 103 kPa for 3 min). Of the methods tested in this study for *Sox* 11 and *Sox* 21 genes, the pretreatment procedure using a pressure cooker proved to be the most effective for both of the probes investigated. In addition, when reactivity seemed to have been lost in tissue blocks that had been prepared some months previously, only the use of pressure cooking could retrieve the staining (5). Although there have only been a few reports of successful in situ hybridization on plastic sections, the results achieved in this study have clearly shown that it is possible to produce good and consistent non-isotopic in situ hybridization if the tissue is embedded in methyl methacrylate. Previously, this plastic has only been reported for isotopic in situ hybridization (15). These results suggest that the use of pressure cooking pretreatment may increase the sensitivity of detection for in situ hybridization protocols, especially if the tissue has been embedded in plastic. Furthermore, it may be possible to combine in situ hybridization and immunocytochemistry using only one pretreatment, resulting in less damage to the tissue and a decrease in time required to perform the techniques.

Several of McMahon and McQuaid's (24) findings contradicted those of other groups. In particular, the study was unique in finding that protease treatment was superior to microwave pretreatment when the two were compared as single protocols for formalin-fixed, paraffin-embedded tissues. However, the study agreed with the majority that a combination of the pretreatments was optimal. In further contrast to other findings, the use of citrate buffer resulted in the least intense signals of all nine buffers tested, and they found that magnesium chloride was the optimal buffer. No other study included this particular solution in their experiments.

Church et al. (5) found that the pressure cooker resulted in the best results for their plastic-embedded tissues. The tissue was deplasticized prior to pretreatment. They reported that enzyme digestion produced better signals than microwave heating for *Sox* 11, but achieved the same intensity of signal for *Sox* 21 when used as single pretreatments. In total, only one of the six investigations utilizing paraffin-embedded tissues found enzyme digestion to be superior to the microwave.

DISCUSSION

The microwave pretreatment method is a rapid, simple, sensitive, and highly reproducible method that will not only be of help to research but will allow the eventual establishment of in situ hybridization as a routine test for diagnostic pathology, a possibility that has been severely limited by the long and complicated protocols and problems of reproducibility associated with the current protocols (1,3,6,16–22). Recent studies have demonstrated that microwave treatment combined with a brief proteinase digestion can enhance signal detection for mRNA and DNA in formalin-fixed, paraffin-embedded tissue sections. It was shown that microwaving in 10 mmol/L citrate buffer, pH 6.0, at a power level of 800 W for 15 minutes, increases the in situ signal using RNA probes in many different tissues (19–21,25,28). Following their experiments, these authors concluded that after suitable pretreatment, such as microwaving for 15 minutes in citrate buffer, detection sensitivity for RNA by in situ hybridization is greatly enhanced (25). In addition, such pretreatment eliminates the need for extensive experimentation with enzymes, durations, etc., to achieve permeation of the tissue sections (19–21,25,28). In addition to increasing target detection sensitivity, the microwave pretreatment method has many other advantages, including preservation of superior morphology, enhanced potential for double labeling, and shortened procedure time (25).

For Lan et al. (19–21), the use of microwave treatment allowed the entire process of in situ hybridization (up to the point of chromogen development) to be completed within 2 hours, making it possible to cut sections and obtain in situ hybridization results within the same day, and replacing the conventional 2- or 3-day protocols. Tornóczky et al. (30) reported that the protocol was significantly simplified by the microwave oven pretreatment. In their studies, in situ hybridization with microwave pretreatment was found to be fast when combined with a nonisotopic method. This facilitates detection of nucleotide sequences in surgical pathology.

Not only does the microwave oven shorten the in situ hybridization time, it has been found to simplify the procedure as well. The study performed by Wilkens et al. (31) clearly demonstrates the striking improvement and simplification in laboratory protocols that can be achieved if microwave pretreatment is performed for in situ hybridization of RNA. Until recently, tissue types, diagnosis, and length of formalin fixation made systematic testing of variable times and/or concentrations of special pretreatment and digestion necessary to obtain optimal results (31). The cumbersome testing of single-case adapted proteinase K digestion for in situ hybridization of RNA can be eliminated by microwave pretreatment (31).

With the new pretreatment protocols, combined in situ hybridization and immunohistochemistry on the same slide becomes possible (12). Additionally, in situ hybridization may be used for otherwise unsuitable tissue samples. For normal samples, it consumes fewer probes and less of each solution for the same levels of target detection (12).

Despite significant advances in the pretreatment for in situ hybridization, there is plenty of room for improvement. In the limited literature available on this topic, there are many discrepancies between groups. In particular, the theory behind the beneficial effect claimed is not clear. It is possible that the energy generated by heating breaks the cross-links between protein molecules, and between protein and nucleotide molecules, and sufficiently frees up target sequences for probe annealing. The loosened molecules may make the enzyme digestion more effective, therefore shortening the required length and strength of digestion. Disintegration of masking architecture would also facilitate probe penetrations and target finding. Whether there is a microwave effect in addition to simple heating remains to be clarified (8–11). Obviously, more work is needed to illustrate the precise mechanism of the beneficial effects of different pretreatment protocols.

SAMPLE PROTOCOL

Based on the available literature and our own experience, a relatively simple protocol for the in situ hybridization procedure is recommended. For hybridization to formalin-fixed and paraffin-embedded sections:

1. Dewax slides in two changes of xylene for 2 minutes each.
2. Rehydrate sections in graded concentrations of ethanol.
3. Wash slides twice in DEPC-treated water.
4. Block endogenous peroxidase by incubating slides in 3% H_2O_2 in methanol for 10 minutes at room temperature.

5. Wash slides for 5 minutes in running tap water and for 5 minutes in DEPC-treated water.

6. Immerse slides in RNase-free 10 mmol/L citrate buffer, pH 6.0.

7. Microwave at a power level of 800 W for three 5-minute periods. After each period, refill the buffer solution to compensate for any evaporation.

8. Keep the slides in the buffer for 30 minutes to cool to room temperature.

9. Wash sections for 15 minutes in DEPC-treated water.

10. Digest the tissue with proteinase K (5 to 30 μg/mL) at 37°C for 2 to 10 minutes in a humid chamber.

11. Wash the tissue in DEPC-treated water 3× for 2 minutes each time.

12. Dehydrate in graded ethanols and air-dry.

13. Prepare the hybridization solution with biotinylated probe:

50% dextran sulfate	250 μL
EDTA (1 mmol/L)	120 μL
20× SSC	100 μL
Formamide	450 μL
Herring sperm DNA	33 μL
DEPC-treated water	47 μL

   Mix well and add probe. Probe final concentration: 0.2 to 1.5 μL.

14. Apply 50 μL of hybridization solution to the section, coverslip, and place in an incubation chamber.

15. Incubate at 42°C for 2 hours. This step may also be performed using a microwave at a power level of 90 W for 20 to 60 minutes with a 2-minute on-and-off cycle.

16. Wash in 2× SSC for 10 minutes at 42°C.

17. Wash in 1× SSC for 10 minutes at 42°C.

18. Wash in 0.5× SSC for 10 minutes at 42°C.

19. Proceed to detection with a biotin detection kit with sufficient background blockage.

20. Wash in distilled water twice for 5 minutes each time.

21. Counterstain and mount.

ACKNOWLEDGMENTS

The authors acknowledge the constructive comments of Brandon Perry.

REFERENCES

1. **Allan, G.M., J.A. Smyth, D. Todd, and M.S. McNulty.** 1993. In situ hybridization for the detection of chicken anemia virus in formalin-fixed, paraffin-embedded sections. Avian Dis. *37*:177-82.
2. **Bourinbaiar, A.S.** 1991. Microwave irradiation stimulated in situ hybridization procedure with biotinylated DNA probe. Eur. J. Morphol. *29*:213-218.
3. **Bourinbaiar, A.S., V.R. Zacharopoulos, and D.M. Phillips.** 1991. Microwave irradiation-accelerated in situ hybridization technique for HIV detection. J. Virol. Methods *35*:49-58.
4. **Burns, W.A. and A. Bretschneider.** 1981. Thin Is In: Plastic Embedding of Tissue for Light Microscopy. ASCP Press, Chicago.
4a. **Cattoretti, G., S. Pileri, C. Parravicini, M.H.G. Becker, S. Poggi, C. Bifulco, G. Key, L. D'Amato, E. Sabat-

tini, E. Feudale, et al. 1993. Antigen unmasking on formalin-fixed, paraffin-embedded tissue sections. J. Pathol. *171*:83-98.

5. **Church, R.J., N.M. Hand, M. Rex, and P.J. Scotting.** 1997. Non-isotopic in situ hybridization to detect chick Sox gene mRNA in plastic-embedded tissue. Histochem. J. *29*:625-629.

6. **Coates, P.J., P.A. Hall, M.G. Butler, and A.J. D'Ardenne.** 1987. Rapid technique of DNA-DNA in situ hybridization on formalin-fixed tissue sections using microwave irradiation. J. Clin. Pathol. *40*:865-869.

7. **Fox, C.H., F.B. Johnson, J. Whiting, and P.P. Roller.** 1985. Formaldehyde fixation. J. Histochem. Cytochem. *33*:845-853.

8. **Gu, J.** 1994. Microwave immunocytochemistry, p. 67-80. *In* J. Gu and G.W. Hacker (Eds.), Modern Methods in Analytical Morphology, Plenum Publishing Corporation, New York.

9. **Gu, J.** 1997. In situ hybridization as an adjunct method with immunohistochemistry, p. 414-421. *In* R. Nakamura (Ed.), Manual of Clinical Laboratory Immunology, 5th ed. American Society of Microbiology Press, Washington, DC.

10. **Gu, J., T.S. Choi, M.M. Whittlesey, S.E. Slap, and V.M. Anderson.** 1995. Recent advances in microwave immunohistochemistry. Scanning *17*:V23-V25.

11. **Gu, J., T.S. Choi, M.M. Whittlesey, S.E. Slap, and V.M. Anderson.** 1997. Microwave immunohistochemistry: advances in temperature control, p. 91-114. *In* Analytical Morphology. Eaton Publishing Company, Natick, MA.

12. **Haas, C.J., A. Hirschmann, A. Sendelhofert, J. Diebold, H. Arnholdt, and U. Lohrs.** 1998. Improvement of nonradioactive DNA in situ hybridization. Biotech. Histochem. *73*:228-232.

13. **Henke, R.P. and N. Ayhan.** 1994. Enhancement of hybridization efficiency in interphase cytogenetics on paraffin-embedded sections by microwave treatment. Anal. Cell Pathol. *6*:319-325.

14. **Hopwood, D.** 1982. Fixation and fixatives, p. 16-28. *In* J.D. Bancroft and A. Stevens (Eds.), Theory and Practice of Histological Techniques, 2nd ed. Churchill Livingstone, Edinburgh.

15. **Jamrich, M., K.A. Mahon, E.R. Gavis, and J.G. Gall.** 1984. Histone RNA in amphibian oocytes visualized by in situ hybridization to methacrylate-embedded tissue sections. EMBO J. *3*:1939-1943.

16. **Khan, G., R.K. Gupta, R.J. Coates, and G. Slavin.** 1993. Epstein-Barr virus infection and *bcl-2* protoncogene expression. Separate events in the pathogenesis of Hodgkin's disease? Am. J. Pathol. *143*:1270-1274.

17. **Kok, L.P. and M.E. Boon.** 1992. Microwave exposure and DNA in situ hybridization, p. 366-371. *In* The Microwave Cookbook for Microscopists, Chapter 25. Coulomb Press, Leiden.

18. **Koshiba, M., K. Ogawa, S. Hamazaki, T. Sugiyama, O. Ogawa, and T. Kitajima.** 1993. The effect of formalin fixation on DNA and the extraction of high-molecular-weight DNA from fixed and embedded tissues. Pathol. Res. Pract. *189*:66-72.

19. **Lan, H.Y., D.J. Nikolic-Paterson, and R.C. Atkins.** 1995. Local macrophage proliferation in experimental Goodpasture's syndrome. Nephrology *1*:151.

20. **Lan, H.Y., W. Mu, Y.Y. Ng, D.J. Mikolic-Paterson, and R.C. Atkins.** 1996. A simple, reliable, and sensitive method for nonradioactive in situ hybridization: use of microwave heating to improve hybridization efficiency and preserve tissue morphology. J. Histochem. Cytochem. *44*:281-287.

21. **Lan, H.Y., D.J. Nikolic-Paterson, W. Mu, and R.C. Atkins.** Local macrophage proliferation in multinucleated giant cell and granuloma formation in experimental Goodpasture's syndrome. Am. J. Pathol. (In press).

22. **Leong, A.S. and J. Milios.** 1993. An assessment of the efficacy of the microwave antigen-retrieval procedure on a range of tissue antigens. Appl. Immunohistochem. *1*:267-274.

23. **Login, G.R., S. Kissell, B.K. Dwyer, and A.M. Dvorak.** 1991. A novel microwave device designed to preserve cell structure in millisecond, p. 329-346. *In* W.B. Snyder, Jr., W.H. Sutton, M.F. Iskander, and D.L. Johnson (Eds.), Microwave Processing of Materials II. Materials Research Society, Pittsburgh.

24. **McMahon, J. and S. McQuaid.** 1996. The use of microwave irradiation as a pretreatment to in situ hybridization for the detection of measles virus and chicken anemia virus in formalin-fixed paraffin-embedded tissue. Histochem. J. *28*:157-164.

25. **Oliver, K.R., R.P. Heavens, and D.J. Sirinathsinghji.** 1997. Quantitative comparison of pretreatment regimens used to sensitize in situ hybridization using oligonucleotide probes on paraffin-embedded brain tissue. J. Histochem. Cytochem. *45*:1707-1713.

26. **Puchtler, H. and S.N. Meloan.** 1985. On the chemistry of formaldehyde fixation and its effects on immunohistochemical reactions. Histochemistry *82*:201-204.

27. **Shi, S.R., M.E. Key, and K.L. Kalra.** 1991. Antigen retrieval in formalin-fixed, paraffin-embedded tissues: an enhancement method for immunohistochemical staining based on microwave oven heating of tissue sections. J. Histochem. Cytochem. *39*:741-748.

28. **Sibony, M., F. Commo, P. Callard, and J.-M. Gasc.** 1995. Enhancement of mRNA in situ hybridization signaled by microwave heating. Lab. Invest. *73*:586-591.

29. **Sperry, A., L. Jin, and R.V. Lloyd.** 1996. Microwave treatment enhances detection of RNA and DNA by in situ hybridization. Diagn. Mol. Pathol. *5*:291-296.

30. **Tornóczky, T., G. Kelényi and L. Pajor.** 1998. EBER oligonucleotide RNA in situ hybridization in EBV associate neoplasms. Pathol. Oncol. Res. *4*:201-205.

31. **Wilkens, L., R. von Wasielewski, M. Werner, M. Nolte, and A. Georgii.** 1996. Microwave pretreatment improves RNA-ISH in various formalin-fixed tissues using a uniform protocol. Pathol. Res. Pract. *192*:588-594.

Multiple Immunoenzyme Staining

7

Hui Y. Lan[1] and David J. Nikolic-Paterson[2]

[1]Department of Medicine, Queen Mary Hospital, University of Hong Kong, Pokfulam, Hong Kong, and [2]Department of Nephrology and Monash University Department of Medicine, Monash Medical Centre, Clayton, Victoria, Australia

INTRODUCTION

The ability to use monoclonal antibodies (mAbs) to detect specific antigens within tissue sections has revolutionized many areas of biologic research and clinical pathology. A logical extension of this technique is the detection of two or more antigens within the same tissue section using different primary antibodies. Double immunoenzymatic staining, often referred to as two-color immunostaining, has great potential, but the technical difficulties associated with this technique have largely prevented its use outside of specialist histopathology laboratories. The two main limitations of multiple immunoenzymatic staining are antibody cross-reactivity and a lack of sensitivity (4).

The detection of tissue antigens by immunoenzymatic staining usually involves a sensitive three-layer method. A primary antibody, often a mouse mAb, specific for the antigen of interest is applied to the tissue section as the first layer. The primary antibody is then detected by a polyclonal anti-mouse antibody is often raised in rabbit or sheep and conjugated to horseradish peroxidase (HRP), alkaline phosphatase (AP), or biotin as the second layer. The third layer is an amplification step in which HRP-conjugated anti-HRP antibody complexes (PAP), AP-conjugated anti-AP antibody complexes (APAAP), or streptavidin-HRP complexes are bound to the tissue, as appropriate, followed by a chromogen reaction to produce a colored precipitate. Antibody cross-reactivity arises when a second round of three-layer immunostaining is performed using a primary antibody raised in the same species as that used in the first round of immunostaining. For example, the application of a second mouse mAb will

Antigen Retrieval Techniques
Edited by Shan-Rong Shi, Jiang Gu, and Clive R. Taylor
©2000 Eaton Publishing, Natick, MA

bind to any free binding sites of the rabbit or sheep anti-mouse IgG antibody used in the first round of staining, resulting in false double positives. Unfortunately, this is a very common problem since most mAbs against human antigens are raised in mice.

A number of strategies have been used in an attempt to block antibody cross-reactivity. First, the primary antibodies can be raised in different species, but this is often impractical or requires the use of polyclonal antibodies, which can present problems with high background staining. Second, isotype-matched irrelevant F(ab) fragments can be used in between the two rounds of three-layer immunostaining to block antibody cross-reactivity (1). This approach is limited in that the F(ab) concentrations need to be titrated for each pair of antibodies used, and that complete blockade of antibody cross-reactivity is difficult when one of the antigens is highly abundant within the tissue. Third, primary mAbs can be conjugated directly to fluorochromes or enzymes (HRP or AP). This has the disadvantage in that one-layer immunoenzymatic staining or direct immunofluorescence is not as sensitive as three-layer staining. One improvement on this approach is to biotin conjugate one primary mAb and detect it with streptavidin-HRP, while the second round of immunostaining uses a digoxigenin (DIG)-conjugated mAb detected using AP-conjugated anti-DIG antibody.

All these approaches to the problem of antibody cross-reactivity suffer from the same difficulty—they need to be set up and optimized for each pair of primary antibodies, they are costly and time-consuming, and they do not provide the same degree of sensitivity as three-layer immunostaining. The ideal solution to this problem would *(i)* be simple and reliable to perform, *(ii)* be generally applicable, *(iii)* remove the need to conjugate primary antibodies, and *(iv)* allow the use of sensitive three-layer immunoenzymatic staining. The solution that encompasses all these features is the use of microwave oven heating to block antibody cross-reactivity (2).

THEORETICAL PRINCIPLE

Microwave oven heating of tissue sections in a salt solution has been shown to enhance antibody binding to a wide range of tissue antigens, a process called antigen retrieval (AR) (9–11). However, microwave oven heating can also be used to block antibody cross-reactivity (2). Microwave treatment is thought to act by increasing the frequency of vibration of water molecules, with lesser effects on other chemical bonds. The effect of microwave heating of sections immersed in an aqueous salt solution is to denature the secondary and tertiary structure of many molecules within the tissue. AR requires that tissues be fixed in aldehyde-based cross-linking fixatives, since the covalent cross-linking bonds limit the degree of denaturation of antigen structure so that antibody access is substantially improved while the antigenic epitope is still recognizable.

The ability of microwave oven heating to denature protein structure can also be used to block antibody cross-reactivity. During the process of immunostaining, an antibody-enzyme complex is bound in a noncovalent fashion (i.e., not cross-linked) to the tissue section. The application of microwave oven heating completely denatures the structure of the native antibody-enzyme complex bound to the tissue so that it no longer has any IgG binding capacity, cannot be recognized by anti-immunoglobulin antibodies, and has no enzymatic activity.

The main limitation of this technique is that at least one of the antigens being stained in a two-color immunostaining protocol must be stable to microwave oven heating. This can be a problem in detecting cell surface antigens, which is discussed further on.

There are two other important considerations for the use of microwave oven heating in multiple immunostaining. First, the insoluble color precipitates formed following the reaction of chromogenic substrates like diaminobenzidine or fast blue are stable to one or more rounds of microwave oven heating. Second, a fortuitous aspect of microwave oven heating is that it denatures endogenous AP within the tissue. This removes the necessity to use levamisole in the AP reaction buffer. This is particularly useful when staining tissues with very high levels of endogenous AP, such as kidney and gut, in which it is difficult to inhibit endogenous AP activity fully using levamisole.

BASIC METHOD

This protocol has been written for the detection of two or more antigens within rat tissues using mouse mAbs (2). However, it can be easily modified to perform multiple immunostaining in human tissues (12) or those from other species.

Tissue Fixation

Tissues need to be fixed in a cross-linking fixative. For frozen samples, we fix tissues by immersion in 2% to 4% paraformaldehyde-lysine-periodate for 4 hours at 4°C followed by three changes in 7% sucrose in phosphate-buffered saline (PBS) over a 36-hour period at 4°C, embedding in Tissue-Tek OCT compound (Miles, Elkhart, IN, USA) and storage at -80°C. For paraffin samples, tissues are fixed in 4% or 10% neutral buffered formalin for 4 to 24 hours, dehydrated, and embedded in paraffin. It is important to avoid prolonged periods of fixation since this causes the loss of antigens of interest and reduces the ability of microwave oven heating to facilitate antigen retrieval.

First Round of Immunostaining

Cryostat or paraffin sections are washed in PBS and then preincubated with serum [10% fetal calf serum (FCS), 10% normal rabbit or goat serum in PBS] to block non-specific antibody binding to the tissue for 20 min. Sections are drained and then incubated with the first mouse mAb (diluted in 1% FCS, 1% normal rabbit or goat serum in PBS) for 60 minutes. After washing (3 times) in PBS, endogenous peroxidase activity is blocked by dehydration of the sections through graded alcohol and then incubation in 0.3% H_2O_2 in methanol for 20 minutes. After washing in PBS, sections are incubated sequentially with HRP-conjugated rabbit or goat anti-mouse IgG and then mouse PAP for 30 minutes. The HRP is then developed with diaminobenzidine and H_2O_2 to produce a brown precipitate.

Blocking Antigen Cross-Reactivity Using Microwave Oven Heating

It is important that sections be attached through adhesion to silanated slides to prevent their detachment during microwave treatment. Slides are placed in a polypropylene rack and immersed in a 1-L polypropylene beaker containing 400 mL of 0.01 mol/L sodium citrate buffer, pH 6.0. The beaker is covered with polyethylene plastic wrapping, and a single 10-minute period of microwave oven heating is used. We have tested a range of different staining methods and found that a single 10-minute period of microwave oven heating is sufficient to block antibody cross-reactivity completely

(2). Any commercially available microwave set to maximum can be used, although the power output of some models does vary. We routinely use an oven with an operating frequency of 2450 MHz and 800 W power output.

Second Round of Immunostaining

There are two effects of microwave oven heating that need to be considered when performing the second round of immunostaining. First, the potential for nonspecific antibody to stick to the tissue is significantly increased. Therefore, it is essential to perform a second round of serum block on the tissue sections. Sometimes we include a second block step using 5% bovine serum albumin to solve this problem. Second, antibody access to the target antigen is greatly improved. This allows a much lower concentration of the primary antibody to be used and is particularly helpful for reducing nonspecific staining. This point is often overlooked and has caused apparently contradictory results in the literature, such as the controversy surrounding the use of the PC-10 mAb against the proliferating cell nuclear antigen (PCNA) (3,6,8).

Sections are washed in PBS, and a serum block is performed as described above. They are then drained and incubated with the second mouse mAb for 60 minutes. After washing (3 times) in PBS, sections are incubated sequentially with AP-conjugated rabbit or goat anti-mouse IgG and then mouse APAAP for 30 minutes. The APAAP is then developed with fast blue BB salt to produce a blue color. Note that microwave treatment inactivates endogenous AP, so that levamisole is not required in the AP reaction solution.

Third Round of Immunostaining

Three-color immunostaining can be performed using this technique. Sections are given a second round of microwave treatment to block antibody cross-reactivity, pre-incubated as above, and then incubated with a third mouse mAb. A three-layer APAAP method can be repeated and the AP developed with fast red to produce a different color. Alternatively, gold-conjugated anti-mouse IgG followed by silver enhancement can be used to provide a dense black stain, which can easily be distinguished from brown and blue stains.

Staining Controls

It is important to incorporate a number of controls to check the specificity and sensitivity of multiple immunostaining. The best control is to perform single-color immunostaining with each primary mAb side by side with multiple immunostaining on serial sections to confirm that the multiple immunostaining represents a simple addition of the individual mAb staining patterns in terms of both distribution and intensity of stain. Another control is to use an irrelevant primary mAb during the first, second, or third round of staining.

DETECTION OF CYTOPLASMIC, NUCLEAR, AND EXTRACELLULAR ANTIGENS

The technique of microwave-based multiple immunostaining is most readily applied to the detection of antigens that are well preserved by tissue fixation and stable to one or more rounds of microwave oven heating. In general, cytoplasmic, nuclear, and extracellular antigens are well preserved by cross-linking fixatives and stable to microwave oven heating. Indeed, microwave oven heating is frequently used to enhance immunostaining of such antigens. This is very convenient since a single round of microwave oven heating can both block antibody cross-reactivity and perform AR. A second important aspect is that antigens that are stable to microwave treatment can generally withstand at least 20 minutes of microwave heating. This allows two or three rounds of microwave oven heating to be used in a protocol for two- or three-color immunostaining without a loss in sensitivity of antigen detection.

An example of two-color immunostaining of cytoplasmic and nuclear antigens is shown in Figure 1(a). Normal rat gut tissue was microwaved for AR, stained for cytoplasmic fibroblast growth factor-2 (FGF-2) using a three-layer PAP method, microwaved a second time to block antibody cross-reactivity, and then stained for PCNA within the cell nuclei by a three-layer APAAP method. Three-color immunostaining is shown in Figure 1(b). Diseased rat kidney tissue was stained for cytoplasmic FGF-2 and CD68 antigens, followed by staining of PCNA within cell nuclei. Microwave oven heating was used between each of the three rounds of immunostaining, and all three colors are clearly discernible within the section.

To obtain the best results from multiple immunostaining, it is important to select chromogen substrates that produce color products that are easily distinguished from each other. It is also preferable to stain antigens located in different cellular compartments, such as the cytoplasm and nucleus, or antigens expressed in different cell types. It can be difficult to perform double immunostaining when two antigens are expressed within the same compartment of the same cell, especially if one antigen is present in greater abundance than the other. This is a limitation of the chromogenic substrates themselves, caused by the relatively diffuse deposition of the colored precipitates, rather than a limitation of microwave oven heating as a method of blocking antibody cross-reactivity. In this particular circumstance, it may be preferable to use two-color immunofluorescence with directly conjugated primary antibodies. The two fluorochromes can be examined individually or in combination with the appropriate use of filters.

DETECTION OF CELL SURFACE ANTIGENS

Immunostaining of cell surface antigens poses a number of technical difficulties. These antigens, which are immersed within a lipid environment, are frequently destroyed by the high temperatures used in the process of paraffin embedding. Therefore, most studies use tissues fixed in 2% to 4% paraformaldehyde and then snap frozen. The application of microwave oven heating to cryostat sections also destroys most cell surface antigens. Therefore, in any two-color immunostaining protocol, it is essential to stain for the cell surface antigen prior to the microwave oven heating step.

An example of detection of a cell surface antigen as part of a three-color immunostaining protocol is shown in Figure 1(c). In this case the CD45 antigen was stained on the cell surface of leukocytes in a section of diseased rat lung tissue before microwave treatment was used to block antigen cross-reactivity followed by detection of the macrophage cytoplasmic CD68 antigen and PCNA in cell nuclei. A high-power field of a triple-stained tissue (Figure 1d), shows the clear distinction of three antigens within different compartments of the same cell; CD45 antigen on the cell surface,

CD68 antigen in the cytoplasm, and PCNA in the nucleus. This illustrates the ability of microwave oven heating to block antibody cross-reactivity completely.

Although most mAbs raised against cell surface molecules cannot stain paraffin-embedded tissues or cryostat tissue sections after microwave oven heating, this does not apply to all mAbs. Indeed, due to commercial incentive, a wide range of mAbs are now available that can recognize cell surface antigens in routine formalin-fixed,

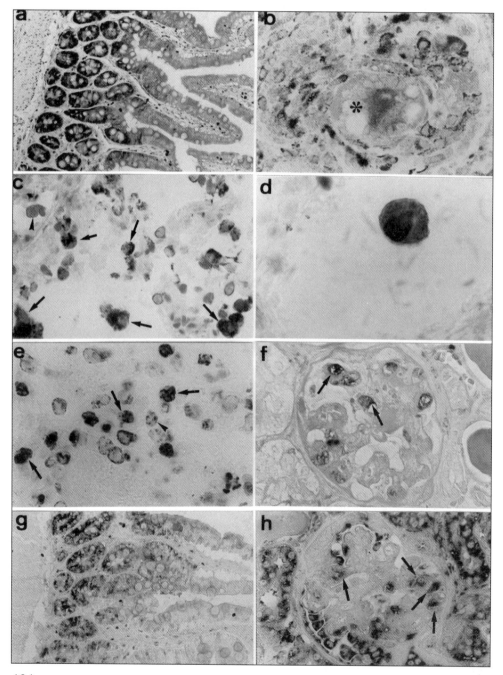

paraffin-embedded human pathology specimens, even after microwave treatment. Based on empirical observation, we propose that such mAbs recognize linear peptide epitopes that are still accessible in a denatured antigen. In contrast, mAbs raised against conformational epitopes fail to recognize antigens when they are denatured by microwave treatment. For example, a mAb raised against a peptide of the cell surface epidermal growth factor receptor actually requires microwave oven heating to detect receptor expression on glomerular epithelial cells, implying that the epitope is not available in the native receptor structure, but that it became accessible in the denatured molecule (7). Thus, careful mAb selection can circumvent the problem of microwave destruction of cell surface antigens in some cases.

COMBINATION OF IMMUNOSTAINING WITH NUCLEIC ACID DETECTION

The use of microwave oven heating for blocking antibody cross-reactivity is not limited to the performance of multiple rounds of tissue antigen immunostaining. This technique can be used to combine immunostaining with other techniques, such as detection of proliferating and apoptotic cells and of mRNA by nonradioactive in situ hybridization.

Figure 1. Examples of multiple immunoenzymatic staining. (a) Paraffin section of normal rat gut. The tissue was microwaved to enhance detection of fibroblast growth factor-2 (FGF-2) using a three-layer PAP method developed with diaminobenzidine (DAB) to give a brown color. A second round of microwave oven heating was used to block antigen cross-reactivity. This was followed by staining for nuclear expression of the proliferating cell nuclear antigen (PCNA) using a three-layer APAAP method and developed with fast blue. The section was counterstained with periodic acid-Schiff (PAS) reagent to display the tissue structure. An association between FGF-2 expression and local proliferation in gut epithelial cells can be seen. (b) Paraffin section of a granulomatous lesion from a diseased rat kidney (crescentic glomerulonephritis). The tissue was microwaved to enhance detection of FGF-2 (three-layer PAP, DAB/brown). After a second round of microwave oven heating, the macrophage cytoplasmic CD68 antigen was stained (three-layer APAAP, fast blue). After a third round of microwave oven heating, nuclear expression of PCNA was stained using a two-layer immunogold reaction with silver enhancement to give a black color. The section shows FGF-2 production by macrophage multinucleated giant cells (*) and many fibroblast-like cells; FGF-2 production is associated with cell proliferation within the lesion. (c) Cryostat section of diseased rat lung (Goodpasture's syndrome) stained for a cell surface antigen on T cells (three-layer PAP, DAB/brown), microwaved, stained for the macrophage cytoplasmic CD68 (three-layer APAAP, fast blue), microwaved, and stained for nuclear PCNA (three-layer APAAP, fast red). This panel demonstrates the presence of locally proliferating macrophages (arrows) and T cells (arrowhead) within the lesions. (d) Cryostat section of diseased rat lung (Goodpasture's syndrome) showing a triple-stained macrophage. The section was stained for the CD45 leukocyte common cell surface antigen (three-layer APAAP, fast blue), microwaved, stained for the macrophage cytoplasmic CD68 (three-layer APAAP, fast red), microwaved, and stained for nuclear PCNA (three-layer PAP, DAB silver/black). (e) Paraffin section from a rat with kidney disease that had been injected 24 hours earlier with bromodeoxyuridine (BrdU). The section was microwaved to enhance immunostaining for the macrophage cytoplasmic CD68 (three-layer PAP, DAB/brown), and then microwaved to block antigen cross-reactivity and to enhance immunostaining of BrdU incorporated into DNA (three-layer APAAP, fast blue). Proliferating CD68+/BrdU+ macrophages are shown by arrows, while a CD68+ macrophage with DNA fragmentation (apoptotic body) defined by BrdU staining is shown by an arrowhead. (f) Paraffin section of diseased rat kidney. TUNEL staining for apoptotic cells was performed using digoxigenin-labeled nucleotides detected with an AP-conjugated anti-digoxigenin antibody and developed to produce a purple color. After microwave oven heating, the section was stained for the macrophage cytoplasmic CD68 antigen (three-layer PAP, DAB/brown) and counterstained with PAS. A number of double-stained TUNEL+/CD68+ apoptotic macrophages can be seen within the glomerulus (arrows). (g) A paraffin section of normal rat gut. In situ hybridization using a digoxigenin-labeled riboprobe for FGF-2 was detected using an AP-conjugated anti-digoxigenin antibody and developed to produce a purple color. The section was microwaved, stained for PCNA (three-layer APAAP, fast blue), and counterstained with PAS. Note that the staining pattern is similar to that seen for double immunostaining of FGF-2 and PCNA shown in panel (a). (h) Paraffin section from diseased rat kidney. In situ hybridization using a digoxigenin-labeled riboprobe for macrophage migration inhibitory factor (MIF) was developed to produce a purple color. The section was microwaved, stained for the macrophage cytoplasmic CD68 antigen (three-layer PAP, DAB/brown), and counterstained with PAS. Expression of MIF mRNA by tubular and glomerular epithelial cells is seen, as well as MIF mRNA expression by CD68+ macrophages (arrows). Magnification 100× (a, g), 400× (b, c, e, f, h), and 1000× (d). **(See color plate A7).**

In these cases, microwave oven heating is used to block potential antibody cross-reactivity between the immunostaining reaction and the other detection system being employed.

During a study of local macrophage proliferation in kidney disease, we found that microwave oven heating provides a useful AR method for detection of bromodeoxyuridine (BrdU) within tissue sections (3). The gold standard technique for detecting cell proliferation in animals is to inject them with the thymidine analog, BrdU, which is specifically incorporated into DNA during the S-phase of the cell cycle. Detection of labeled cells within tissue sections requires denaturation of DNA to allow antibody access to the incorporated BrdU. This denaturation step is usually performed using harsh chemicals such as 0.1 mol/L HCl or NaOH or heating in a 95% formamide solution. We found that 10 minutes of microwave oven heating provides excellent DNA denaturation and antibody access to the incorporated BrdU within cell nuclei. Figure 1(e) shows an example of rat kidney disease in which an animal was killed 1 day after injection with BrdU. Macrophages were identified by staining the cytoplasmic CD68 antigen, and BrdU was stained after microwave oven heating. Interestingly, both proliferating and apoptotic macrophages can be seen. Thus, macrophages that were going through S-phase when the BrdU was injected were found to undergo apoptosis just 1 day later. This implies that proliferating macrophages within the damaged kidney undergo only one or two cell divisions before dying through apoptosis.

In situ terminal deoxyribonucleotide transferase (TdT)-mediated dUTP nick-end labeling (TUNEL) using digoxigenin-labeled nucleotides is a popular method for the detection of apoptotic cells within tissue sections. This technique uses the TdT enzyme to incorporate digoxigenin-labeled nucleotides into the DNA of apoptotic cells; the DNA is then detected by an AP-conjugated anti-digoxigenin antibody and developed with nitro blue tetrazolium chloride and 5-bromo-4-chloro-3-indolyl-phosphate (NBT/X-phosphate). Once the TUNEL staining has been completed, the tissue can be microwave treated to enable immunostaining to be performed without possible antibody cross-reactivity with the anti-digoxigenin antibody. The combination of TUNEL and immunostaining allows the phenotype of apoptotic cells to be established. An example is shown in Figure 1(f), in which combined TUNEL and immunostaining for CD68-positive macrophages clearly identify the presence of apoptotic macrophages in diseased rat kidney (5). Indeed, the detection of apoptotic macrophages in the diseased rat kidney using combined TUNEL and CD68 immunostaining is consistent with the detection of apoptotic macrophages shown in Figure 1(e).

Nonradioactive in situ hybridization is widely used for the detection of mRNA expression within tissue sections. Although there are many different methods of performing nonradioactive in situ hybridization, the most popular uses digoxigenin-labeled probes detected by an AP-conjugated anti-digoxigenin antibody and developed with NBT/X-phosphate. Microwave oven heating can be used after in situ hybridization to block any potential antibody cross-reactivity with a later immunostaining step. The combination of in situ hybridization and immunostaining of tissue antigens is particularly useful for identifying the cell type(s) expressing the gene of interest. Examples of combined in situ hybridization and immunostaining are shown in Figure 1 (g) and (h).

CONCLUSION

The application of microwave oven heating has changed double and triple immunoenzymatic staining from a complex and difficult technique used in only the most advanced histopathology laboratories into a relatively simple technique that can be easily mastered in any laboratory. The strengths of this technique are that it is simple, reliable, and sensitive and can be applied in most types of multiple immunostaining. This technique is far simpler than other approaches to blocking antibody cross-reactivity such as raising primary antibodies in different species, purifying and conjugating primary antibodies, or the use of irrelevant F(ab) immunoglobulin fragments. Three other major advantages of this technique are *(i)* a single step of microwave oven heating can both block antibody cross-reactivity and facilitate AR; *(ii)* microwave oven heating allows immunostaining to be combined with nucleic acid detection systems such as TUNEL staining of apoptotic cells and nonradioactive in situ hybridization; and *(iii)* microwave heating preserves excellent tissue morphology, which can be seen by the use of histologic stains such as periodic acid-Schiff (Figure 1). The ability of microwave oven heating to inactivate endogenous AP also simplifies the staining method by removing the need to include levamisole in subsequent staining rounds. The only limitation of the technique occurs when the antigen is destroyed by microwave oven heating.

In summary, this simple, reliable, and sensitive technique of multiple immunostaining is likely to become a routine method performed in many laboratories. This has great potential for biologic research and clinical diagnosis.

REFERENCES

1. **Carl, S.A.L., I. Gillete-Ferguson, and D.G. Ferguson.** 1993. An indirect immunofluorescence procedure for staining the same cryosection with two mouse monoclonal primary antibodies. J. Histochem. Cytochem. *41*:1273-1278.

2. **Lan, H.Y., W. Mu, D.J. Nikolic-Paterson, and R.C. Atkins.** 1995. A novel, simple, reliable and sensitive method of multiple immunoenzymic staining: use of microwave oven heating to block antibody cross-reactivity and retrieve antigens. J. Histochem. Cytochem. *43*:97-102.

3. **Lan, H.Y., D.J. Nikolic-Paterson, W. Mu, and R.C. Atkins.** 1995. Local macrophage proliferation in progressive glomerular and tubulointerstitial injury in experimental anti-GBM glomerulonephritis. Kidney Int. *48*:753-60.

4. **Lan, H.Y., W. Mu, D.J. Nikolic-Paterson, and R.C. Atkins.** 1996. The application of microwave techniques in multiple immunostaining and in situ hybridisation. Nephrology (2 Suppl) *1*:S116-S121.

5. **Lan, H.Y., H. Mitsuhashi, Y.-Y. Ng, D.J. Nikolic-Paterson, N. Yang, W. Mu, and R.C. Atkins.** 1997. Macrophage apoptosis in rat crescentic glomerulonephritis. Am. J. Pathol. *151*:531-538.

6. **Lynch, D.A.F., A.M.T. Clarke, P. Jackson, A.T.R. Axon, M.F. Dixon, and P. Quirke.** 1994. Comparison of labelling by bromodeoxyuridine, MIB-1, and proliferating cell nuclear antigen in gastric mucosal biopsy specimens. J. Clin. Pathol. *47*:122-125.

7. **Nikolic-Paterson, D.J., G.H. Tesch, H.Y. Lan, K. Nukii, R. Foti, and R.C. Atkins.** 1995. EGF and EGF-receptor expression in rat anti-Thy-1 mesangial proliferative nephritis. Nephrology *1*:83-93.

8. **Rose, D.S.C., P.H. Maddox, and C.D. Brown.** 1994. Which proliferation markers for routine immunohistology? A comparison of five antibodies. J. Clin. Pathol. *47*:1010-1014.

9. **Shi, S.-R., M.E. Key, and K.L. Kalra.** 1991. Antigen retrieval in formalin-fixed, paraffin-embedded tissues: an enhancement method for immunohistochemical staining based on microwave oven heating of tissue sections. J. Histochem. Cytochem. *39*:741-748.

10. **Shi, S.-R., B. Chaiwun, L. Young, R.J. Cote, and C.R. Taylor.** 1993. Antigen retrieval technique utilizing citrate buffer or urea solution for immunohistochemical demonstration of androgen receptor in formalin-fixed paraffin sections. J. Histochem. Cytochem. *41*:1599-1604.

11. **Tesch, G.H., W. Mu, Y.-Y. Ng, R.C. Atkins, and H.Y. Lan.** 1995. Enhancement of immunodetection of cytokines and cytokine receptors in tissue sections using microwave treatment. Cell Vision, Analytical Morphology *2*:435-439.

12. **Yang, N., N.M. Isbel, D.J. Nikolic-Paterson, Y. Li, R. Ye, R.C. Atkins, and H.Y. Lan.** 1998. Local macrophage proliferation in human glomerulonephritis. Kidney Int. *54*:143-151.

Microwave-Stimulated Antigen Retrieval in Neuroscience

8

Paul Evers and Harry B.M. Uylings

Graduate School for Neurosciences Amsterdam, Netherlands Institute for Brain Research, Amsterdam, The Netherlands

INTRODUCTION

Most human brain tissue is preserved by immersion in a formaldehyde solution. The formaldehyde fixative is a solution that penetrates relatively quickly into brain tissue, but its fixating properties are rather slow (14). Brain tissue is therefore often left in the fixative for some weeks or even months. Also, for storage, the tissue is put in a formaldehyde solution, sometimes for years. During this fixation formaldehyde reacts with the proteins in the tissue. The tertiary and quarternary structure of the proteins alters, which impedes the accessibility of antibodies (7,14,26). This phenomenon is often called "masking of the tissue antigen." This masking is an important problem, especially when monoclonal antibodies, which recognize only one epitope, are applied. Fortunately, it has proved to be a reversible process, meaning that the alterations in the proteins can, at least partially, be undone, and thus the accessibility for antibodies be restored. Many techniques have been developed to unmask the proteins: washing the tissue or sections in water or buffer for very long periods (18,34) or pretreatment of the sections with enzymes (2), formic acid (21), periodic acid (22), guanidine HCl (6), or ultrasound (33). Often these techniques give good results, but only for a limited amount of antibodies.

In the early nineties, heating of the tissue sections in an aqueous solution proved to be an important factor in unmasking the antigens. For this purpose, a conventional oven (38), pressure cooker (28), microwave oven (38), or autoclave (44) can be used. When these heating methods were compared, the use of a microwave oven proved to be the best way to retrieve many antigens (20,38,50). Comparisons made between the conventional enzyme predigestion technique and the microwave oven revealed that

Antigen Retrieval Techniques
Edited by Shan-Rong Shi, Jiang Gu, and Clive R. Taylor
©2000 Eaton Publishing, Natick, MA

heating in the microwave oven gives better results (4,27,29,32). Since the introduction of the microwave-stimulated antigen retrieval (MW-AR) technique in 1991 by Shi et al. (38), many researchers all over the world have made great efforts to optimize this technique. Most of the work was done on paraffin sections [in pathologic laboratories (3,4,17,30,39,40,42,48,49,54), but also for in situ hybridization (24,46,47)] and also on cryostat and vibratome sections in neuroscience (1,8,10–12,15,16,19,25,27,31, 35–37,45,53,55–57; Table 1). After the introduction of the MW-AR technique, it soon became clear that fast heating to high temperatures and the pH of the AR solution in which the tissue was heated played an important role in unmasking the proteins. However, which temperature and AR solution should be used for optimal results remained a matter of trial and error. Reviews summarizing all the results obtained were written in which the need for a standard method of working in all cases was emphasized (5,13,43,51). Unfortunately, until now it has not been possible to find this standard method, although the use of a retrieval solution with a high pH seems to work in most cases (3,12,32,40,41; Figures 1 and 2). In this review we describe the present state of the art, emphasizing the application of MW-AR in neuroscience.

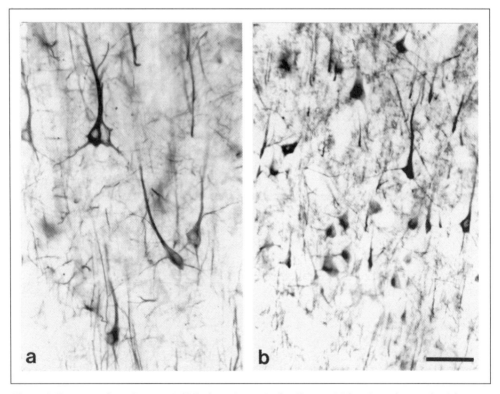

Figure 1. Human prefrontal cortex (middle frontal gyrus) of a 69-year-old female patient, stained for non-phosphorylated neurofilament protein (a) and microtubule-associated protein-2 (b) after 6 months of formaldehyde fixation and microwave pretreatment with TBS, pH 9.0. Without AR, only some vaguely stained somata would be visible. Scale bar = 50 μm.

Table 1. Antigens Successfully Retrieved by Microwave Irradiation in Neuroscience Research

Neuronal and axonal markers
    Neurofilament protein (12,27,32,56; Figure 1a)
    Microtubule-associated protein-2 (MAP-2) (12; Figure 1b)
    PGP9.5 (27)
    Synaptophysin (27,41,54)
    NeuN (55)

Glial markers
    Glial fibrillary acidic protein (GFAP) (8,27,56)
    Carbonic anhydrase type II (27)

Microglial markers
    CD68 (27)
    Ferritin (27)
    HLA-DR (27,31)

Calcium binding proteins
    Calbindin D 28-K (12; Figure 2a)
    Parvalbumin (12; Figure 2b)
    Calretinin (12,15; Figure 2c)

Neuropeptides
    MG-160 (25,35,36)
    Vasopressin (57)
    Vasoactive intestinal protein (VIP) (57)
    Interleukin-1 (19)
    Interleukin-1 receptor antagonist (19)
    Neuropepide Y (12,31)
    Polypeptide 7B2 (16)

Neurotransmitter receptors
    γ-Aminobutyric acid A (GABA$_A$) (15)

Enzymes
    Prohormone convertase 1 and 2 (PC1 and PC2) (16)
    Calcineurin, Ca^{2+}/calmodulin-dependent protein phosphatase (53)

Proliferation markers
    Proliferating cell nuclear antigen (56)

Dementia markers
    Tau protein kinase I/glycogen synthase kinase-3β (45)
    Tau-2 (27)
    Ubiquitine (27)
    β-Crystallin (27)
    β-Amyloid (precursor) protein (31,37)

Tumor markers
    MIB-1/Ki-67 (1,3,4,29,32,39,41,54)
    Medulloblastomas (56)

Endothelial markers
    CD34 (27)

CRITICAL FACTORS INFLUENCING THE QUALITY OF ANTIGEN RETRIEVAL

Temperature and Irradiation Time

High temperatures have been shown to be one of the critical factors in AR. Microwave irradiation produces oscillating electric fields that make small bipolar molecules, such as water, rotate. This movement produces heat in the tissue that is irradiated. The produced heat is the factor that is of importance for the retrieval of the antigen. Other sources of heat, such as an autoclave, pressure cooker, or conventional oven, have also been applied more or less successfully (28,38,44). The advantages of the microwave oven are the production of heat in a quick and reproducible way and the fact that the technique can be applied in a simple and relatively cheap household appliance. The time of irradiation mainly depends on the temperature used. Nearly all investigators have come to the conclusion that, in general, a temperature of at least 90°C is required to obtain good results. Cooking the tissue (sections) in a retrieval solution appears to be even better. When these high temperatures are used, an irradiation time of 10 to 15 minutes is usually sufficient (12,43).

Retrieval Solution and pH Values

The second very important factor in AR is the solution in which the technique is performed. In the beginning, it was thought that the chemical composition of the solution played an important role. When introducing the technique, Shi et al. (38) stated

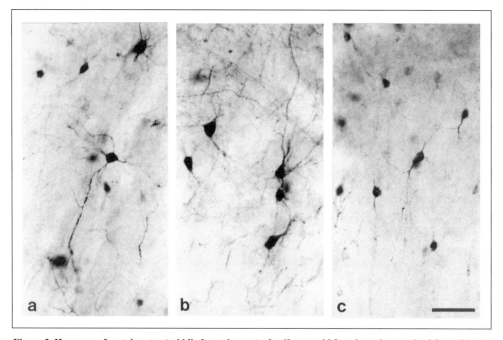

Figure 2. Human prefrontal cortex (middle frontal gyrus) of a 69-year-old female patient, stained for calbindin (a), parvalbumin (b), and calretinin (c) after 6 months of formaldehyde fixation and microwave pretreatment with TBS, pH 9.0. Without AR, calbindin and parvalbumin would only show somata and no dendrites, whereas calretinin would not stain at all. Scale bar = 50 μm.

that a solution containing heavy metal salts gave the best results. They recommended lead thiocyanate or zinc sulfate, which are rather toxic chemicals. Later, these toxic solutions were replaced by a solution of 4% aluminum chloride (4,11,30).

In determining which factor is of importance, it became clear that it is not the chemical composition, but the pH of the solution that plays a critical role (11). It became possible to use relatively harmless solutions like buffers. Many investigators, applying the technique on paraffin sections, got and still get satisfactory results using a citrate buffer of pH 6.0 (5,30,31,37,45,47,53–55). When we applied the technique on whole blocks of brain tissue before vibratome sectioning, we originally found that for our antigens (the nonphosphorylated part of the neurofilament and microtubule-associated protein), lower pH values were required. Optimal results were obtained using citrate buffers with pH values of 2.5 and 4.5, respectively (10). Because we wanted to perform both stainings on sections of the same tissue block, this turned out to be a very inconvenient finding. It was clear that one method that works for all or most antigens was desirable. Beckstead (3) and Shi et al. (40) found that the use of high pH values could be the solution for this problem. Many antigens were tested in a pH range from 1.0 to 10.0. Although some of the antigens only stained well after low pH treatment, and some others had an optimum at a more neutral pH level, it appeared that most antigens give good staining results when they are pretreated in a retrieval solution with a high pH of 8.0 to 10.0. These findings were later confirmed by us (12). Using Tris-buffered saline (TBS) with a pH of 9.0, it was possible to obtain very good staining results for different antigens in vibratome sections of the same MW-pretreated tissue block [phosphorylated and nonphosphorylated parts of the neurofilament and microtubule-associated protein-2 (Figure 1), calbindin, parvalbumin, calretinin (Figure 2), and neuropeptide Y (NPY)].

PROTOCOLS

The following protocols for antigen retrieval in brain tissue are according to Evers et al. (12,13).

Materials and Reagents

- Superfrost-plus slides
- Microwave oven
- 3-amino-propyltriethoxysilane
- Poly-L-lysine
- Tris
- Sodium chloride

Paraffin-Embedded Tissue

1. Attach the paraffin sections to slides coated with an adhesive such as 3-amino-propyltriethoxysilane or poly-L-lysine (Sigma, St. Louis, MO, USA). The use of Superfrost-plus slides (Menzel-Gläser, Braunschweich, Germany), which have a positive charge, is also recommended.
2. After deparaffination and hydration, place the slides in a plastic staining jar con-

taining approximately 200 mL of AR solution. TBS, pH 9.0 is recommended.

3. Put the jar in a microwave oven, which is set on full power (700 W). The retrieval solution is kept boiling for two cycles of 5 minutes. Between these boiling times the amount of evaporated solution can be replenished.
4. After heating, remove the jar from the microwave oven and allow it to cool for at least 15 minutes.
5. Rinse the slides in normal TBS, and proceed with the standard immunohistochemical staining procedure.

Nonembedded Tissue Slices before Vibratome Sectioning

1. Cut a tissue slice, approximately 5 mm thick, from the region of interest.
2. Rinse the slice with water (change regularly) for several hours to wash away the formaldehyde fixative.
3. Immerse the slice overnight in the AR solution (TBS, pH 9.0, is recommended).
4. The following morning, place the slice in a plastic container holding approximately 200 mL of retrieval solution, and place the container in a microwave oven for 10 to 15 minutes at full power (700 W), divided into two cycles of 5 or 7.5 minutes to check the fluid level. (We ourselves use a household microwave oven, Miele Electronics 696.)
5. After heating, remove the jar from the oven and allow it to cool for 15 minutes.
6. Rinse the slice in TBS, pH 7.6.
7. Start cutting the vibratome sections.
8. Proceed with the immunohistochemical staining procedure.

Free-Floating Vibratome Sections (Not Advised for Low-pH Retrieval Solutions)

1. Cut the vibratome sections, and collect them in plastic vials of 10 mL.
2. Wash in AR solution for 1 hour (TBS, pH 9.0, is recommended).
3. Cover the plastic vials with gauze caps, and fill them completely with retrieval solution.
4. Put the vials in a plastic container also filled with retrieval solution to prevent complete evaporation of the 10-mL solution in the vials during irradiation in the microwave oven.
5. Put the container in the microwave oven for 10 minutes at full power (700 W).
6. Allow the container to cool for 15 minutes.
7. Take the vials out of the container, and start the standard immunohistochemical staining procedure.

APPLICATIONS IN NEUROSCIENCE AND NEUROPATHOLOGY

Neuronal and Axonal Markers

In 1994, neuronal intermediate filament proteins were successfully retrieved by Yachnis and Trojanowski (56). They boiled their formalin- and Bouin's solution-fixed paraffin sections for 5 minutes in distilled water. Later in 1995, McQuaid et al. (27) used a citrate buffer, pH 7.8, as the retrieval solution for neurofilament proteins, and in 1997 Pileri et al. (32) were successful using Tris-HCl, pH 8.0, and EDTA + NaOH, pH 8.0, as retrieval solutions. In our study, we came to the conclusion that a buffer with a higher pH (TBS, pH 9.0) is more optimal for these proteins (12; Figure 1a). We (12) have also used TBS, pH 9.0, to retrieve microtubule-associated protein-2 (MAP-2; Figure 1b). In 1994, synaptophysin was successfully retrieved by Von Wasielewski et al. (54) using a citrate buffer of pH 6.0 as the AR solution. For this antigen, an AR solution with a high pH also proved to be very successful. McQuaid et al. (27) used a citrate buffer, pH 7.8. Shi et al. (41) were successful in using a Tris-HCl buffer, pH 9.5; when 5% urea was added to the Tris-HCl buffer (pH 9.2), the results were even better. Neuronal marker PGP9.5 was also retrieved by McQuaid et al. (27) using a citrate buffer, pH 7.8. A newly developed neuronal marker, NeuN, can be retrieved by citrate buffer, pH 6.0 (55). As far as we know from the literature, AR solutions with a high pH have not been tested on the last two antigens mentioned.

Glial Markers

Glial fibrillary acidic protein (GFAP) was retrieved for the first time by Yachnis and Trojanowski (56) using distilled water as the AR solution. In 1996, DeHart et al. (8) described the retrieval of GFAP in cryostat sections by using a 10 mmol/L citrate buffer + 0.04% Triton® X-100, pH 6.0, which had not been possible previously. An AR solution with a high pH of 9.0 has not yet been applied but might be important to study. This can be concluded from the work of McQuaid et al. (27). They stained for GFAP using a citrate buffer, pH 7.8, as the AR solution. Other glial and microglial markers that have been successfully retrieved are carbonic anhydrase type II, CD68, ferritin, and HLA-DR. These markers have all been retrieved by McQuaid et al. (27) using citrate buffer, pH 7.8, as the AR solution. The retrieval of HLA-DR was also described by Newman and Gentleman (31), who were successful using a citrate buffer of pH 6.0. AR solutions with a higher pH have not yet been tested for these antigens. Vimentin has been frequently studied in many postnatal tissues using a variety of AR solutions (pH 2.75–9.2). In all these studies, vimentin staining was improved (4,5,20,29,32,38,41,48,50,54). Vimentin has also been used in prenatal brain tissue to demonstrate early astrocytes. As far as we know from the literature, no AR for vimentin has been examined in prenatal brain tissue.

Calcium Binding Proteins

Our study (12; Figure 2) proves that an AR solution with a high pH (TBS, pH 9.0) gives an optimal result for the calcium binding proteins calbindin D 28-K, parvalbumin, and calretinin. Fritschy et al. (15) described a good result for the retrieval of calretinin using a citrate buffer of pH 4.5. It is not clear whether or not they also tested other buffers with different pHs on this antigen. Our personal findings are that the use of AR solutions with low pHs of 2.5 and 4.5 is less optimal for calbindin D 28-K and parvalbumin.

Neuropeptides

The intrinsic membrane sialoglycoprotein of the medial cisternae of the Golgi apparatus, MG-160, was successfully retrieved by Lucassen et al. (25) and Salehi et al. (35,36). They used a 1% zinc sulfate solution (pH 6.0) as the AR solution on paraffin sections of the hypothalamus of patients with Alzheimer's disease. The same procedure was also used by Zhou et al. (57) to retrieve vasopressin and vasoactive intestinal polypeptide. Whether or not these antigens can be retrieved with high-pH AR solutions has not yet been described. Interleukin-1 and Interleukin-1 receptor antagonist were retrieved by Huitinga et al. (19). They investigated the paraventricular nucleus and nucleus supraopticus of the hypothalamus in patients with multiple sclerosis. Staining of both antigens was clearly improved when the sections were pretreated with TBS, pH 7.6, as the AR solution. Polypeptide 7B2 was retrieved by Gabreëls et al. (16) by using a citrate buffer of pH 6.0. The effect of high pH AR solutions on the latter three antigens has also not yet been described. In 1997, NPY was retrieved in paraffin sections by Newman and Gentleman (31) using a 10 mmol/L citrate buffer of pH 6.0. We ourselves stained free-floating vibratome sections successfully for NPY without AR (9,52). After applying our AR technique (TBS, pH 9.0) on whole tissue blocks before vibratome sectioning, we found that NPY staining was also much more improved than without AR (12).

Neurotransmitter Receptors

Fritschy et al. (15) tested a variety of buffers (pH 2.2–9.5) as the AR solution, to find a way to retrieve the γ-aminobutyric acid $(GABA)_A$ receptor. Citrate buffer of pH 4.5 gave the best results when the free-floating cryostat sections were boiled in this solution for 150 to 180 seconds.

Enzymes

Calcineurin, a Ca^{2+}/calmodulin-dependent protein phosphatase (52), prohormone convertase 1 and 2 (16), and tau-protein kinase I/glycogen synthase kinase-3β (45) have been successfully retrieved using a citrate buffer of pH 6.0. Whether other AR solutions were tested for retrieval of these antigens was not mentioned.

Proliferation Markers

Proliferating cell nuclear antigen was retrieved by Yachnis and Trojanowski in 1994 (56) by boiling their formaldehyde- and Bouin's solution-fixed sections in distilled water. The effects of other AR solutions on this antigen have not yet been reported.

Dementia Markers

McQuaid et al. (27) tested a variety of AR solutions (unfortunately the pH was not mentioned for all the solutions) on three antigens, among which was tau-2. Citrate buffer of pH 7.8 and 0.01 mol/L urea (pH 6.0) gave the best results. They chose the citrate buffer in an attempt to retrieve many other antigens. They have also successfully retrieved ubiquitine and β-crystallin using a citrate buffer of pH 7.8 as the AR solution. Another antigen that is of interest in Alzheimer's disease research and that is often masked by prolonged fixation is β-amyloid protein. This antigen was retrieved by Sherriff et al. in 1994 (37) and by Newman and Gentleman in 1997 (31). Both groups used a citrate buffer of pH 6.0 as the AR solution. McQuaid et al. (27) tried to retrieve this antigen with a citrate buffer of pH 7.8. They were less successful and found that pretreatment with formic acid gave a far superior result. An AR solution with a high pH (pH 9.0) was not examined.

146

Tumor Markers

One of the most frequently investigated antigens in examinations of brain tumors is MIB-1/Ki-67. The earliest reports mentioned good results using a citrate buffer of pH 6.0 as the AR solution (1,3,4,29,54). Later on, buffers with a high pH, like Tris-HCl (3,41), urea (3,4,39), glycine-HCl (39), and EDTA + NaOH (32), all of which have a pH between 8.0 and 10.0, proved to be very useful as AR solutions for the MIB-1/Ki-67 antigen. Pediatric primitive neuroectodermal tumors, also called medulloblastomas, were successfully retrieved by Yachnis and Trojanowski (56) by boiling the sections in distilled water.

Endothelial Markers

The endothelial marker CD34 was also tested by McQuaid et al. (27). A citrate buffer of pH 7.8 and 0.01 mol/L urea (pH unknown) gave the best results.

In summary, citrate buffers of pHs 6.0 and 7.8 have proved to be AR solutions in which many antigens can be retrieved, but certainly not all antigens. Unfortunately, good comparisons between different AR solutions have only been made in a few reports. It is therefore possible that many of the antigens retrieved by using citrate buffers can also be retrieved (perhaps even better) by buffers with a high pH of about 9.0. The molarity of the solution, which varies between 0.01 and 0.1 mol/L, does not seem to be that important. The optimal irradiation time lies between 5 and 15 minutes. This may depend on the temperature (11), but Ainley and Ironside (1) stated that over-irradiation may destroy many epitopes and may induce nonspecific staining. The most successful results are obtained by an irradiation time of 2×5 minutes for paraffin sections and 2×7.5 minutes for tissue blocks.

CONCLUDING REMARKS

In the past 7 years, much good work has been done in an attempt to optimize the MW-AR technique. Unfortunately, as described above, there is still no optimal method to retrieve all antigens in (brain) tissue that has been fixed in formaldehyde for too long. Although Beckstead (3), Pileri et al. (32), Shi et al. (40), and we ourselves (12) recommend the use of a solution with a high pH, this does not mean that, if the result with a certain antigen is negative, MW-AR is impossible. Starting AR with a buffer of pH 9.0 gives the best chance of a good result. However, if the result is negative, it is advisable to use a test battery like the one decribed by Shi et al. (42,43). With this test battery, three temperature levels (mid-high, high, and super-high) are combined with three pH levels (low, neutral, and high). Using this test, one should keep in mind that the lower temperatures might call for longer irradiation times.

A problem that initially occurred when applying the MW-AR technique to free-floating vibratome sections was shrinkage and curling of the sections (10). This made it impossible to get the sections homogeneously stained, and presented problems when they were mounted onto glass slides afterward. The problem was solved by applying the MW-AR technique to whole tissue blocks before sectioning. However, if more than one antigen has to be retrieved, and it is known that the antigens require different AR procedures, a problem still exists. Recently, it appeared that this problem only occurs when an AR solution with a low pH is used. If the technique is applied to free-floating sections in a more neutral (45) or basic environment (authors' unpublished observations), hardly any problems occur with regard to shrinkage and curling of the sections.

Although false-positive reactions after MW treatment have never been described, it is recommended to include a negative control section (omitting the first antibody) and a section of a similar tissue type that shows the optimal staining after a sufficient short fixation period.

An additional advantage of microwaving is that endogeneous peroxidase reactivity is blocked by the microwave pretreatment, which renders the blocking step with hydrogen peroxide superfluous. Moreover, Lan et al. (23) noted that MW treatment between sequential rounds of staining denatures bound antibody molecules, thereby completely blocking cross-reactivity. This makes it possible to perform double staining while using primary antibodies raised in the same species.

MW-AR often diminishes background staining and allows the use of higher dilutions of primary antibodies (see examples in Reference 12).

Although high-tech laboratory microwave ovens that allow exact control over temperature, power, etc., have now been specially developed, it is also possible to obtain very good results using a relatively simple and cheap household microwave oven. However, it is advisable to use an oven with a turning table. In most microwave ovens, so-called hot and cold spots can be found. These spots may have a great influence on the results of the technique. This problem is resolved by using an oven with a turning table.

ACKNOWLEDGMENTS

The authors would like to thank Mr. G. van der Meulen for his photographic assistance and Ms. O. Pach for correcting the English.

REFERENCES

1. **Ainley, C.D. and J.W. Ironside.** 1994. Microwave technology in diagnostic neuropathology. J. Neurosci. Methods *55*:183-190.
2. **Battifora, H. and M. Kopinski.** 1986. The influence of protease digestion and duration of fixation on the immunostaining of keratins. J. Histochem. Cytochem. *34*:1095-1100.
3. **Beckstead, J.H.** 1994. Improved antigen retrieval in formalin-fixed, paraffin-embedded tissues. Appl. Immunohistochem. 2:274-281.
4. **Cattoretti, G., S. Pileri, C. Parravicini, M.H.G. Becker, S. Poggi, C. Bifulco, G. Key, L. d'Amato, E. Sabattini, E. Feudale et al.** 1993. Antigen unmasking on formalin-fixed, paraffin-embedded tissue sections. J. Pathol. *171*:83-98.
5. **Cattoretti, G. and A.J.H. Suurmeijer.** 1995. Antigen unmasking on formalin-fixed paraffin-embedded tissues using microwaves: a review. Adv. Anat. Pathol. 2:2-9.
6. **Costa, P.P., B. Jacobsson, V.P. Collins, and P. Biberfeld.** 1986. Unmasking antigens determinants in amyloid. J. Histochem. Cytochem. *34*:1683-1685.
7. **Dapson, W.D.** 1993. Fixation for the 1990's: a review of needs and accomplishments. Biotech. Histochem. *68*:75-82.
8. **DeHart, B.W., R.K. Kan, and J.R. Day.** 1996. Microwave superheating enhances immunocytochemistry in the freshly frozen rat brain. Neuroreport 7:2691-2694.
9. **Delalle, I., P. Evers, I. Kostović, and H.B.M. Uylings.** 1997. Laminar distribution of neuropeptide Y-immunoreactive neurons in human prefrontal cortex during development. J. Comp. Neurol. 379:515-522.
10. **Evers, P. and H.B.M. Uylings.** 1994. Effects of microwave pretreatment on immunocytochemical staining of vibratome sections and tissue blocks of human cerebral cortex stored in formaldehyde fixative for long periods. J. Neurosci. Methods *55*:163-172.
11. **Evers, P. and H.B.M. Uylings.** 1994. Microwave-stimulated antigen retrieval is pH and temperature dependent. J. Histochem. Cytochem. *42*:1555-1563.

12. Evers, P. and H.B.M. Uylings. 1997. An optimal antigen retrieval method suitable for different antibodies on human brain tissue stored for several years in formaldehyde fixative. J. Neurosci. Methods 72:197-207.

13. Evers, P., H.B.M. Uylings, and A.J.H. Suurmeijer. 1998. Antigen retrieval in formaldehyde-fixed human brain tissue. Methods 15:133-140.

14. Fox, C.H., F.B. Johnson, J. Whiting, and P.P. Roller. 1985. Formaldehyde fixation. J. Histochem. Cytochem. 33:845-853.

15. Fritschy, J-M., O. Weinmann, A. Wenzel, and D. Benke. 1998. Synapse-specific localization of NMDA and GABA_A receptor subunits revealed by antigen-retrieval immunohistochemistry. J. Comp. Neurol. 390:194-210.

16. Gabreëls, B.A.Th.F., D.F. Swaab, D.P.V. de Kleijn, N.G. Seidah, J.-W. van de Loo, W.J.M. van de Ven, G.J.M. Martens, and F.W. van Leeuwen. 1998. Attenuation of the polypeptide 7B2, prohormone convertase PC2 and vasopressin in the hypothalamus of some Prader-Willi patients: indications for a processing defect. J. Clin. Endocrinol. Metab. 83:591-599.

17. Hazelbag, H.M., L.J.C.M. v.d. Broek, E.B.L. van Dorst, G.J.A. Offerhaus, G.J. Fleuren, and P.C.W. Hogendoorn. 1995. Immunostaining of chain-specific keratins on formalin-fixed, paraffin-embedded tissues: a comparison of various antigen retrieval systems using microwave heating and proteolytic pre-treatments. J. Histochem. Cytochem. 43:429-437.

18. Helander, K.G. 1994. Kinetic studies of formaldehyde binding in tissue. Biotech. Histochem. 69:177-179.

19. Huitinga, I., M.J.F. van der Cammen, B. Fisser, and D.F. Swaab. 1998. Detectie van cytokines in paraffine-ingebed formaline-gefixeerd hersenweefsel van multiple sclerose patienten. Histotech. Cyto-visie 5:19-22.

20. Igarashi, H., H. Sugimura, K. Maruyama, Y. Kitayama, I. Ohta, M. Suzuki, M. Tanaka, Y. Dobashi, and I. Kino. 1994. Alteration of immunoreactivity by hydrated autoclaving, microwave treatment, and simple heating of paraffin-embedded tissue sections. APMIS 102:295-307.

21. Kitamoto, T., K. Ogomori, J. Tateishi, and S.B. Prusiner. 1987. Formic acid pretreatment enhances immunostaining of cerebral and systemic amyloids. Lab. Invest. 57:230-236.

22. Kwaspen, F., F. Smedts, J. Blom, A. Pronk, M.J. Kok, M. van Dijk, and F. Ramaekers. 1995. Periodic acid as a nonenzymatic enhancement technique for the detection of cytokeratin immunoreactivity in routinely processed carcinomas. Appl. Immunohistochem. 3:54-63.

23. Lan, H.Y., W. Mu, D.J. Nikolic-Paterson, and R.C. Atkins. 1995. A novel, simple, reliable and sensitive method for multiple immunoenzyme staining: use of microwave oven heating to block antibody crossreactivity and retrieve antigens. J. Histochem. Cytochem. 43:97-102.

24. Lan, H.Y., W. Mu, Y.Y. Ng, D.J. Nikolic-Paterson, and R.C. Atkins. 1996. A simple, reliable, and sensitive method for nonradioactive in situ hybridization: use of microwave heating to improve hybridization efficiency and preserve tissue morphology. J. Histochem. Cytochem. 44:281-287.

25. Lucassen, P.J., R. Ravid, N.K. Gonatas, and D.F. Swaab. 1993. Activation of the human supraoptic and paraventricular nucleus neurons with aging and in Alzheimer's disease as judged from increasing size of the Golgi apparatus. Brain Res. 632:105-113.

26. Mason, J.T. and T.J. O'Leary. 1991. Effects of formaldehyde fixation on protein secondary structure: a calorimetric and infrared spectroscopic investigation. J. Histochem. Cytochem. 39:225-229.

27. McQuaid, S., R. McConnell, J. McMahon, and B. Herron. 1995. Microwave antigen retrieval for immunocytochemistry on formalin-fixed, paraffin-embedded post mortem CNS tissue. J. Pathol. 176:207-216.

28. Miller, R.T. and C. Estron. 1995. Heat-induced epitope retrieval with a pressure cooker-suggestions for optimal use. Appl. Immunohistochem. 3:190-193.

29. Momose, H., P. Mehta, and H. Battifora. 1993. Antigen retrieval by microwave irradiation in lead thiocyanate. Appl. Immunohistochem. 1:77-82.

30. Munakata, S. and J.B. Hendricks. 1993. Effect of fixation time and microwave oven heating time on retrieval of the Ki-67 antigen from paraffin-embedded tissue. J. Histochem. Cytochem. 41:1241-1246.

31. Newman, S.J. and S.M. Gentleman. 1997. Microwave antigen retrieval in formaldehyde-fixed human brain tissue, p. 145-152. In R.C. Rayne (Ed.), Methods in Molecular Biology, Vol. 72. Neurotransmitter Methods. Humana Press, Totowa, NJ.

32. Pileri, S.A., G. Roncador, C. Ceccarelli, M. Piccioli, A. Briskomatis, E. Sabattini, S. Ascani, D. Santini, P.P. Piccaluga, O. Leone et al. 1997. Antigen retrieval techniques in immunohistochemistry: comparison of different methods. J. Pathol. 183:116-123.

33. Podkletnova, I. and H. Alho. 1993. Ultrasound-amplified immunohistochemistry. J. Histochem. Cytochem. 41:51-56.

34. Puchtler, H. and S.N. Meloan. 1985. On the chemistry of formaldehyde fixation and its effects on immunohistochemical reactions. Histochemistry 82:201-204.

35. Salehi, A., P.J. Lucassen, C.W. Pool, R. Ravid, N.K. Gonatas, and D.F. Swaab. 1994. Decreased neuronal activity in the nucleus basalis of Meynert in Alzheimer's disease as suggested by the size of the Golgi apparatus. Neuroscience 59:871-880.

36. Salehi, A., R. Ravid, N.K. Gonatas, and D.F. Swaab. 1995. Decreased activity of hippocampal neurons in Alzheimer's disease is not related to the presence of neurofibrillary tangles. J. Neuropathol. Exp. Neurol. 54:704-709.

37. Sherriff, F.E., L.R. Bridges and P. Jackson. 1994. Microwave antigen retrieval of b-amyloid precursor protein immunoreactivity. Neuroreport 5:1085-1088.

38. **Shi, S.-R., M.E. Key, and K.L. Kalra.** 1991. Antigen retrieval in formalin-fixed, paraffin-embedded tissues: an enhancement method for immunohistochemical staining based on microwave oven heating of tissue sections. J. Histochem. Cytochem. *39*:741-748.

39. **Shi, S.-R., B. Chaiwun, L. Young, A. Imam, R.J. Cote, and C.R. Taylor.** 1994. Antigen retrieval using pH 3.5 glycine-HCl buffer or urea solution for immunohistochemical localization of Ki-67. Biotech. Histochem. *69*:213-215.

40. **Shi, S.-R., S.A. Imam, L. Young, R.J. Cote, and C.R. Taylor.** 1995. Antigen retrieval immunohistochemistry under the influence of pH using monoclonal antibodies. J. Histochem. Cytochem. *43*:193-201.

41. **Shi, S.-R., R.J. Cote, L. Young, S.A. Imam, and C.R. Taylor.** 1996. Use of pH 9.5 Tris-HCl buffer containing 5% Urea for antigen retrieval immunohistochemistry. Biotech. Histochem. *71*:190-196.

42. **Shi, S.-R., R.J. Cote, C. Yang, C. Chen, H.-J. Xu, W.F. Benedict, and C.R. Taylor.** 1996. Development of an optimal protocol for antigen retrieval: a "test battery" approach exemplified with with reference to the staining of retinoblastoma protein (pRB) in formalin-fixed paraffin sections. J. Pathol. *179*:347-352.

43. **Shi, S.-R., R.J. Cote, and C.R. Taylor.** 1997. Antigen retrieval immunohistochemistry: past, present, and future. J. Histochem. Cytochem. *45*:327-343.

44. **Shin, R-W., T. Iwaki, T. Kitamoto, and J. Tateishi.** 1991. Hydrated autoclave pretreatment enhances TAU immunoreactivity in formalin-fixed normal and Alzheimer's disease brain tissues. Lab. Invest. *64*:693-702.

45. **Shiurba, R.A., E.T. Spooner, K. Ishiguro, M. Takahashi, R. Yoshida, T.R. Wheelock, K. Imahori, A.M. Cataldo, and R.A. Nixon.** 1998. Immunocytochemistry of formalin-fixed human brain tissues: microwave irradiation of free-floating sections. Brain Res. Prot. *2*:109-119.

46. **Sibony, M., F. Commo, P. Callard, and J.-M. Gasc.** 1995. Enhancement of mRNA in situ hybridization signal by microwave heating. Lab. Invest. *73*:586-591.

47. **Sträter, J., A.R. Günthert, S. Brüderlein, and P. Möller.** 1995. Microwave irradiation of paraffin-embedded tissue sensitizes the TUNEL method for in situ detection of apoptotic cells. Histochemistry *103*:157-160.

48. **Suurmeijer, A.J.H. and M.E. Boon.** 1993. Optimizing keratin and vimentin retrieval in formalin-fixed, paraffin-embedded tissue with the use of heat and metal salts. Appl. Immunohistochem. *1*:143-148.

49. **Taylor, C.R., S.-R. Shi, B. Chaiwun, L. Young, S.A. Imam, and R.J. Cote.** 1994. Strategies for improving the immunohistochemical staining of various intranuclear prognostic markers in formalin-paraffin sections. Hum. Pathol. *25*:263-270.

50. **Taylor, C.R., S.-R. Shi, C. Chen, L. Young, C. Yang, and R.J. Cote.** 1996. Comparative study of antigen retrieval heating methods: microwave, microwave and pressure cooker, autoclave, and steamer. Biotech. Histochem. *71*:263-270.

51. **Taylor, C.R., S.-R. Shi, and R.J. Cote.** 1996. Antigen retrieval for immunohistochemistry. Status and need for greater standardization. Appl. Immunohistochem. *4*:144-166.

52. **Uylings, H.B.M. and I. Delalle.** 1997. Morphology of neuropeptide Y-immunoreactive neurons and fibers in human prefrontal cortex during prenatal and postnatal development. J. Comp. Neurol. *379*:523-540.

53. **Usuda, N., H. Arai, H. Sasaki, T. Hanai, T. Nagata, T. Muramatsu, R.L. Kinkaid, and S. Higuchi.** 1996. Differential subcellular localization of neural isoforms of the catalytic subunit of calmodulin-dependent protein phosphatase (calcineurin) in central nervous system neurons: imunohistochemistry on formalin-fixed paraffin sections employing antigen retrieval by microwave irradiation. J. Histochem. Cytochem. *44*:13-18.

54. **Von Wasielewski, R., M. Werner, M. Nolte, L. Wilkens, and A. Georgii.** 1994. Effects of antigen retrieval by microwave heating in formalin-fixed tissue sections on a broad panel of antibodies. Histochemistry *102*:165-172.

55. **Wolf, H.K., R. Buslei, R. Schmidt-Kastner, P.K. Schmidt-Kastner, T. Pietsch, O.D. Wiestler, and I. Blümcke.** 1996. NeuN: a useful neuronal marker for diagnostic histopathology. J. Histochem. Cytochem. *44*:1167-1171.

56. **Yachnis, A.T. and J.Q. Trojanowski.** 1994. Studies of childhood brain tumors using immunohistochemistry and microwave technology: methodological considerations. J. Neurosci. Methods *55*:191-200.

57. **Zhou, J.-N., M.A. Hofman, and D.F. Swaab.** 1996. Morphometric analysis of vasopressin and vasoactive intestinal polypeptide neurons in the human suprachiasmatic nucleus: influence of microwave treatment. Brain Res. *742*:334-338.

Section III

Application of Antigen Retrieval Technique in Pathology

Antigen Retrieval for Detection of Steroid Hormone Receptors

9

Louis P. Pertschuk and Constantine A. Axiotis

Department of Pathology, State University of New York Health Science Center at Brooklyn and the Kings County Hospital Center, Brooklyn, NY, USA

INTRODUCTION

For many years pathologists and clinicians have been searching for parameters to better prognosticate disease course in women with early breast cancer. Only a few recognized and valid prognostic markers exist. These include stage of disease and tumor grade. The stage of disease is dependent on tumor size and extent of lymph node involvement. The percentage of tumor cells in S-phase and steroid hormone receptor measurements as determined by ligand-binding assays are also recognized prognostic markers. Many of the other proposed prognostic tests have either failed to perform accurately or remain controversial. The only assays that foretell whether or not the patient will respond to hormone therapies are steroid hormone receptor studies.

ANTIGEN RETRIEVAL FOR ESTROGEN RECEPTORS

Historical Perspective

Following the report by Beatson (4) that a number of women with advanced breast cancer showed a significant amelioration of symptoms after ovariectomy, it was discovered, many years later, that some tumors contained an estrogen binding protein designated estrophilin or estrogen receptor (ER), while other tumors did not (13,42). This was of major clinical importance since the presence of ER appeared to correlate with response to endocrine therapies. This would indicate to the clinician that the primary therapeutic modality should be hormonal rather than chemical.

Initially, ER determinations were made by ligand-binding assays performed on

Antigen Retrieval Techniques
Edited by Shan-Rong Shi, Jiang Gu, and Clive R. Taylor
©2000 Eaton Publishing, Natick, MA

cytosol derived from tumor homogenates. Using such methods, i.e., the dextran-coated charcoal (DCC) and sucrose gradient assay (SGA), it was found that about 70% of breast cancer patients have neoplasms containing ER and that approximately 70% of the latter tumors show a significant, measurable response to hormonal therapies. Unfortunately 30% of ER-positive patients do not respond to such therapies. In addition, 85% to 90% of ER-negative women evidence disease progression when treated with hormones (reviewed in Reference 15). Most physicians and biochemists considered DCC/SGA to be the ultimate gold standard for measuring ER, since initial findings were made with these methods. Furthermore, results obtained by Scatchard plot analysis expressed in fmoles/mg protein were alluring, suggesting great accuracy.

The Estrogen Receptor

The gene coding for ER is complex and includes more than 140 kb of DNA and 8 exons. It consists of a DNA binding domain, an N-terminal domain, and a hormone-dependent COOH domain. A number of modified ERs have been described, including truncations, point mutations, polymorphisms, and abnormal or alternative splicing (reviewed in References 8 and 17). Such changes may result in a nonfunctioning molecule responsible for some ER-positive patients who fail endocrine therapies.

The mechanism whereby estrogen is able to exert its effects is now well known. The steroid is small and lipid soluble and is thus able to pass freely through cell membranes, across the cytoplasm (perhaps with the help of heat shock proteins), and into the nucleus, where it binds to its receptor. There it forms a dimer and becomes activated. The activated molecule binds to DNA sites adjacent to target genes, which are either stimulated or inhibited. Transcription and eventual alterations in cell growth and function follow (reviewed in Reference 43).

Disadvantages of Ligand-Binding Assay Procedures

Since all ligand-binding assays are performed on tissue homogenates, no assays can evaluate certain parameters likely to be of prognostic importance. Such parameters include tumor cell receptor heterogeneity and the contribution to the total ER content made by benign mammary tissue components inadvertently included in the specimen submitted. The former parameter is of importance in prognosticating endocrine response, as is shown by the fact that patients with tumors ER positive by DCC yet containing less than 10% positive cells by histochemistry fail hormonal treatment, while the latter may be responsible for falsely positive biochemical results. Heterogeneity is also evident in processed tissue sections studied by various image analysis systems (reviewed in Reference 38), and, as we detail below, staining homogeneity (as determined by imaging) is of great importance in predicting endocrine response in processed frozen sections. There is no current biochemical equivalent to image analysis for assessing ER hererogeneity.

Early Histochemical and Immunohistochemical Methods

In an attempt to improve on ligand-binding procedures, a number of histochemical methods were devised using various ligands and antiestrogen antibodies (reviewed in Reference 21). These methods never gained acceptance. However, following the development of highly specific antiestrophilin antibodies by Geoffrey Greene and his associates (10,11,14), controversy concerning histochemical methods ceased. One of these antibodies, H222Spγ (H222), recognizes an epitope near the binding site of the N-terminal domain of ER. H222 was commercialized by Abbott Laboratories (North Chicago, IL, USA) and successfully utilized by numerous workers in correlative biochemical studies with endocrine response (reviewed in References 2 and 26). This ER immunocytochemical assay was abbreviated ER-ICA.

Estrogen Receptor Immunocytochemical Assay on Frozen Sections

Our laboratory was fortunate to have developed a close working relationship with Dr. Greene at the Ben May Institute for Cancer Research, University of Chicago, as well as with a premier receptor assay laboratory, under the direction of the late William McGuire at the University of Texas Health Science Center at San Antonio. As a consequence, we had the opportunity to perform a large number of assays using ER-ICA and to obtain biochemical and clinical correlations with ER by DCC prior to commercialization of the assay (18,20).

Another monoclonal anti-ER antibody developed by Dr. Greene was designated D75P3 (D75). This antibody recognizes a different epitope on the N-terminal domain of ER (10,11). In a comparison of results between H222 and D75 in over 230 specimens, we noted significant differences (unpublished study). There was concordance in only 76% of cases. D75 failed to detect antigen in 15% of cases positive with H222, and H222 failed to detect antigen in 26% of cases positive with D75. It was obvious that since each antibody detected a different epitope, and with such discordant results, one could anticipate that there would be differences in the ability of each to prognosticate endocrine response. In our hands, H222 gave the best predictive information when frozen tissue was examined. However, D75 had the advantage of working quite well on paraffin sections while H222 did not (6,40).

Image Analysis and Estrogen Receptor Immunocytochemical Assay

There was concern because many ER-ICA-positive cases failed endocrine therapy. It was therefore decided to examine the sections with a sophisticated image analysis system to see whether such methods could throw light on this problem. In collaboration with Dr. Robert J. Sklarew at the Imaging Laboratories of the New York Medical College (Valhalla, NY), we investigated the value of image analysis in the detection of ER by H222 (36–38). Several patterns of ER positivity were identified. In summary, cases with multiple and skewed ER peaks were found most likely to fail endocrine therapy, whereas patients with monoclonal ER peaks were significantly more likely to respond. It is hypothesized that monoclonal peaks represent an intact and functional ER whereas skewed curves or multiple peaks exemplify altered or mutant forms of ER. In the latter patients the antigenic epitopes, still present, resulted in a positive immunocytochemical assay, but the receptor itself was nonfunctional. Many other workers have utilized image analysis to quantify breast cancer ER and progesterone receptor (PgR) (reviewed in Reference 38), but their methodologies were controversial, with nearly all limiting their study to comparisons with other methods of assay rather than with endocrine response.

Estrogen Receptor Detection in Routinely Prepared Tissue

A major drawback to ER-ICA was the requirement that the substrate be freshly frozen. Many community hospitals do not possess the equipment needed for flash freezing and ultracold storage. Furthermore, if tissue is sent to a reference center for either biochemical or histochemical studies, there is the danger of an in-transit thaw. ER is a temperature-sensitive protein, so much so that freshly cut cryostat sections become ER negative if exposed to ambient temperatures for more than 10 seconds prior to fixation. In addition, as diagnostic techniques improve and smaller and smaller tumors are excised, there often is insufficient tissue left for specialized studies after histopathologic examination is complete. The ability to study the very same paraffin block of tissue as is utilized for diagnosis (for ER and other tumor markers) is of great importance in such cases. Also, if patients originally diagnosed with breast cancer before the era of steroid receptor assay developed a recurrence or metastasis, there was no way to determine receptor content unless the archival tissue block could be utilized.

Because of these disadvantages, a number of workers sought ways to perform ER immunohistochemistry on formalin-fixed, paraffin-embedded sections. Varying degrees of success were encountered, often employing enzymatic pretreatment of the section before processing (reviewed in Reference 21). A major problem was that H222 did not work very well on routinely processed tissue. Furthermore, the processing methods of hospitals vary considerably, especially as to times of tissue fixation. In addition, different batches of the various enzymes employed for pretreatment differed markedly in their enzymatic activity. As a consequence, what worked well in one author's laboratory could not be readily reproduced in others.

Antigen Retrieval

Among the significant contributions resulting from antigen retrieval techniques (and having a direct bearing on patient care) are those permitting the detection of steroid hormone receptors in tumor tissue from women with breast cancer. At the time antigen retrieval (AR) methods were first reported (33), the state of affairs in regard to immunohistochemical ER assay procedures was as described above, i.e., the need for frozen specimens as the assay substrate was paramount.

In 1993, the first report was published utilizing antigen retrieval for the immunodetection of ER (3,12). This was followed by several papers detailing similar procedures (9,30,32,39). However, in only one (9) were assay results correlated with hormone response, although all reported concordance with DCC and/or with ER-ICA.

Although concordance of assay results between various methods is necessary, more important correlations had to be made with clinical endocrine response and disease-free interval. After all, these were the reasons for developing steroid hormone receptor assays in the first place. Therefore, following publication of antigen retrieval methods, samples of breast cancer from a group of 74 women were assayed in our laboratory using the newly described method (24). These specimens, collected over the years, were from patients with advanced disease and documented endocrine response and initially had been assayed by both DCC and ER-ICA. Paraffin sections from archival blocks were dewaxed and subjected to high-intensity microwaves for 15 minutes in citrate buffer (pH 6.0) followed by standard streptavidin-biotin complex (ABC) processing. Initially we used the antibody ER1D5 (Dako, Carpenteria, CA, USA). ER1D5 is a mouse immunoglobulin G1 monoclonal antibody that reacts with the A/B region of the N-terminal domain of ER and with the 67-kd polypeptide ER chain obtained by transformation of *Escherichia coli* and transfection with COS cells containing plasmid vectors expressing ER (3). Later, we reexamined this series of cases using AR and ER88

(BioGenex, San Ramon, CA, USA), and this time employed an Optimax automated cell staining system (BioGenex). ER88 is an anti-ER antibody that reacts with native 68-kd human ER as assessed by Western blot and immunoprecipitation analyses.

A comparison of ER by DCC, ER-ICA, (H222), ER1D5, and ER88 in relation to prediction of endocrine response in this series of 74 patients may be summarized as follows: ER1D5 gave the best prognostic information ($P = 0.0001$), followed by ER-ICA ($P = 0.001$), and ER88 ($P = 0.004$), while ER by DCC was not prognostic ($P = 0.99$).

The use of automation for ER immunohistochemical processing provides an opportunity for standardization of the assay procedure, allowing comparison of results between institutions. Furthermore, it makes little difference whether the specimen is fixed for 4 hours or for 48 hours, since the AR technique permits identification of ER under both circumstances. It also appears that there is little need for routine ER image analysis when ER1D5 or ER88 is employed, although this requires further investigation as it is still possible that image analysis may fine tune these assays.

During comparative studies of paraffin-embedded and frozen sections, a number of curiosities were noted. Some specimens that were ER positive when frozen were negative after fixation, while others, initially positive, became ER negative. Several explanations for these variations can be considered. In the first place, different antibodies were employed that recognize different ER epitopes. Furthermore, since steroid receptors are temperature sensitive, it is possible that a delay between removal from the patient and freezing could result in receptor loss. On the other hand, immediate placing of the specimen in formalin, as is commonly done in securing biopsy specimens, prevents receptor degradation. Repeated freeze-thawing of specimens might also have resulted in antigen loss and a negative ER-ICA, as could tumor cell ER heterogeneity. It is of more than usual interest that most of the patients who were ER positive with ER-ICA and DCC, yet negative with ER1D5, failed hormonal therapy. These findings suggest that the epitope targets of the latter antibody are of greater importance in modulating endocrine response than the target of H222 or the biochemical measurement of specific binding alone.

Allred (2) and his colleagues have obtained similar results using antigen retrieval and another anti-ER antibody (6F11) on routinely processed specimens. In a study of 1900 breast cancer cases, they noted a 15% difference in disease-free survival at 5 years when the specimen was ER positive. In a subset of 500 patients treated hormonally, this difference increased to 25%. In another study originating in the Mayo Clinic, 316 women with breast cancer were evaluated with antigen retrieval and ER1D5, and significant concordance was found with both disease-free interval and overall survival (1).

Current Status of Estrogen Receptor Immunohistochemistry

A note of caution must be injected at this point, as has been noted by several workers (2,7,26). In spite of the above studies and the fact that more than 1000 breast cancer patients have been reported for whom ER immunohistochemistry has been correlated with endocrine response (reviewed in References 2 and 26), these studies involved different antibodies, substrates, and techniques. Some authors used frozen or paraffin-embedded sections, while others utilized aspirated cells, tumor imprints, or scrapings. Furthermore, the antibodies employed included H222, H226, D75, ER1D5, and 6F11, among others. As a consequence, no standard acceptable way to perform the assay is available at this time, nor is it clear which antibody, or method, provides the best prognostic information. In addition, the number of cases available cannot compare with the thousands of cases studied by ligand-binding assays. A great deal more work needs to be done before ER immunohistochemistry can join the ranks of the few accepted prognostic breast cancer markers. This should not be a problem since retrospective study of archival tissue with antigen retrieval methods is now possible.

Estrogen Receptor Immunocytochemistry in Endometrial Carcinoma

ER immunohistochemistry is also of importance in endometrial carcinoma, another estrogen-dependent tumor. In this neoplasm, the problems of the biochemists are even more complicated than in breast cancer, since myometrium, hyperplastic and normal endometrial glands, and endometrial stroma may all contain receptor proteins in addition to tumor. This, of course, is no problem for the immunohistopathologist viewing a tissue section who can readily distinguish these various components. In a study of 78 cases of endometrial carcinoma (in frozen section), a positive ER correlated significantly with DCC, but only ER-ICA was found to be predictive of survival (25).

ANTIGEN RETRIEVAL AND PROGESTERONE RECEPTORS

Progesterone Receptor Immunohistochemistry in Breast Cancer

Human PgR is composed of A and B fragments. Some of the initial anti-PgR antibodies recognized only one of these fragments. Since PgR is coded for by a functional ER, it was felt that ER/PgR-positive patients should stand a better chance of responding to endocrine therapies than women with ER-positive/PgR-negative cancers. Using ligand-binding techniques, this was indeed found to be the case. More importantly, PgR-positive patients had a significantly longer disease-free interval after surgery and a better overall survival (reviewed in Reference 16).

Following the development of anti-ER antibodies, Greene and his colleagues raised several antibodies against PgR. Two such monoclonals, designated KD 68 and JZB 39, recognize both A and B PgR subunits (27).

In our hands, in over 600 cases, only 45% of breast cancer patients are PgR positive. Furthermore, although cases that are ER/PgR positive by immunohistochemistry respond to endocrine therapies more often than those that are ER positive/PgR negative, this is not of statistical significance. However, PgR positivity with JZB 39 was associated with a significantly longer disease-free interval and overall survival (19,20). Similar results were obtained with KD 68 in a smaller number of cases, with the latter antibody possessing greater specificity and sensitivity in relation to endocrine response.

In comparing results of KD 68 and JZB 39 in frozen breast cancer sections, differences were again apparent. This was not surprising as each antibody recognizes a separate epitope on the receptor molecule. In 433 cases, there was a variance in positivity of 11%. JZB 39 was positive in 13 cases negative with KD 68, while KD 68 was positive in 34 cases negative with JZB. This indicates that both epitopes are not always available for detection and that each antibody might have different prognostic ability. However, KD 68 has the distinct advantage of performing very well on formalin-fixed, paraffin-embedded sections without any need for special pretreatment or for AR. Therefore, results with KD 68 in frozen tissue can be safely extrapolated to paraffin-embedded sections.

Progesterone Receptor in Endometrial Carcinoma

We studied a group of women with endometrial carcinoma using KD 68 without any pretreatment of the (paraffin-embedded) tissue sections and found a good correlation with PgR by DCC/SGA (5). Unfortunately, KD 68, which is available in kit form (Abbott, No. Chicago, IL, USA), is presently too expensive for routine use in the clinical laboratory.

Using antigen retrieval, we have employed two other anti-PgR antibodies in paraffin-embedded sections that react with both the A and B subunits of PgR: PR 88 (Bio-Genex) and NCL-PGR (clone 1A6; Novocastra, Newcastle-upon-Tyne, UK). Processing with 1A6 was performed manually while the Optimax automated processor was used for PR 88. PR88 is said to react with purified human PgR in enzyme-linked immunosorbent assay (ELISA) and Western blot analyses.

Once again, several cases that were PgR positive in frozen section remained positive in paraffin, and some cases initially positive were negative after fixation. It is likely that the same explanations given for ER differences apply to the PgR variations.

Neither 1A6 nor PR 88 appears to be of value, in our hands, in prognosticating results of endocrine therapy in the cases studied to date. In the 74 women with breast cancer and documented endocrine response noted above, PgR positivity with either antibody only minimally improved the prognosis of successful endocrine response in ER-positive cases ($P > 0.18$) and when PgR results were analyzed alone, no significant correlation was found ($P = 0.22$). This is in sharp contrast to the predictive improvement apparent with ER1D5 in paraffin.

Allred (2) and his co-workers also employed 1A6 in a study of their 1900 breast cancer cases; in the subset treated hormonally, they noted a difference in survival of 25%. Currently, we are looking to see whether PR 88 is of value in predicting disease-free interval and overall survival utilizing archival paraffin blocks from 100 women presenting with stage I and II disease and followed for up to 20 years.

Current Status of Progesterone Receptor Immunohistochemistry

The available published information regarding PgR immunohistochemistry has been reviewed recently (2,26). In general, significantly less information is available about PgR than about ER. It is obvious that a great deal more work needs to be done before we know which antibody gives the best prognostic information and the ideal way to perform the assay in paraffin sections. It is apparent that PgR immunohistochemistry in paraffin cannot, as yet, be an accepted prognostic test for breast cancer.

ANTIGEN RETRIEVAL AND ANDROGEN RECEPTORS

Historical Perspective

Prostate cancer is an androgen-dependent disease, just as breast and endometrial carcinoma are estrogen-dependent diseases. Accordingly, it is logical to assume that identification of the androgen receptor (AnR) by biochemistry or immunohistochemistry might be of aid to the clinician in predicting response to additive or ablative hormonal treatment and disease-free survival. However, biochemists had great difficulty in developing suitable assays for the measurement of AnR in the prostate for reasons similar to those encountered in endometrial carcinoma. Prostate tissue may contain

AnR in stroma, vessels, and benign as well as malignant glands, and there is no way to separate the AnR contribution of each component in a homogenized specimen. It would seem therefore, an ideal situation for immunohistochemistry. Unfortunately, when specific anti-AnR antibodies became available, initial reports were confusing. Some studies reported correlation of AnR immunohistochemistry with tumor grade, while others did not. Some papers found an association with endocrine response and disease-free interval, while others found no such association. Several obstacles were apparent. Unlike breast cancer, in which only 70% of tumors are ER positive, the vast majority of prostate cancers (approximately 85%–90%) are AnR positive histochemically. Furthermore, tumors obviously androgen resistant or insensitive nonetheless remained AnR positive (reviewed in Reference 28).

Androgen Receptor Immunohistochemistry in Prostate Cancer

The antibody PG-21 was raised against a synthetic peptide containing the first 21 amino acids of the N-terminal of rat AR (29) and was provided by Geoffrey Greene and Gail Prins, the latter at the University of Illinois. Initially 63 cases of prostate cancer, stored in liquid nitrogen, were studied. All patients had continuous follow-up including evaluation of endocrine response, disease-free interval, and overall survival (22).

A significant association between assay results and AnR positivity was found, but many AnR-positive patients failed therapy. There was also a good association with disease-free interval: AnR-negative patients experienced a poor overall survival. Following publication of an antigen retrieval method for AnR by Shi et al. (34), we employed this method to examine a group of 90 men with prostate cancer using formalin-fixed, paraffin-embedded tissue. Patients were followed as described (22). Sections were deparaffinized and microwaved in citrate buffer (pH 6.0) for 30 minutes and then reacted with PG-21 in an ABC system. Frozen tissue from each case was assayed for AnR by DCC in the laboratory of Dr. Hannah Rosenthal at the former Roswell Park Memorial Institute in Buffalo, NY (23).

AnR by ICA did not correlate with AnR by DCC, perhaps illustrating the difficulties associated with the biochemical assay of AnR. AnR by ICA nonetheless correlated with endocrine response and showed a striking concordance with overall survival. There were 15 AnR-negative patients, and all were dead by 24 months.

Differences between AnR in frozen and formalin-fixed, paraffin-embedded tissue sections were also noted. There was a considerably higher percentage of AnR-negative cases in the series of cases studied when frozen. We attributed this to loss of receptor protein during prolonged storage, possibly from repeated freeze-thaw cycles or from too long a delay before initial freezing. It also appeared that specimens removed by electrocautery experienced some receptor loss. Cases that were clearly negative when frozen were AnR positive in paraffin, probably because fixation prevented receptor degradation. No case that was positive when frozen was negative after fixation, perhaps because only one anti-AnR antibody was employed.

Image Analysis and Androgen Receptor Analysis by Immunohistochemistry

In the examination of routinely prepared prostate cancer sections, it was once again evident that there were too many AnR-positive cases progressing on endocrine treatments. Indeed, positive and negative predictive values only approached significance ($P = 0.09$). In light of our experience with image analysis and ER-ICA in breast cancer, processed sections from all the 45 AnR-positive cases in the study were subjected to image analysis by Dr. Sklarew at the New York Medical College. Several patterns of positivity were again identified. More importantly, as in breast cancer, patients with unimodal AnR peaks were most likely to respond to endocrine treatment, while all 13 men with highly skewed AnR peaks progressed. Among the responding patients, 17 of 18 exhibited unimodal peaks, while 16 of 17 men who were stabilized on hormonal therapy exhibited multimodal peaks but with very well-defined distributions. The positive predictive value of AnR, with imaging, was 100%, and the negative predictive value was 93% (28; $P < 0.0001$). This contrasts with the positive and negative predictive values without image analysis, which were 71% and 62%, respectively. We are currently engaged in a long-term study to see whether AnR can predict disease-free survival in men with early-stage prostate cancer.

Similar experiences with imaging AnR in prostate cancer have been reported by others. Sadi and Barrack (31) analyzed 17 cases of men with advanced disease and found that staining homogeneity and unimodal peaks were associated with a favorable endocrine response. Tilley et al. (41) studied 30 cases and found that average staining intensity per cell could predict outcome. It is of interest that both authors utilized different imaging systems and different AnR antibodies and yet obtained similar results. Sadi and Barrack (31) hypothesize that a skewed AnR pattern represents genetic instability in the tumor and is associated with a poor outcome. It might equally represent mutant varieties of AnR that still retain antigenicity although they are no longer functional.

We have recently examined bone marrow biopsies from a group of 21 men with metastatic prostate cancer using PG-21 after antigen retrieval. These cases were processed in the laboratory of Dr. Prins and sent to us for interpretation. Three patients were AnR negative, while the remainder showed an AnR distribution that varied from 10% to 95% positive cells. Since all bone biopsies were decalcified prior to initial sectioning, it is apparent that AnR immunohistochemistry permits identification with ease in bone metastases. The percentage of AnR-positive cases (86%) is very similar to the percentage of positive cases in our larger biopsy series. The presence of normal marrow elements in the biopsies did not hinder identification of receptor.

To learn whether imaging patterns are associated with AnR mutations, we are in the process of comparing imaging with molecular determinations of genetic alterations performed on freshly frozen tissue.

Currently, we routinely perform AnR immunohistochemistry in all newly diagnosed prostate cancer patients at our Center, to determine whether loss of AnR will predict those patients with early stage disease whose disease will recur at an early date. This is a long-term study that will take several more years to complete.

It is obvious that confirmation of our results in prostate cancer must be obtained from other institutions and in a larger number of cases before the assay can be accepted as a useful clinical tool. However, unlike breast cancer, for which DCC/SGA is available, there is no acceptable biochemical method for assaying AnR. The future, therefore, looks bright for this method. The major disadvantage is that in order to benefit from the assay's maximum prognostic ability, image analysis is presently required, with the additional expense entailed.

SIMILARITIES AND DIFFERENCES IN RECEPTOR LOCALE IN ENDOCRINE TARGETS

There are many similarities in steroid hormone receptors in breast and prostate cancer, the most important being that both are endocrine-responsive tumors and that receptor locale is invariably nuclear. Furthermore, in both diseases, monoclonal receptor peaks by imaging are associated with endocrine response. There are, however, differences. In the breast, stromal ER/PgR is not seen even in benign cellular tumors such as fibroadenoma. Receptor in the nuclei of endothelial cells of vessels in the breast is never observed. The only locale in the breast is epithelium. In the prostate, in addition to epithelium, stromal nuclei are nearly always positive for AnR, and receptor is occasionally seen in nuclei of the endothelium. Of interest is the fact that while ER is present in the smooth muscle vasculature and endothelium of ovarian and uterine arteries, the vessels within the myometrium are receptor negative. This finding suggests that in some way, blood flow to these endocrine targets is under control of steroids. Antigen retrieval techniques will permit detailed studies of these similarities and differences in archival specimens.

CONCLUSION

While ER immunohistochemistry is close to being an acceptable test for prognosticating endocrine response in breast cancer, this cannot be currently said for PgR immunohistochemistry. The results of AnR immunostaining in prostate cancer, particularly in association with image analysis, are exciting and await further confirmation. At the present time only disease stage, tumor grade, and perhaps ploidy are currently of prognostic value in this common malignancy, and there is no other way to predict hormone response.

ACKNOWLEDGMENTS

This work was supported in part by Grant Nos. CA23623 (to L.P.P.) and CA66532 (to C.A.A.) from the National Cancer Institute.

REFERENCES

1. **Alberts, S.R., J.N. Ingle, P.R. Roche, S.S.Cha, L.E. Wold, G.H. Farr, Jr., J.E.Krook, and H.S. Wieand.** 1996. Comparisons of estrogen receptor determinations by a biochemical ligand-binding assay and immunohistochemical staining with monoclonal antibody ER1D5 in females with lymph node positive breast carcinomas entered on two prospective clinical trials. Cancer 78:764-772.
2. **Allred, D.C.** Prognostic indicators in breast cancer. Presented at the US and Canadian Academy of Pathology meeting, Orlando, FL, March 5th, 1997.
3. **al Saati, T., S. Clamens, E. Cohen-Knafo, J.C. Faye, H. Prats, J.H. Coindre, J. Wofflart, P. Caveriviere, F. Bayard, and G. Delsol.** 1993. Production of monoclonal antibodies to human estrogen receptor protein (ER) using recombinant ER (RER). Int. J. Cancer 55:651-654.
4. **Beatson, G.T.** 1896. On the treatment of inoperable cases of carcinoma of the mamma: suggestion for a new method of treatment with illustrative cases. Lancet 2:104-106.
5. **Brustein, S., R. Fruchter, G.L. Greene, and L.P. Pertschuk.** 1989. Immunocytochemical assay of progesterone receptors in paraffin-embedded specimens of endometrial carcinoma and hyperplasia: a preliminary evaluation. Mod. Pathol. 2:449-455.
6. **De Rosa, C.M., L. Ozzello, G.L. Greene, and D.V. Habif.** 1987. Immunostaining of estrogen receptor in paraffin sections of breast carcinomas using monoclonal antibody D75P3: effects of fixation. Am. J. Surg. Pathol. 11:943-950.
7. **Elias, J.M. and S. Masood.** 1995. Estrogen receptor assay: are we all doing it the same way? A survey. J Histotechnol. 18:95-96.
8. **Fuqua, S.A.W.** 1996. Estrogen and progesterone receptors and breast cancer, p. 261-271. In J.R. Harris, M.E. Lippman, M. Morrow, and S. Hellman (Eds.), Diseases of the Breast. Lippincott-Raven, Philadelphia-New York.
9. **Goulding, H., S. Pinder, P. Cannon, D. Pearson, R. Nicholson, D. Snead, J. Bell, C.W. Elston, J.F. Robertson, and R.W. Blamey.** 1995. A new immunohistochemical antibody for the assessment of estrogen receptor status on

routine, formalin-fixed tissue samples. Hum. Pathol. 26:291-294.

10. **Greene, G.L., F.W. Fitch, and E.V. Jensen.** 1980. Monoclonal antibodies to estrophilin: probes for the study of estrogen receptor. Proc. Natl. Acad. Sci. USA 77:157-161.

11. **Greene, G.L., C. Nolan, J.P. Engler, and E.V. Jensen.** 1980. Monoclonal antibodies to human estrogen receptor. Proc. Natl. Acad. Sci. USA 77:5115-5119.

12. **Hendricks, J.B. and E.J. Wilkinson.** 1993. Comparison of two antibodies for evaluation of estrogen receptors in paraffin-embedded tumors. Mod. Pathol. 6:765-770.

13. **Jensen, E.V. and E.R. DeSombre.** 1973. Estrogen receptor interaction. Estrogenic hormones effect transformation of specific receptor proteins to a biologically functional form. Science 182:126-134.

14. **King, W.J. and G.L. Greene.** 1984. Monoclonal antibodies localize oestrogen receptor in the nuclei of target cells. Nature 307:745-747.

15. **McGuire, W.L., P.P. Carbone, M.E. Sears, and G.C. Escher.** 1975. Estrogen receptors in human breast cancer: an overview, p. 1-8. In W.L. McGuire, P.P. Carboce, and E.P. Vollmer (Eds.), Estrogen Receptors in Human Breast Cancer. Raven Press, New York.

16. **McGuire, W.L., J.-P. Raynaud, and E.-E. Baulieu.** 1977. Progesterone receptors: introduction and overview, p. 1-8. In W.L. McGuire, J.-P. Raynaud, and E.-E. Baulieu (Eds.), Progesterone Receptors in Normal and Neoplastic Tissue. Raven Press, New York.

17. **McGuire, W.L., G.C. Chamness, and S.A.W. Fuqua.** 1991. Estrogen receptor variants in clinical breast cancer. Mol. Endocrinol. 5:1571-1577.

18. **Pertschuk, L.P., K.B. Eisenberg, A.C. Carter, and J.G. Feldman.** 1985. Immunohistological localization of estrogen receptors in breast cancer with monoclonal antibodies: correlation with biochemistry and clinical endocrine response. Cancer 55:1515-1518.

19. **Pertschuk, L.P., J.G. Feldman, K.B. Eisenberg, A.C. Carter, W.L. Thelmo, W.P. Cruz, S.M. Thorpe, I.J. Christensen, B.B. Rasmussen, C. Rose, and G.L. Greene.** 1988. Immunocytochemical detection of progesterone receptor in breast cancer with monoclonal antibody. Cancer 62:342-349.

20. **Pertschuk, L.P., D.S. Kim, K. Nayer, J.G. Feldman, K.B. Eisenberg, A.C. Carter, T.R. Zheng, W.L. Thelmo, J. Fleisher, and G.L. Greene.** 1990. Immunocytochemical estrogen and progestin receptor assays in breast cancer with monoclonal antibodies. Cancer 66:1663-1670.

21. **Pertschuk, L.P.** 1990. Immunocytochemical assay of estrogen receptors in breast cancer: a review of the literature. Ch. 2, p. 11-23. In L.P. Pertschuk (Ed.), Immunocytochemistry for Steroid Receptors. CRC Press, Boca Raton.

22. **Pertschuk, L.P., R.J. Macchia, J.G. Feldman, K.A. Brady, M. Levine, D.S. Kim, K.B. Eisenberg, G.S. Prins, and G.L. Greene.** 1994. Immunocytochemical assay for androgen receptors. A prospective study of 63 cases with long-term follow-up. Ann. Surg. Oncol. 1:495-503.

23. **Pertschuk, L.P., H. Schaeffer, J.G. Feldman, R.J. Macchia, Y.-D. Kim, K.B. Eisenberg, L.V. Braithwaite, C.A. Axiotis, G.S. Prins, and G.L. Greene.** 1995. Immunostaining for prostate cancer androgen receptor in paraffin identifies a subset of men with a poor prognosis. Lab. Invest. 73:302-305.

24. **Pertschuk, L.P., J.G. Feldman, Y.-D. Kim, L. Braithwaite, F. Schneider, A.S. Braverman, and C.A. Axiotis.** 1996. Estrogen receptor immunocytochemistry in paraffin embedded tissues with ER1D5 predicts breast cancer endocrine response more accurately than H222Sp in frozen sections or cytosol-based ligand-binding assays. Cancer 77:2514-2519.

25. **Pertschuk, L.P., S. Masood, J. Simone, J.G. Feldman, R.G. Fruchter, C. Axiotis, and G.L. Greene.** 1996. Estrogen receptor immunocytochemistry in endometrial carcinoma: a prognostic marker for survival. Gynecol. Oncol. 63:28-33.

26. **Pertschuk, L.P. and C.A. Axiotis.** 1999. Steroid hormone receptor immunohistochemistry in breast cancer: past, present and future. Breast J. 5:3-12.

27. **Press, M.F. and G.L. Greene.** 1988. Localization of progesterone receptor with monoclonal antibodies to the human progesterone receptor. Endocrinology 122:1165-1175.

28. **Prins, G.S., R.J. Sklarew, and L.P. Pertschuk.** 1998. Image analysis of androgen receptor immunostaining in prostate cancer accurately predicts response to hormonal therapy. J. Urol. 159:641-649.

29. **Prins, G.S., L. Birch, and G.L. Greene.** 1991. Androgen receptor localization in different cell types of the adult rat prostate. Endocrinology 129:3187-3189.

30. **Saccani, J.G., S.R. Johnston, J. Salter, S. Detre, and M. Dowsett.** 1994. Comparison of new histochemical assay for oestrogen receptor in paraffin wax embedded breast carcinoma tissue with quantitative enzyme immunoassay. J. Clin. Pathol. 47:900-905.

31. **Sadi, M. and E. Barrack.** 1993. Image analysis of androgen receptor immunostaining in metastatic prostate cancer. Cancer 71:2576-2580.

32. **Sannino, P. and S. Shousha.** 1994. Demonstration of oestrogen receptors in paraffin wax sections of breast carcinoma using the monoclonal antibody 1D5 and microwave oven processing. J. Clin. Pathol. 47:90-92.

33. **Shi, S.-R., M.E. Key, and K.J. Kalra.** 1991. Antigen retrieval in formalin-fixed, paraffin-embedded tissues: an enhancement method for immunohistochemical staining based upon microwave oven heating of tissue sections. J. Histochem. Cytochem. 39:741-748.

34. **Shi, S.-R., B. Chaiwun, L. Young, R.J. Cote, and C.R. Taylor.** 1993. Antigen retrieval technique utilizing citrate buffer or urea solution for immunohistochemical demonstration of androgen receptor in formalin-fixed, paraffin

sections. J. Histochem. Cytochem. *41*:1599-1604.

35. **Shi, S.-R., J. Gu, K.L. Kalra, T. Chen, R.J. Cote, and C.R. Taylor.** 1994. Antigen retrieval technique: a novel approach to immunohistochemistry on routinely processed tissue sections. Cell Vision 2:6-22.

36. **Sklarew, R.J. and L.P. Pertschuk.** 1987. Quantitation of the immunocytochemical assay for estrogen receptor protein (ER-ICA) in human breast cancer by television imaging. J. Histochem. Cytochem. *35*:1253-1259.

37. **Sklarew, R.J., S.C. Bodmer, and L.P. Pertschuk.** 1990. Quantitative imaging of immunocytochemical (PAP) estrogen receptor staining patterns in breast cancer sections. Cytometry *11*:359-378.

38. **Sklarew, R.J., S.C. Bodmer, and L.P. Pertschuk.** 1991. Comparison of microscopic imaging strategies for evaluating immunocytochemical (PAP) steroid receptor heterogeneity. Cytometry *12*:207-220.

39. **Szekeres, J.B., Y. Lutz, A. Le Tourneau, and M. Delaage.** 1994. Steroid hormone receptor immunostaining on paraffin sections with microwave heating and trypsin digestion. J. Histotechnol. *17*:321-324.

40. **Thorpe, S.M., B.B. Rasmussen, W.J. King, E.R. DeSombre, R.M. Blough, H.T. Mouridsen, N. Rossing, and K.W. Andersen.** 1986. Steroid hormone receptors as prognostic indicators in primary breast cancer. Breast Cancer Res. Treat. *7*(Suppl):91-98.

41. **Tilley, W., S. Lim-Tio, D. Horsfall, J. Aspinall, V. Marshall, and J. Skinner.** 1994. Detection of discrete androgen receptor epitopes in prostate cancer by immunostaining: measurement by color video image analysis. Cancer Res. *54*:4096-4102.

42. **Toft, D. and J. Gorski.** 1966. A receptor molecule for estrogens: isolation from the uterus and preliminary characterization. Proc. Natl. Acad. Sci. USA *35*:1574-1581.

43. **Wahli, W. and E. Martinez.** 1991. Superfamily of steroid nuclear receptors: positive and negative regulators of gene expression. FASEB J. *5*:2243-2249.

Application of the Antigen Retrieval Technique in Experimental Pathology: From Human to Mouse

10

Giorgio Cattoretti and Qing Fei

Department of Pathology, Columbia University College of Physicians and Surgeons, New York, NY, USA

INTRODUCTION

In the last 50 years, surgical pathology has witnessed amazingly rapid changes in available knowledge and techniques applicable to everyday routine diagnostics. The benefits of applied and basic research are reflected in modern concepts of the approach to human tissues by a surgical pathologist (29). Immunohistochemistry and in situ hybridization can be taken as an example and a paradigm of such changes. After the early days of single-fluorochrome fluorescence microscopy on frozen sections, using antiimmunoglobulin polyclonal antibodies, we are now in the era of genetic mapping of routine specimens by a diversified multicolor approach, which includes high-efficiency immunohistochemistry, in situ hybridization, interphase karyotyping, and single-cell molecular analysis (5). In immunohistochemistry, the recent development of antigen retrieval (AR) (32; discussed in detail elsewhere in this book) has given us a wealth of reagents to be used for diagnostic or research.

The Human Genome Project, the plan to map the entire human genome, has fueled most of these changes, by providing tools to understand the cause and the mechanism of human diseases. To prove experimentally the role of newly discovered genes in human pathology, scientist have turned to in vivo models, by altering genes in nonhuman animal germlines (mostly mice) and observing the consequences (1,2). This approach has been defined as reverse genetics (3): while human genetics identifies genes from the observation of human pathology, reverse genetics introduces mutations in mouse genes and observes the biologic consequences.

The number of new genes discovered every month is astonishing and increasing; therefore we expect that mouse models of disease will increase exponentially as well (6).

Antigen Retrieval Techniques
Edited by Shan-Rong Shi, Jiang Gu, and Clive R. Taylor
©2000 Eaton Publishing, Natick, MA

As many of the readers may have experienced, surgical pathologists are often asked by colleagues to examine their transgenic or knockout mice. Usually the request comes from a highly specialized laboratory and is addressed to a highly specialized pathologist, in the (sometimes wrong) assumption that this latter can "read" in the mouse the expected pathology, being skilled in diagnosing those entities in humans. The pathologist applies the specialized techniques he uses in his daily work to a new material, whose only advantage is that an affected mouse can be compared with a healthy littermate (ethically impossible in humans).

This chapter introduces the problems of this entirely new field and considers some solutions, with a focus on hematopathology. Because of the ease in handling and the morphologic detail of formalin-fixed, paraffin-embedded tissues, all immunohistochemical techniques and examples will be fixed specimens, with a particular attention to AR.

CHOICE OF REAGENTS

Polyclonal and monoclonal antibodies are widely available for diagnostic use in humans. Although polyclonal antibodies were used first, before the advent of the hybridoma technique, they did not become obsolete. On the contrary, once a gene is mapped and sequenced, an antibody can be quickly generated by immunizing a rabbit or a goat with a synthetic peptide, whose sequence is generated after the nucleotide sequence. This is quicker and cheaper than making a monoclonal antibody, which can always be made later on. The expression and distribution of the gene product can be traced in tissues with such a polyclonal antibody; the chance that it will stain fixed and embedded tissue is higher than with a monoclonal antibody.

Working with nonhuman tissues in immunohistochemistry poses the problem of reactivity of the secondary antibodies with endogenous immunoglobulins. As long as the primary antibody is made in a species different from the sample species, absorption or affinity purification solves the problem. Rabbit or goat polyclonal antibodies are therefore welcome in experimental pathology.

The number of antibodies produced against human proteins is enormous. Mouse monoclonal antibodies are preferred because of their availability and reproducibility.

The immunodominant sequences are often conserved among mammalian species, and many mouse monoclonal antibodies react with mouse proteins as well. Their use on mouse tissues raises the problems of cross-reactivity with endogenous immunoglobulins. The best solution is to tag the antibody with a hapten (biotin, fluorescein) not present in mouse tissue or able to bind a reported molecule [avidin-horseradish peroxidase (HRP) or alkaline phosphatase (AP)], so that only the tagged antibody can be detected. These are more efficient and readily available solutions rather than provide direct enzyme conjugation of the primary antibody. However, few of the mouse monoclonal antibodies reacting with mouse are conjugated, and it is unusual to do in-house conjugation of a large amount of primary antibody.

Complex solutions have been published, to overcome the inevitable cross-reactivity (9,16,24), and there are commercially available proprietary kits for blocking (DAKO, Carpinteria, CA, USA; Zymed, South San Francisco, CA, USA).

An alternative is to exploit the level of sensitivity of the immunohistochemistry on fixed and embedded tissues. Young nonimmunized laboratory mice raised in sterile, pathogen-free barriers have lower endogenous immunoglobulin levels than older ani-

Table 1. Mean Immunoglobulin Serum Concentration in Barrier-Reared Mice[a]

Isotype	Mean concentration (μg/mL) ± SD
IgM	406 ± 162
IgA	496 ± 274
IgG1	872 ± 454
IgG2a	898 ± 680
IgG2b	1143 ± 536
IgG3	458 ± 165

[a]Average concentration (μg/mL) of immunoglobulin isotypes in 5- to 12-week-old, barrier-reared S129/C57B1(F1) mice.

mals raised in conventional housing (4). In addition, each immunoglobulin isotype contributes to a fraction of the total immunoglobulin levels (Table 1), e.g., IgG1, the most frequent isotype of mouse monoclonal antibody, contributes up to one-fifth of all mouse serum immunoglobulins. Based on this observation, we used primary mouse IgG1 monoclonal antibodies on mouse tissue sections, counterstained with an isotype-specific biotin-conjugated secondary antibody (goat anti-mouse IgG1 heavy chain). The results are much cleaner than a conventional anti-mouse heavy and light chain antibody (Figure 1), the only endogenously reactive cells being the rare IgG1+ plasma cells. The cleaner background is due to the relatively greater amount of the exogenously added mouse IgG1 monoclonal antibody than the endogenous IgG1 immunoglobulin levels, to be detected by the secondary antibody.

The use of rat monoclonal antibodies will overcome all these problems, and investigators and companies are currently developing reagents in the rat that are suitable for mouse analysis. One example is the detection of proliferating cells in mouse tissue. Traditionally, S-phase in laboratory animals has been detected by DNA analog administration [bromodeoxyuridine (BrdU)] in vivo, followed by detection with an anti-BrdU antibody. Because the anti-BrdU antibodies were made in the mouse, the same problem outlined above applies when they are used in tissues. Ki-67 is the gold standard for proliferating cell detection in fixed, embedded tissues (19), but many monoclonal and polyclonal anti-human Ki-67 antibodies do not recognize mouse Ki-67.

Polyclonal rabbit antibodies specific for murine Ki-67 are available. There are also two mouse monoclonal antibodies, produced against recombinant Ki-67 sequences, that also recognize murine Ki-67: MIB-5 (21) and MM1 (Novocastra, Newcastle-U-Tyne, UK). The former is excellent for cell cycle analysis by flow cytometry (Cattoretti, unpublished data). The second, excellent on human tissues, may react with additional nuclear epitopes on mouse specimens (Cattoretti, unpublished data). Both are mouse IgG1. Recently, Gerdes et al. (14), who produced the original Ki-67 clone, generated a rat anti-murine Ki-67 antibody (TEC-3) that does not recognize human Ki-67 and reacts with fixed mouse tissue (Figure 2). This reagent, which is mouse specific and does not recognize human Ki-67, will be a useful reagent for cell proliferation in mouse tissues.

There is an even quicker and cheaper method to trace a protein in cells, by tagging the protein with an exogenous short sequence for which an antibody already exists. A nucleotide sequence, coding for a short peptide, is joined at the 5′ or 3′ ends of the gene sequence, in frame, so that in transfected cells, the protein is now produced with the peptide attached. The tag is then traced in cells and, if a mouse with the tag in its genome is produced, in tissues.

As an example, a novel gene (MUM-1/IRF4) (17) was found to be involved in the t(6;14)(p25;q32) chromosomal translocation in human myeloma. The translocation deregulates MUM-1 expression by changing its promoter. To investigate the consequences of enforced expression of this gene, we generated transgenic mice in which MUM-1 is driven by an IgM heavy chain promoter (manuscript in preparation). To trace the expression of human MUM-1 in mouse tissue and to distinguish it from the mouse homolog, the human transgene was tagged with a 10-amino-acid-long peptide (EQKLISEEDL), derived from the human c-myc gene and not expressed in mouse c-myc or mouse MUM-1. As shown in Figure 3, we were able to detect selectively the exogenous transgenic protein in mouse tissue by using the 9E10 anti-myc IgG1 mon-

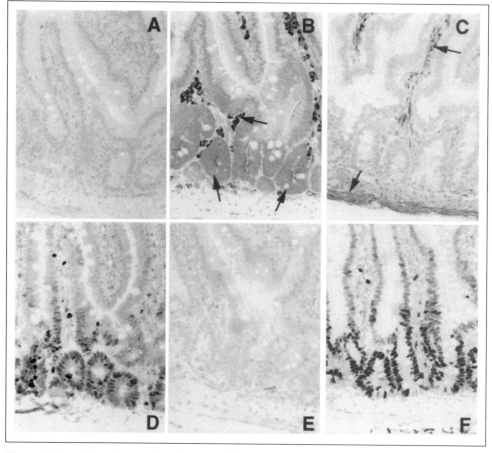

Figure 1. Comparison of mouse tissue immunostaining with rabbit polyclonal and mouse monoclonal antibodies. (A) Negative control (mouse irrelevant IgG1) followed by goat anti-mouse IgG1. (B) Negative control (mouse irrelevant IgG1) followed by goat anti-mouse heavy and light immunoglobulin chains. Note background staining on epithelium and lamina propria plasma cells (arrows). (C) Mouse anti-mouse desmin IgG1 antibody followed by goat anti-mouse IgG1. Note smooth muscle fibers (arrows). (D) Rabbit anti-mouse Ki-67 polyclonal antibody, followed by goat anti-rabbit Ig immunoglobulin. (E) Negative rabbit serum control followed by anti-rabbit Ig. (F) Mouse anti-mouse Ki-67 IgG1 (MIB-5), followed by goat anti-mouse IgG1. All sections are consecutive.

oclonal antibody and to distinguish it from mouse MUM-1, for which an antibody was already available.

VALIDATION OF SPECIFICITY

Primary validation of an antibody includes proof of its specificity by biochemical analysis of positive and negative controls by Western blot and/or immunoprecipitation, tissue distribution analysis, and population analysis to rule out polymorphisms. In the era of molecular biology, cells transfected with the gene or with an empty construct as control are the gold standard for antibody specificity (8). In addition, the generation of a mouse with a germline-deleted gene provides the ultimate tool to verify the specificity of an antibody directed against that gene product (37). As shown in Figure 4, an antibody directed against the N terminus of the BCL-6 protein stains germinal centers in a wild-type mouse but fails to detect any signal in mice in which the entire BCL-6 gene has been deleted.

If we use a well-characterized antibody against human determinants on mouse tissue, we face additional problems: differential gene expression between mouse and human (20) and epitope mimicry. Two examples are give here.

Intermediate filaments are a limited variety of ubiquitous proteins with selective tissue expression (25). In hematopathology, antikeratin antibodies are used to highlight thymic epithelium and a subset of fibroblasts in lymph nodes (11). In humans and mice, an antikeratin mouse monoclonal antibody (K8.13) detects the thymic

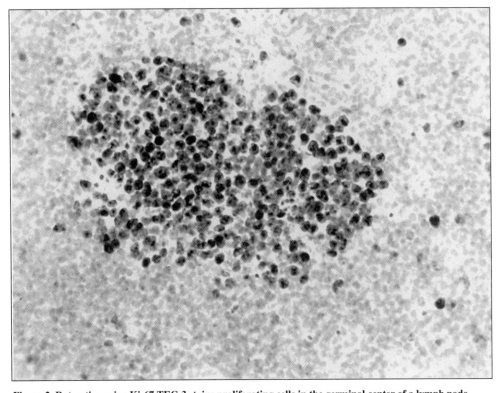

Figure 2. Rat anti-murine Ki-67 TEC-3 stains proliferating cells in the germinal center of a lymph node.

epithelium and several other epithelia. However, nodal fibroblasts in mice are keratin negative. Antidesmin antibodies label all lymph nodal fibroblasts in mice (Figure 5) and only a subpopulation in humans (11).

PGP9.5 is a protein expressed in neuroendocrine human tissue and described in follicular dendritic cells. The reason for this latter reactivity is unclear (22,23). In mice, rabbit anti-human PGP9.5 has identical reactivity on neural tissue but is negative on follicular dendritic cells. This may be due to a cross-reactive epitope that is human restricted.

The pathologist who may wish to use reagents validated for human use on mouse tissue must be prepared to revalidate their reactivity, exactly as has been done for humans.

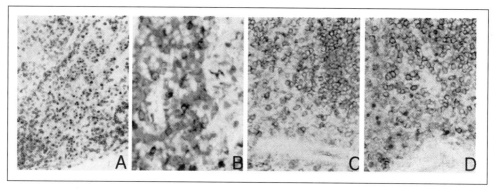

Figure 3. Double immunostaining for MUM-1/IRF-4, transgenic MUM-1, and lineage markers in mouse tissue. (A and B) Sections from a wild-type mouse lymph node. (C and D) Sections from transgenic MUM-1. (A) MUM-1 stains in brown the nuclei of B220-negative (blue) plasma cells. (B) MUM-1-positive plasma cells (brown) are not stained by the antimacrophage antibody Mac-2 (blue). (C) Negative control mouse IgG1 negative stain (in blue) on a B220-stained (brown) lymph node. (D) myc-tagged transgenic MUM-1 is recognized (blue nuclei) by 9E10 (mouse IgG1 monoclonal antibody) in B220-negative (brown) plasma cells. **(See color plate A8).**

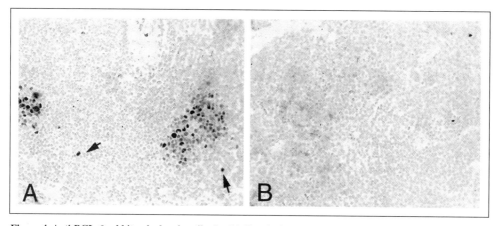

Figure 4. Anti-BCL-6 rabbit polyclonal antibody. (A) Germinal center cells and rare scattered interfollicular cells (arrows) are stained in wild-type spleen. (B) In BCL-6 knockout mice, in which the whole gene has been ablated, the same antibody does not stain any cells.

THE ANTIGEN RETRIEVAL TECHNIQUE

Discovery of the AR technique has changed the antibody-unfriendly paraffin section to a field in which multiple targets can be detected, with the added advantage of superior morphologic detail. Not only can we delineate the phenotype of single cells in the tissue, but we also know its gene repertoire expression and its dynamic life just before the specimen was fixed. In surgical pathology, analysis of the growth fraction of tumors is now part of the clinical evaluation.

The reason for the success of Ki-67 is that it is restricted to proliferating cells, and the tissue does not need preincubation with thymidine or thymidine analogs in vitro in order to detect the growth fraction (labeling index). However, in animals one can use nucleotide analogs such as BrdU to label proliferating cells.

The analysis of proliferating cells tagged with BrdU in tissues poses interesting problems of detection and double staining with lineage-specific markers. Traditionally, BrdU detection is applied to cell suspensions and cultures. Two methods are available (reviewed in Reference 26), both of which involve denaturing or enzymatic digestion, in order to expose the pieces of DNA that incorporate the nucleotide analog. Both methods accommodate with difficulty a second staining with additional cell markers. Ethanol fixation is a poor fixative for many low-molecular-weight proteins and peptides.

We used the BrdU detection in tissue sections as a model to improve the AR technique. BrdU detection in dewaxed, fixed tissues with or without DNase treatment leads

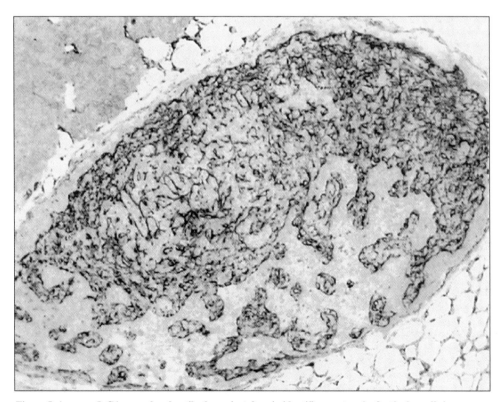

Figure 5. A mouse IgG1 monoclonal antibody against desmin identifies a network of reticular cells in a mouse lymph node. An immunodeficient mouse, depleted of lymphoid cells, has been used to enhance the stromal staining.

to poor and poorly reproducible results (Figure 6). However, after conventional AR treatment (EDTA 0.01 mol/L, pH 7.5), incorporated BrdU is readily detected. This may signify that high-temperature treatment in the presence of calcium chelators exposes the artifical epitope by separating it from the DNA strand and does it more efficiently than DNase alone. This may also occur because DNase cannot reach and cut efficiently the DNA in fixed and embedded tissue. We then tested whether the combined use of AR and DNase treatment was additive. Stronger anti-BrdU staining was obtained after combined use, although the increase was less dramatic than from DNase to AR (Figure 6).

Reports on the use of DNase to improve nuclear antigen staining were published long before the AR era (31,33). If the hypothesis that AR allows better access of antibodies and enzymes to their target is correct and if DNase treatment contributes independently to this, then staining for nuclear DNA-bound proteins should be increased by combined AR and DNase staining. We tested this hypothesis by staining for Ki-67, estrogen receptor (ER), and cyclin D1 in eight breast carcinoma cases on a multitissue block. While Ki-67 and ER did not differ in blind evaluation of DNase or non-DNase-treated AR-treated slides, cyclin D1 staining was reproducibly improved by the sequential treatment. We are now using this procedure for diagnostic immunohistochemistry, and we routinely observe specific nuclear staining in endogenous control cells (epithelia, fibroblasts) in every stained sample.

We applied this combined technique successfully to mouse tissue, to detect two enzymes involved in DNA recombination in lymphoid cells, RAG-1 and RAG-2 (36). In DNase/AR-treated tissues, RAG-1 and RAG-2 were detected in the thymus and bone marrow of wild-type animals and in v-abl-induced pre-B-cell lymphomas (kindly provided by K. Calame, Columbia University, New York, NY) (Figure 7).

BUILDING A PANEL OF DIAGNOSTIC ANTIBODIES FOR MOUSE EXPERIMENTAL PATHOLOGY

Reports on rodent tissue staining for diagnostic purposes have been scanty, and most of the publications have dealt with either technical advances in staining (12,13,15, 16,35) or detection of selected proteins, within highly specialized basic science publications. Reports on the use of specific antibody classes in routine specimens for diagnostic use are rare (10,18,27,28,34).

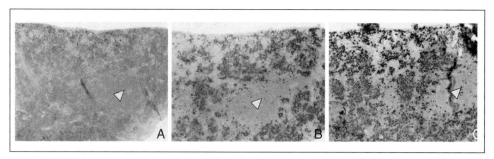

Figure 6. Serial sections of a spleen from a BrdU-injected mouse are stained with an IgG1 anti-BrdU murine monoclonal antibody followed by goat anti-mouse IgG1. (A) The section was treated with DNase I before staining. (B) The section was treated with AR before staining. (C) The section was first treated with AR and then digested with DNase I before immunostaining. The sections are centered on a quiescent primary follicle (triangles) and contain numerous proliferating erythroid precursors in the red pulp.

172

The impact of novel mouse pathology, newly generated from unknown genes, encounters a relatively underdeveloped diagnostic murine surgical pathology. It is also difficult to build up a body of knowledge about immunohistochemistry in rodents, given the dispersion of this information.

In Table 2 we provide a partial list of commercially available antibodies that have been tested on routinely fixed mouse tissue to diagnose cell lineage and differentiation of hematopoietic and nonhematopoietic cells. For the mouse immunologist, the germinal center is a fascinating entity, which historically has been recognized by staining with a lectin derived from *Arachis hypogaea*, the peanut agglutinin (PNA) (30). Obtaining a good batch of peroxidase-conjugated PNA has taken quite a few days for every immunologist, the staining being highly capricious (G.J. Thorbecke, personal communication). We borrowed the intuition of Burroni et al. (7) and used an anti-PNA biotin-conjugated goat polyclonal antibody to stain AR-treated paraffin sections, with reproducible results (Figure 8). By using this and the other reagents listed, we can reproducibly assess proliferation, differentiation, and lineage of most hematopoietic subsets in formalin-fixed, paraffin-embedded mouse tissue.

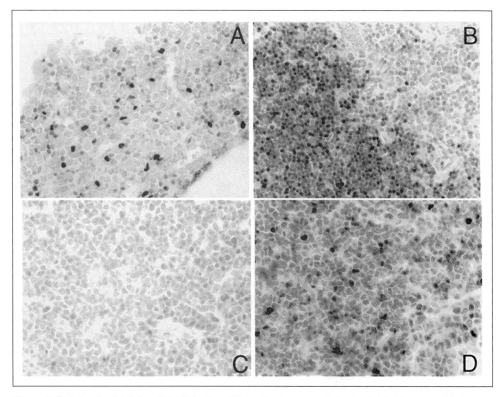

Figure 7. Staining for RAG-1 and RAG-2. (A and B) Nuclear immunostaining for RAG-2 in scattered bone marrow B-cell precursors (A) and the thymic cortex (B) but not medulla. (C) Negative rabbit control on a v-abl-induced pro-B lymphoma. (D) RAG-1 antibody stains the nuclei of scattered cells in the same specimen.

Table 2. Antibodies Effective in Murine Formalin-Fixed, Paraffin-Embedded Tissues[a]

Antibody	Species	Reactivity	Reference/source
CD3ε	Rabbit	All T cells	DAKO, Carpinteria, CA
CD3ζ	Mouse IgG1	All T cells	Santa Cruz Biotechnology, Santa Cruz, CA
B220	Rat	All B cells	PharMingen, San Diego, CA
Mac-2	Rat	All macrophages, epithelia	G.J. Thorbecke
IgD	Sheep	B cells	ICN, Costa Mesa, CA
IgM	Goat	B cells	Southern Biotechnology Associates (SBA), Birmingham, AL
IgA	Goat	B cells	SBA
IgE	Goat	B cells	ICN
Ig isotypes (γ1, γ2α, γ2β, γ3)	Goat	B cells	SBA
κ, λ	Goat	B cells	SBA
CD138 syndecan	Rat	Plasma cells, epithelia	PharMingen
BCL-6	Rabbit	Germinal center B cells	Santa Cruz Biotechnology
BCL-6 (P1F6)	Mouse IgG1	Germinal center B cells	Novocastra (Vector, Burlingame, CA)
Peanut agglutinin (PNA)	Lectin	Germinal center B cells	Sigma, St. Louis, MO
Anti-PNA	Goat	Antilectin	Vector
RAG-1	Rabbit	Lymphoid precursors	PharMingen
RAG-2	Rabbit	Lymphoid precursors	PharMingen
TdT	Rabbit	Lymphoid precursors	Supertechs, Rockville, MD
CD28	Goat	Pan-T-cell reactivity	Santa Cruz Biotechnology
CTLA-4	Goat	Subset of T cells	Santa Cruz Biotechnology
CD40	Goat	Dendritic cells, B cells	Santa Cruz Biotechnology
CD43	Rat	All T cells	PharMingen
von Willebrand factor (vWF)	Rabbit	Megakaryocytes	DAKO
Glycophorin (TER117)	Rat	Erythroid cells	PharMingen
Myeloperoxidase	Rabbit	Myeloid cells	DAKO
Major basic protein	Rabbit	Eosinophils	G. Gleich
Lysozyme	Rabbit	Kidney	DAKO
Cytokeratin (K8.13)	Mouse IgG1	All epithelia	Sigma
Desmin	Mouse IgG1	Muscle cells	DAKO
PGP9.5	Rabbit	Neuroendocrine cells, nerves	Novocastra
Ki-67	Rabbit	Proliferating cells	Novocastra
MIB-5 (Ki-67)	Mouse IgG1	Proliferating cells	Immunotech, Miami, FL
TEC-3 (Ki-67)	Rat	Proliferating cells	J. Gerdes
Cyclin A	Rabbit	Proliferating cells	Santa Cruz Biotechnology
Cyclin B1	Rabbit	Subpopulation of proliferating cells	Santa Cruz Biotechnology
Cyclin D1	Rabbit	Scattered cells	Santa Cruz Biotechnology
p53 (CM5)	Rabbit	p53	Novocastra

[a]The method was microwave oven antigen retrieval treatment, except trypsin was used for major basic protein.

PROTOCOLS

Protocol for Immunohistochemistry on Fixed, Paraffin-Embedded Mouse Sections

Materials and Reagents

- 100 mmol/L EDTA, pH 7.5, stock solution: dilute 1:100 in double-distilled water (DDW)
- TBS-T Tris-buffered saline (TBS) 0.05 mol/L, pH 7.5, containing 0.01% Tween® 20)
- Acetate buffer, pH 5.5 (52.5 mL of 0.1 mol/L acetic acid solution + 196.5 mL of a 0.1 mol/L Na acetate solution; bring to 500 mL)
- Tris-HCl 0.1 mol/L, pH 9.2 (1:10 from a 1 mol/L stock solution)
- Deoxyribonuclease I (DNase type II; Sigma, St. Louis, MO, USA; D-4527) 5 U/mL in TBS, pH 7.5
- NaN_3 10% stock solution (100×) in double-distilled water
  Caution: Highly toxic and explosive under acidic conditions.
- 30% (wt/wt) H_2O_2 stock solution (100×)
- Xylene or Hemo-De (Fisher, Pittsburgh, PA, USA)
  Caution: Xylene is toxic.
- Ethanol, absolute
- Aminoethylcarbazole (AEC) (20-mg tablets; Sigma; A-6926) dissolved in 2.5

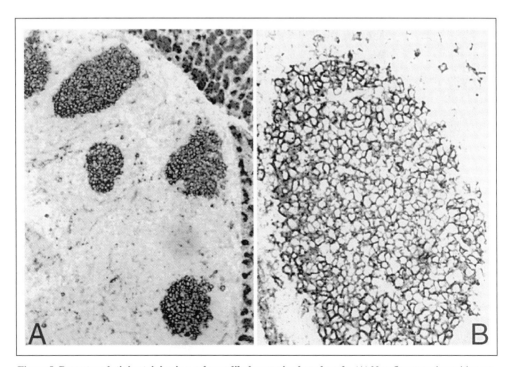

Figure 8. Peanut agglutinin staining in a submandibular murine lymph node. (A) Note five strongly positive germinal centers, as well as scattered positive stromal cells and salivary gland (top right). (B) Higher magnification of a germinal center.

mL *NN*-dimethyl formamide, immediately prior to use
- Naphtol as BI phosphate (Sigma; N2250) 20 mg (stock solution 40 mg/mL in *NN*-dimethyl formamide, anhydrous, kept at -20°C)
- Fast blue BB diazonium salt (Sigma; F3378), 10 mg
- Glycerol-gelatin mounting medium
- Adhesive-coated glass slides (e.g., Fisher; Superfrost Plus no. 12-550-15)
- WVR/Baxter slide staining holder S7636 or radiotransparent slide holder

Procedure for Immunoperoxidase Stain

1. Cut sections at 4-μm, use a clean water bath with distilled water, and let the sections dry upright to facilitate adhesion between the section and the charged glass surface. Optional: use 1 teaspoon of Elmer's glue per water bath. Optional: bake at 60°C for 1 hour. Do not use a microwave oven to dry the slides because the temperature cannot be controlled.

2. Deparaffinize the slides with two 5-minute incubations of clean xylene or Hemo-De, followed by three washes with absolute ethanol. Then gradually bring to distilled water.

3. Place the sections in a radiotransparent slide holder. Immerse slides and holder in 1 mmol/L EDTA, pH 7.5 (from a 100 mmol/L stock) in a beaker. Cover with a piece of Saran wrap in which you have made holes. Put in a microwave oven and bring to a boil at maximum power (8 min for 800 mL). Let boil for 15 minutes at a reduced power so the liquid continues to simmer. Cool at room temperature for 30 minutes to 1 hour. Transfer to TBS.

4. DNase treatment (optional; perform at this point). Warm the slides to 37°C in phosphate-buffered saline (PBS). Incubate in deoxyribonuclease I at 37°C for 30 minutes, followed by two washes in TBS.

5. Wash twice with TBS-T. Apply nonspecific binding blocking serum (1% human serum in TBS) for 10 minutes.

6. Blot the slides without washing, and apply the primary antibody in a moist chamber at room temperature for 1 to 18 hours.

7. Wash twice with TBS-T.

8. Add the biotin-conjugated secondary antibody (typically 100 μL) and incubate for 45 minutes. The secondary antibody, preferably raised in horse or donkey, should be absorbed against human and mouse serum; if not, add 1% human and 1% mouse serum before use.

   Caution: If you are planning to do a double staining that includes a mouse monoclonal primary antibody, omit the mouse serum. If you plan to do double staining with a mouse and a rat monoclonal antibody, you may use a rat-absorbed anti-mouse secondary antibody first and then a mouse-absorbed anti-rat secondary antibody.

   Most reagents are used at 1:100 or 1:200 dilution.

9. Wash twice with TBS-T.

10. Block endogenous peroxidase by incubating in 0.1% NaN_3 and 0.3% H_2O_2 in TBS-T for 30 minutes. This procedure is optional. Wash three times.

11. Add the HRP-conjugated avidin (typically 100 μL, dilution 1:300–500 in TBS-T), and incubate for 20 minutes.

12. Wash three times with TBS-T.

13. Develop with AEC, diluted in 50 mL of acetate buffer, to which 25 μL of 30%

(wt/wt) H_2O_2 has been added. Keep away from direct sunlight. Filter the developing solution with a 45-μm filter (optional). Carefully avoid excessive background staining and reach full development if planning to do double staining (see below).

14. When staining is complete (usually less than 1 h), wash thoroughly in tap water. Counterstain and mount in water-soluble mounting medium (glycerol gelatin).

Procedure for Double Immunohistochemistry: Double Indirect Immunoalkaline Stain

You should not use antigens located on the same structure (nucleus, membrane, or cytoplasm), since the success of this double-staining procedure is based on the complete development of the first stain, which should mask the structure stained first. Therefore, you should be able to use two antibodies raised in the same species. However, better results are obtained if two different species are used.

Perform the first stain up to step 13. Do not counterstain.

14. Apply the second primary antibody in a moist chamber at room temperature for 1 to 18 hours.
15. Wash twice with TBS-T.
16. Add the AP-conjugated secondary antibody (typically 100 μL), and incubate for 45 minutes. The secondary antibody should be absorbed against human and mouse serum; if not, add 1% human and mouse serum before use. Most rabbit anti-goat AP or goat anti-rabbit AP can be used 1:200 in TBS-bovine serum albumin (BSA) NaN_3.
17. Wash twice with TBS-T.
18. Add the AP-conjugated tertiary antibody directed against the species of the secondary antibody (typically 100 μL), and incubate for 15 minutes. The tertiary antibody should be absorbed against human serum; if not, add 1% human serum before use. Most goat anti-mouse AP or goat anti-rabbit AP can be used 1:200 in TBS-BSA NaN_3. This tertiary antibody step can be omitted if the secondary antibody gives enough signal.
19. Wash three times with TBS-T.
20. Develop with fast blue BB dissolved in Tris-HCl 0.1 mol/L, pH 9.2, buffer, containing 20 mg of Naphtol AS-BI phosphate. Filter with a 45-μm filter (optional). Keep away from direct sunlight. Levamisole, an endogenous alkaline phosphatase inhibitor, is not necessary on boiled sections, because the endogenous enzyme is inactivated.
21. When staining is complete (usually less than 1 h), wash thoroughly in tap water. Preferably postfix in formalin for 4 to 5 hours before mounting in water-soluble mounting medium (glycerol gelatin). Do not counterstain, unless you can afford a very light hematoxylin hue in the nuclei.

Procedure for Peanut Agglutinin Immunoperoxidase Stain

Proceed through steps 1 through 3 as described above. Omit step 4.

5. Wash twice with TBS-T. Apply nonspecific binding blocking serum (1% human serum in TBS) for 10 minutes.
6. Blot the slides without washing, and apply the biotin-conjugated peanut agglu-

tinin (Sigma; L6135; 5 µg/mL), in a moist chamber at room temperature for 1 to 18 hours.

7. Wash twice with TBS-T.
8. Add the biotin-conjugated goat anti-PNA secondary antibody (Vector, Burlingame, CA, USA; 1:300; typically 100 µL), and incubate for 45 minutes.
9. Wash twice with TBS-T.
10. Block endogenous peroxidase by incubating in 0.1% NaN_3 and 0.3% H_2O_2 for 30 minutes. This procedure is optional. Wash three times.
11. Add the HRP-conjugated avidin (typically 100 µL, dilution 1:300–500 in TBS-T), and incubate for 20 minutes.
12. Wash three times with TBS-T.
13. Develop with AEC, as above, and counterstain, or proceed to double staining.

ACKNOWLEDGMENTS

We thank Riccardo Dalla Favera for generous help and support on this project. Steve Tronick (Santa Cruz Biotechnology), James Champlin (Immunotech), Alan M. Stall (Pharmingen), Gerald J. Gleich (Mayo Clinic), Jeannette Thorbecke (New York University), and Johannes Gerdes (MIB, Borstel, FRG) gave generous gifts of precious reagents. Ruby and Chery provided excellent technical support. G.C. is a Leukemia Society of America Special Fellow.

REFERENCES

1. **Bedell, M.A., N.A. Jenkins, and N.G. Copeland.** 1997. Mouse models of human disease. Part I: techniques and resources for genetic analysis in mice. Genes Dev. *11*:1-10.
2. **Bedell, M.A., D.A. Largaespada, N.A. Jenkins, and N.G. Copeland.** 1997. Mouse models of human disease. Part II: recent progress and future directions. Genes Dev. *11*:11-43.
3. **Berg, P.** 1993. Co-chairman's remarks: reverse genetics: directed modification of DNA for functional analysis. Gene *135*:261-264.
4. **Bos, N.A., H. Kimura, C.G. Meeuwsen, H. De Visser, M.P. Hazenberg, B.S. Wostmann, J.R. Pleasants, R. Benner, and D.M. Marcus.** 1989. Serum immunoglobulin levels and naturally occurring antibodies against carbohydrate antigens in germ-free BALB/c mice fed chemically defined ultrafiltered diet. Eur. J. Immunol. *19*:2335-2339.
5. **Brandtzaeg, P.** 1998. The increasing power of immunohistochemistry and immunocytochemistry. J. Immunol. Methods *216*:49-67.
6. 1998. Building a global mouse house [editorial]. Nat. Genet. *18*:299-300.
7. **Burroni, D., M. Cintorino, L. Leoncini, P. Tosi, and C. Ceccarini.** 1988. Site-specific monoclonal antibodies against peanut agglutinin (PNA) from Arachis hypogaea. Immunohistochemical study of tissue-cultured cells and of 27 cases of Hodgkin's disease. Am. J. Pathol. *131*:351-360.
8. **Cattoretti, G., C.C. Chang, K. Cechova, J. Zhang, B.H. Ye, B. Falini, D.C. Louie, K. Offit, R.S. Chaganti, and R. Dalla-Favera.** 1995. BCL-6 protein is expressed in germinal-center B cells. Blood *86*:45-53.
9. **Eichmuller, S., P.A. Stevenson, and R. Paus.** 1996. A new method for double immunolabelling with primary antibodies from identical species. J. Immunol. Methods *190*:255-265.
10. **Flotte, T.J., T.A. Springer, and G.J. Thorbecke.** 1983. Dendritic cell and macrophage staining by monoclonal antibodies in tissue sections and epidermal sheets. Am. J. Pathol. *111*:112-124.
11. **Franke, W.W. and R. Moll.** 1987. Cytoskeletal components of lymphoid organs. I. Synthesis of cytokeratins 8 and 18 and desmin in subpopulations of extrafollicular reticulum cells of human lymph nodes, tonsils, and spleen. Differentiation *36*:145-163.
12. **Fung, K.M., A. Messing, V.M. Lee, and J.Q. Trojanowski.** 1992. A novel modification of the avidin-biotin complex method for immunohistochemical studies of transgenic mice with murine monoclonal antibodies. J. Histochem. Cytochem. *40*:1319-1328.
13. **Gendelman, H.E., T.R. Moench, O. Narayan, and D.E. Griffin.** 1983. Selection of a fixative for identifying T cell subsets, B cells, and macrophages in paraffin-embedded mouse spleen. J. Immunol. Methods *65*:137-145.

14. Gerdes, J., U. Schwab, H. Lemke, and H. Stein. 1983. Production of a mouse monoclonal antibody reactive with a human nuclear antigen associated with cell proliferation. Int. J. Cancer *31*:13-20.

15. Hermiston, M.L., C.B. Latham, J.I. Gordon, and K.A. Roth. 1992. Simultaneous localization of six antigens in single sections of transgenic mouse intestine using a combination of light and fluorescence microscopy. J. Histochem. Cytochem. *40*:1283-1290.

16. Hierck, B.P., L.V. Iperen, A.C. Gittenberger-De Groot, and R.E. Poelmann. 1994. Modified indirect immunodetection allows study of murine tissue with mouse monoclonal antibodies. J. Histochem. Cytochem. *42*:1499-1502.

17. Iida, S., P.H. Rao, M. Butler, P. Corradini, M. Boccadoro, B. Klein, R.S. Chaganti, and R. Dalla-Favera. 1997. Deregulation of MUM1/IRF4 by chromosomal translocation in multiple myeloma. Nature Genet. *17*:226-230.

18. Iyonaga, K., M. Takeya, T. Yamamoto, M. Ando, and K. Takahashi. 1997. A novel monoclonal antibody, RM-4, specifically recognizes rat macrophages and dendritic cells in formalin-fixed, paraffin-embedded tissues. Histochem. J. *29*:105-116.

19. Key, G., M.H. Becker, B. Baron, M. Duchrow, C. Schluter, H.D. Flad, and J. Gerdes. 1993. New Ki-67-equivalent murine monoclonal antibodies (MIB 1-3) generated against bacterially expressed parts of the Ki-67 cDNA containing three 62 base pair repetitive elements encoding for the Ki-67 epitope. Lab. Invest. *68*:629-636.

20. Kinzler, K.W. and B. Vogelstein. 1996. Breast cancer. What's mice got to do with it? [news; comment]. Nature *382*:672.

21. Kubbutat, M.H., G. Key, M. Duchrow, C. Schluter, H.D. Flad, and J. Gerdes. 1994. Epitope analysis of antibodies recognising the cell proliferation associated nuclear antigen previously defined by the antibody Ki-67 (Ki-67 protein). J. Clin. Pathol. *47*:524-528.

22. Langlois, N.E., G. King, R. Herriot, and W.D. Thompson. 1994. Non-enzymatic retrieval of antigen permits staining of follicle centre cells by the rabbit polyclonal antibody to protein gene product 9.5. J. Pathol. *173*:249-253.

23. Langlois, N.E., G. King, R. Herriot, and W.D. Thompson. 1995. An evaluation of the staining of lymphomas and normal tissues by the rabbit polyclonal antibody to protein gene product 9.5 following non- enzymatic retrieval of antigen. J. Pathol. *175*:433-439.

24. Lu, Q.L. and T.A. Partridge. 1998. A new blocking method for application of murine monoclonal antibody to mouse tissue sections. J. Histochem. Cytochem. *46*:977-984.

25. Moll, R., W.W. Franke, D.L. Schiller, B. Geiger, and R. Krepler. 1982. The catalog of human cytokeratins: patterns of expression in normal epithelia, tumors and cultured cells. Cell *31*:11-24.

26. Penit, C. and F. Vasseur. 1993. Phenotype analysis of cycling and postcycling thymocytes: evaluation of detection methods for BrdUrd and surface proteins. Cytometry *14*:757-763.

27. Perez-Martinez, C., R.A. Garcia-Fernandez, M.C. Ferreras-Estrada, A. Escudero-Diez, J. Espinosa-Alvarez, and M.J. Garcia-Iglesias. 1998. Optimization of the immunohistochemical demonstration of keratins in paraffin wax-embedded mouse skin. J. Comp. Pathol. *119*:177-181.

28. Ramos-Vara, J.A., M.A. Miller, E. Lopez, N. Prats, and L. Brevik. 1994. Reactivity of polyclonal human CD3 antiserum in lymphoid tissues of cattle, sheep, goats, rats and mice. Am. J. Vet. Res. *55*:63-66.

29. Rosai, J. 1997. Pathology: a historical opportunity [editorial]. Am. J. Pathol. *151*:3-6.

30. Rose, M.L., M.S. Birbeck, V.J. Wallis, J.A. Forrester, and A.J. Davies. 1980. Peanut lectin binding properties of germinal centres of mouse lymphoid tissue. Nature *284*:364-366.

31. Said, J.W., I.P. Shintaku, and G.S. Pinkus. 1988. Immunohistochemical staining for terminal deoxynucleotidyl transferase (TDT). An enhanced method in routinely processed formalin-fixed tissue sections. Am. J. Clin. Pathol. *89*:649-652.

32. Shi, S.R., R.J. Cote, and C.R. Taylor. 1997. Antigen retrieval immunohistochemistry: past, present, and future. J. Histochem. Cytochem. *45*:327-343.

33. Shintaku, I.P. and J.W. Said. 1987. Detection of estrogen receptors with monoclonal antibodies in routinely processed formalin-fixed paraffin sections of breast carcinoma. Use of DNase pretreatment to enhance sensitivity of the reaction. Am. J. Clin. Pathol. *87*:161-167.

34. Tsubura, A., T. Hatano, S. Hayama, and S. Morii. 1991. Immunophenotypic difference of keratin expression in normal mammary glandular cells from five different species. Acta Anat. *140*:287-293.

35. Whiteland, J.L., S.M. Nicholls, C. Shimeld, D.L. Easty, N.A. Williams, and T.J. Hill. 1995. Immunohistochemical detection of T-cell subsets and other leukocytes in paraffin-embedded rat and mouse tissues with monoclonal antibodies. J. Histochem. Cytochem. *43*:313-320.

36. Yamamoto, A., M. Atsuta, and K. Hamatani. 1992. Restricted expression of recombination activating gene (RAG-1) in mouse lymphoid tissues. Cell Biochem. Funct. *10*:71-77.

37. Ye, B.H., G. Cattoretti, Q. Shen, J. Zhang, N. Hawe, R. de Waard, C. Leung, M. Nouri-Shirazi, A. Orazi, R.S. Chaganti, et al. 1997. The BCL-6 proto-oncogene controls germinal-centre formation and Th2- type inflammation. Nat. Genet. *16*:161-170.

Antigen Retrieval Procedures for Cell Proliferation Markers

11

Anthony S.-Y. Leong and Farid S. Zaer

Hunter Area Pathology Services and The Discipline of Anatomical Pathology, University of Newcastle, Australia

INTRODUCTION

Abnormal cell proliferation appears to be a precursor and perhaps a predictor of tumorigenesis (43). The rate of tumor growth is determined by the difference in the rates of proliferation and tumor cell death, the latter through necrosis and apoptosis. Cell proliferation kinetics is thus an important biologic variable in neoplastic and nonneoplastic tissues and a useful adjunct to the histologic classification and grading of tumors. A variety of techniques employed in the assessment of cell proliferation have demonstrated that quantitation of the proliferative activity in malignant tumors can predict clinical outcome (7), and the assessment of this biologic parameter has become of great clinical and pathologic interest (26).

Cells in tissues have only three options: they can grow and divide, remain dormant, or die by programmed cell death or apoptosis. The proliferation cycle consists of the several recognizable phases. The dormant or resting cell is in G_0. To begin dividing, it must be induced to enter G_1, in which the cell increases in size and prepares to copy its DNA. This copying occurs in the next phase, termed the S-phase, and enables the cell to duplicate precisely its complement of chromosomes. After this stage of chromosomal duplication, a second gap period, termed G_2, follows, during which the cell prepares for mitosis or the M-phase, when the enlarged cell finally divides to produce two identical cells. The M-phase is readily recognizable in light microscopy by the presence of mitotic figures. The new cells immediately enter G_1

Antigen Retrieval Techniques
Edited by Shan-Rong Shi, Jiang Gu, and Clive R. Taylor
©2000 Eaton Publishing, Natick, MA

and may go through the full cycle again. Alternatively, they may stop cycling temporarily or permanently. Cyclins, cyclin-dependent kinases (CDKs), and their inhibitors (CDKIs) regulate progression through the cell cycle. Mutations that dysregulate the activity of cyclins and CDKs therefore favor cell proliferation, with mishaps affecting the expression of cyclin D and CDK4 being common events in neoplastic transformation. Also of great interest is the recognition of a concomitant or parallel cycle of physiologic cell death or apoptosis, but this is beyond the scope of this chapter and is not discussed.

This chapter is concerned with the assessment of immunologic markers that identify cells in the proliferation cycle and the use of antigen retrieval (AR) techniques for the demonstration and optimization of these markers. While antibodies to some of the cyclins, CDKs, and CDKIs are now available, many are not immunoreactive following fixation and paraffin embedding. Only markers that are immunoreactive in routinely processed and paraffin-embedded tissues are discussed here. In addition, some applications of these markers in the prediction of tumor outcome are briefly reviewed.

MARKERS OF CELL PROLIFERATION

The counting of mitotic figures is the most established method employed by pathologists to assess proliferative activity in paraffin sections. While simple to perform, mitosis counting is not a standardized or reproducible procedure. The recognition of mitosis is subjective, and furthermore, it only reflects the mitotic or M-phase of the cell cycle. If the M-phase is prolonged, mitotic counts may indicate a deceptively high rate of proliferation in some tumors, such as basal cell carcinoma of the skin. It has also been demonstrated that the number of mitotic figures is inversely related to the interval between removal of the tissue and fixation. Delays in fixation allow the M-phase to proceed to completion with corresponding reduction in the number of mitotic figures.

TRITIATED THYMIDINE UPTAKE AND BROMODEOXYURIDINE INCORPORATION

Better established techniques for measurement of tumor proliferation are the tritiated thymidine labeling or bromodeoxyuridine (BrdU) incorporation techniques. While these procedures provide accurate measurements of cell proliferation, they are laborious, difficult to perform, and not appropriate for diagnostic laboratories. Thymidine is one of the four DNA bases and is incorporated into the nuclear DNA only during S-phase of the cell cycle. Thymidine uptake or the tritiated thymidine labeling index has become the gold standard for measuring cell cycle kinetics, but the requirement for fresh tissue, the loss of tissue viability, and the time required in completing the assessment have hampered its use on a routine basis. Furthermore, thymidine has to be tagged with a radioactive substance, introducing additional problems of handling and disposal. The development of monoclonal antibodies to the thymidine analog BrdU dispenses with the need for autoradiography, but the procedure still requires in vivo or fresh tissue preincubation. The use of exonuclease III after DNase I digestion has been reported to improve sensitivity of staining in fixed cells (71), and heat-induced AR has been applied successfully to enhance sensitivity further for immunohistochemical study of BrdU (77).

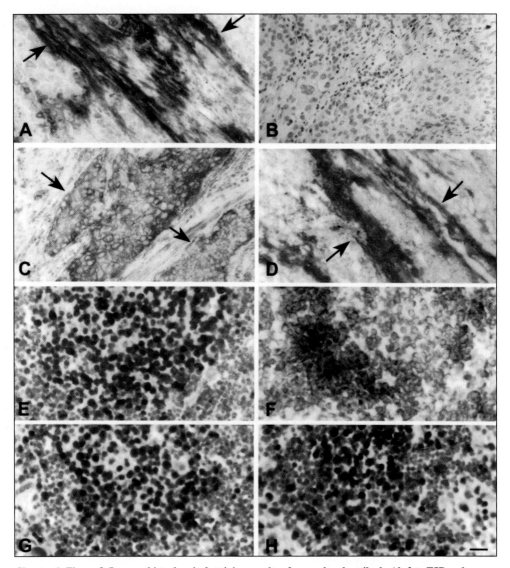

Chapter 1, Figure 8. Immunohistochemical staining results of monoclonal antibody Ab-3 to TSP and monoclonal antibody MIB-1 on frozen tissue sections of bladder cancer and lymph node. The effects of pretreatment with CaCl$_2$ (A–D), and the monoclonal antibody MIB-1 on frozen sections of lymph node showing similar effects of CaCl$_2$ (E–H). (A) Frozen section fixed in 10% neutral buffered formaldehyde (NBF) for 10 min showed strong TSP labeling of extracellular pattern (arrows): no pretreatment (positive control). (B) Frozen section incubated with 50 mmol/L CaCl$_2$ at 4°C overnight, then fixed in 10% NBF. A negative staining result was demonstrated in 50% of total area in the section. (C) Frozen section incubated with CaCl$_2$ at 4°C overnight, and then fixed in 10% NBF. An altered pattern of staining showing cytoplasmic staining of cancer cells (arrows) was showed in 40% of the total area in the tissue section for Ab-3. Such an altered pattern was demonstrated in 4/7 antibodies. (D) Frozen tissue section incubated with 20 mmol/L EDTA after overnight incubation with 50 mmol/L CaCl$_2$ and fixed in 10% NBF for 10 minutes. Restoration of extracellular positive staining (arrows) was demonstrated. (E) Frozen tissue section of lymph node was incubated in distilled water at 4°C overnight and then fixed in acetone, showing strong MIB-1 nuclear staining of the germinal center. (F) Frozen section incubated with 50 mmol/L CaCl$_2$ at 4°C overnight and then fixed in acetone showed a negative result. (G) Frozen section incubated with 20 mmol/L EDTA at 4°C overnight and then fixed in acetone showed slightly decreased nuclear staining. (H) Frozen section incubated with 20 mmol/L EDTA after overnight incubation with 50 mmol/L CaCl$_2$ at 4°C and fixed in acetone showed partial restoration of nuclear staining of MIB-1. AEC was used as chromogen, and hematoxylin was used as the counterstain. Original magnification × 100. Scale bar = 50 μm (A–D) × 200; 25 μm (E–H). Reprinted with permission from Reference 67.

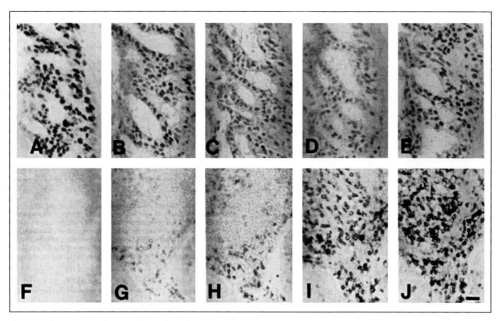

Chapter 2, Figure 1. Comparisons of the intensity of AR immunostaining in routinely formalin-fixed, paraffin-embedded tissue sections. (A–E) A monoclonal antibody (mAb) to ER in breast tissue. (F–J) mAb MT1 in lymph node. Sodium diethylbarbiturate-HCl (SDH) buffer was utilized as the AR solution for both antibodies. (A–E) The pH values of the AR solution were pH 2.0, 3.0, 4.0, 6.0, and 8.0, which correspond to staining intensities of ++++, +++, +, ++, and +++, respectively, for ER with a type B pattern. (F–J) A type C pattern with SDH as the AR solution of pH 2.0, 3.0, 4.0, 6.0, and 8.0 and staining intensities of -, +, ++, +++, and ++++, respectively, for MT1. Some nuclei showed very weak false nuclear staining in F. Diaminobenzidine (DAB) was the chromogen, and hematoxylin was the counterstain. Original magnification 100×. Bar = 20 μm. Reprinted with permission from Reference 38.

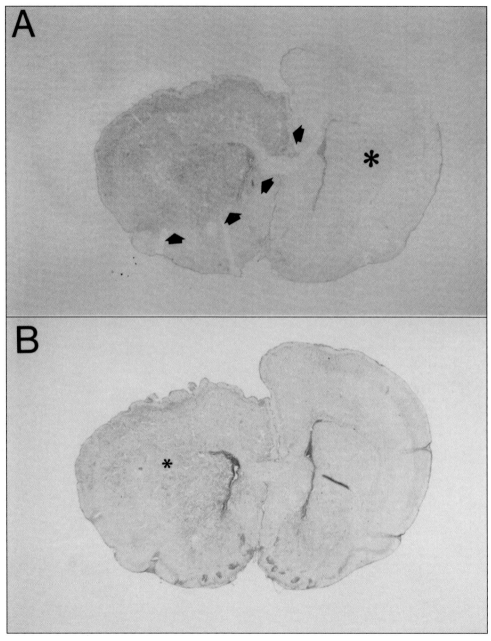

Chapter 4, Figure 1. NMDA-injected rat brain. Pattern of TUNEL-detected DNA fragmentation in adjacent frontal paraffin sections of a 7-day-old rat pup brain 24 h after unilateral injection of the neurotoxin NMDA in the striatum. Brain tissue was perfusion-fixed and subsequently postfixed for 10 days in paraformaldehyde (shown in panel B). Weak TUNEL signal of variable intensity is observed in the ipsilateral side (small asterisk) of the brain, whereas the contralateral side is also weakly positive. Panel A shows a section adjacent to the one shown in panel B, but after microwave pretreatment in pH 3.0 citrate buffer. Clear and increased labeling is now observed, allowing the lesion area to be clearly delineated (arrowheads), whereas nonspecific labeling is absent in the contralateral side (large asterisk). Reprinted with permission from Reference 39.

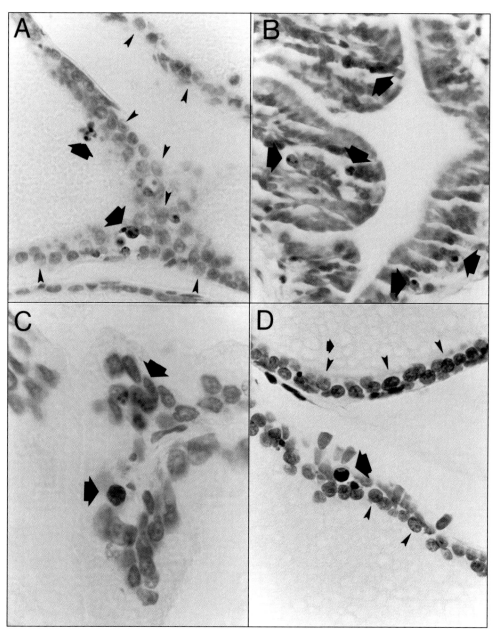

Chapter 4, Figure 2. TUNEL-positive, apoptotic cells in the rat prostate 3 days after castration identified after MW pretreatment and a 50% reduction in standard enzyme and label concentrations. (A) MW pretreatment at pH 3.0 resulted in a clear identification of apoptotic cells (arrows), but with some weak background, also seen in non-apoptotic cells (arrowheads). (B) Background staining is absent following incubation at pH 9.0 and shows clear staining of apoptotic cells (arrows). (C) MW pretreatment at pH 9.0 reveals prominent staining of individual apoptotic cells (arrows), whereas no background staining was apparent. (D) Standard enzyme conditions in combination with MW and PK pretreatment caused all nuclei, including intact ones, to be stained (arrowheads), although a possibly apoptotic nucleus (large arrow) can still be recognized. Small arrows indicate prostate vesicle lumen wall.

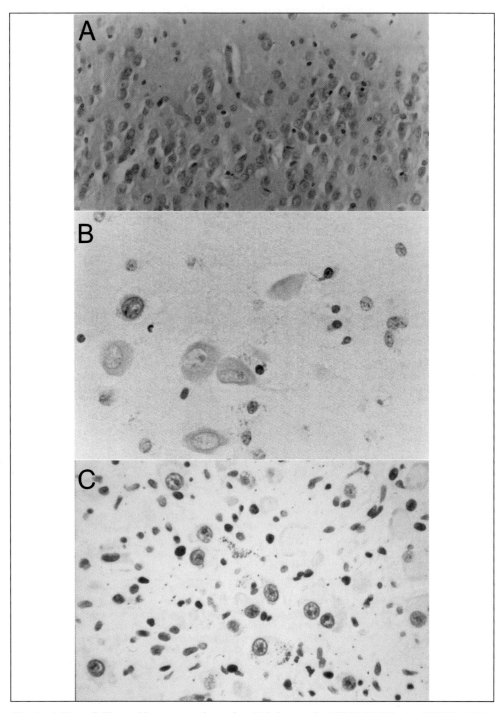

Chapter 4, Figure 3. Human hippocampus tissue of an Alzheimer patient (PMD 4h) following TUNEL. (A) No labeling is observed if no MW pretreatment is applied. (B) In adjacent sections, following a short MW protocol at pH 3.0 in combination with rapid cooling (see text for details), an optimal staining pattern was achieved, as revealed by labeling of only some hippocampal neurons and smaller glia cells, in the absence of background labeling. (C) Almost every nucleus (neuron or glia) has become positive following standard (2× 5 minutes full power) microwave pretreatment of human postmortem brain tissue in pH 3.0 or 6.0 buffer including 15 minutes cooling at room temperature and standard enzyme and label concentrations. Local differences in specific signal can no longer be assessed.

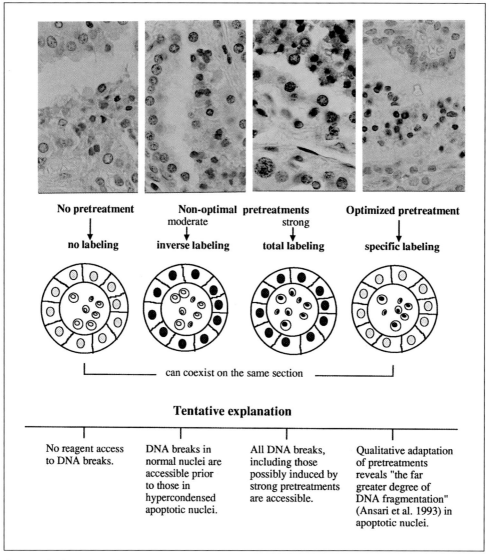

Chapter 4, Figure 4. Possible TUNEL patterns in relation to tissue pretreatment. Tissue fixation, i.e., protein and DNA cross-linking, in addition to extensive condensation of the chromatin during apoptosis, will hamper the TUNEL enzyme mixture components from reaching the fragmented 3′ OH DNA ends that are present in much larger amounts in apoptotic cells than in intact cells. The adaptation of fixation conditions, pretreatment, and enzyme/label concentrations, in addition to a careful monitoring of color development after TUNEL, will allow specific identification of apoptotic cells, before the lower amounts of DNA breaks in nonapoptotic cells becomes detectable. Reprinted with permission from Reference 34.

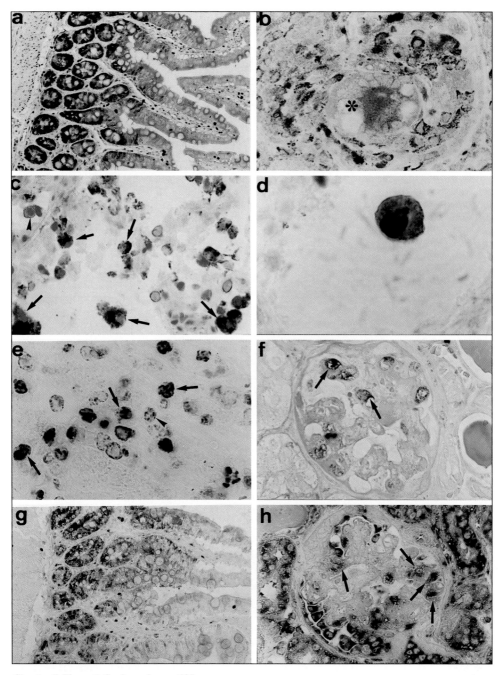

Chapter 7, Figure 1. See legend on p. 135.

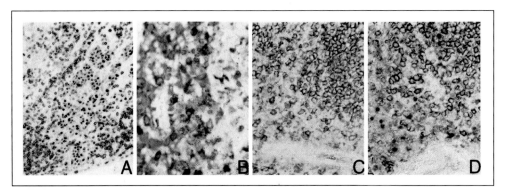

Chapter 10, Figure 3. Double immunostaining for MUM-1/IRF-4, transgenic MUM-1, and lineage markers in mouse tissue. (A and B) Sections from a wild-type mouse lymph node. (C and D) Sections from transgenic MUM-1. (A) MUM-1 stains in brown the nuclei of B220-negative (blue) plasma cells. (B) MUM-1-positive plasma cells (brown) are not stained by the antimacrophage antibody Mac-2 (blue). (C) Negative control mouse IgG1 negative stain (in blue) on a B220-stained (brown) lymph node. (D) myc-tagged transgenic MUM-1 is recognized (blue nuclei) by 9E10 (mouse IgG1 monoclonal antibody) in B220-negative (brown) plasma cells.

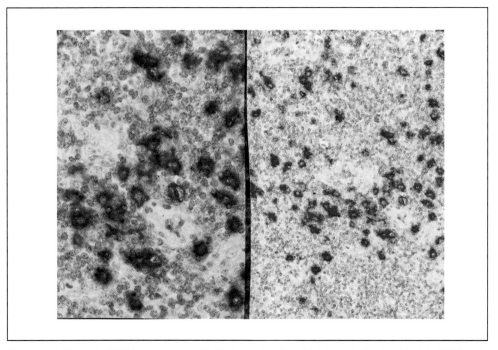

Chapter 14, Figure 2. CD30 is demonstrated in both panels using AR (citrate buffer for 15 min), HRS4 antibody (kind gift of Prof. Pfreundschuh, Hamburg, Germany), and TSA. HRS4 was used at 1/100th of the dilution used in the conventional ABC technique. Typically, CD30-positive blasts were seen in a case of florid Epstein-Barr virus infection.

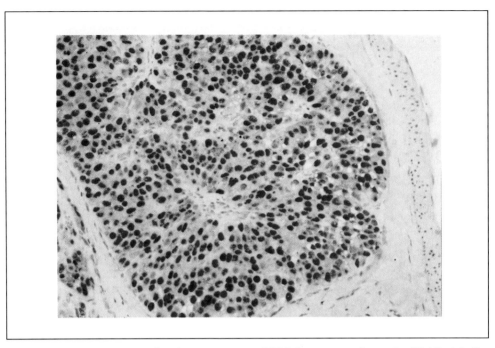

Chapter 14, Figure 3. The expression of estrogen receptor (ER) in breast cancer tissue using AR (citrate buffer for 30 min), the anti-ER-Ab (DAKO), and TSA. Anti-ER-Ab was used at 1/10th of the dilution used in the conventional ABC technique. The strong nuclear staining of ER is highlighted in this intraductal carcinoma.

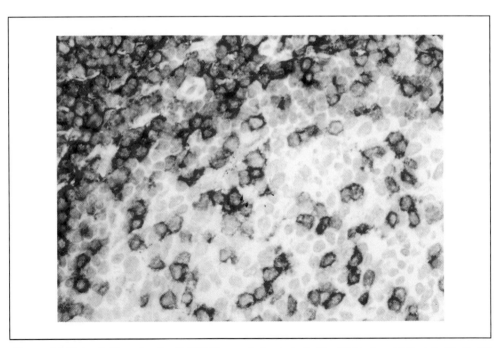

Chapter 14, Figure 4. Monoclonal anti-CD3 (Novocastra) was used after AR treatment (citrate buffer for 20 min and trypsin 0.1% for 5 min) and TSA. CD3-Ab was used at 1/25th of the dilution used in the conventional ABC technique. Strong staining of CD3-positive T cells is seen in the mantle zone of a reactive germinal center; some scattered T cells are seen within the germinal center.

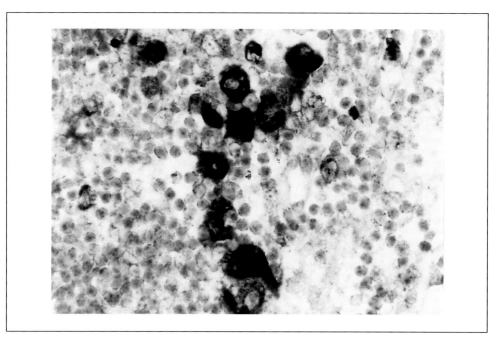

Chapter 14, Figure 5. In situ hybridization of IL-6 using three digoxigenen double-labeled oligonucleotides. Strong cytoplasmic staining of Hodgkin cells and weaker staining of histiocytic cells in a case of Hodgkin's disease. The NBT-BCIP substrate was used. Morphology is not optimal; only proteolytic digestion with proteinase K was used. Although slides are slightly overdigested, there is a good signal-to-noise ratio.

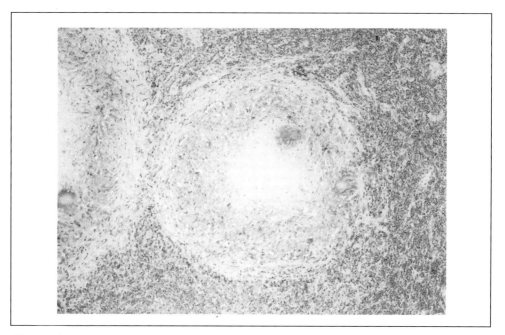

Chapter 14, Figure 6. In situ hybridization of IL-6 using AR (citrate buffer for 15 min) and proteinase K [10 µg/mL] for 5 min), three digoxigenen double-labeled oligonucleotides, and F(ab)$_2$-anti-Dig-POX and TSA. Here a case of tuberculosis was examined. The histiocytic and Langhans giant cells are stained brown. DAB was used as substrate.

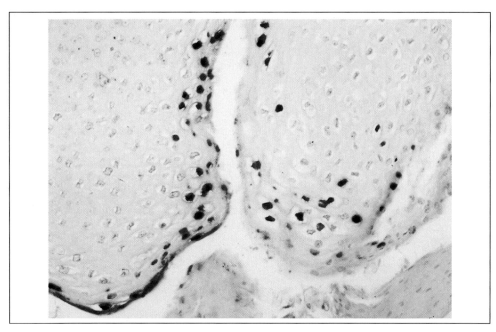

Chapter 14, Figure 8. In situ hybridization of human papillomavirus (HPV) in a case of condyloma acuminatum. AR (citrate buffer for 30 min), three labeled oligonucleotides, and ABC/AP with neufuchsin/naphthol AS BI substrate were used. This is by far the most brilliant contrast; however, the counterstain is weak due to the boiling effect after microwave pretreatment of slides.

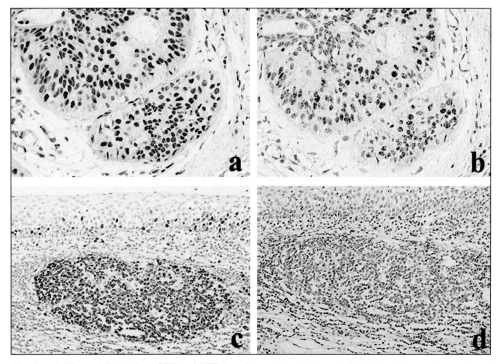

Chapter 15, Figure 1. Detection of ER and MIB-1 antigens. (a) ER, AR with citrate buffer (pH 6.0), (b) ER, TSA method without AR, (c) MIB-1, AR with citrate buffer (pH 6.0), and (d) MIB-1, TSA method without AR. It should be noted that ER can be comparably detected by TSA method, but AR is mandatory for MIB-1 (no staining by TSA method).

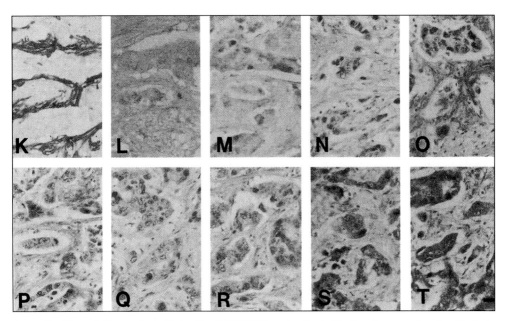

Appendix, Figure 1. Comparison of intensity of AR-IHC by using the test battery for monoclonal antibody to thrombospondin (TSP) on sections of bladder carcinoma. The AR protocols used are arranged in the following order: pH 1.0, 100°C, 20 min (K); pH 1.0, 100°C, 10 min (L); pH 1.0, 90°C, 10 min (M); pH 6.0, 100°C, 20 min (N); pH 6.0, 100°C, 10 min (O); pH 6.0, 90°C, 10 min (P); pH 10.0, 100°C, 20 min (Q); pH 10.0, 100°C, 10 min (R); pH 10.0, 90°C, 10 min (S); no AR pretreatment (T). The strongest extracellular labeling of TSP was found by using an AR solution at pH 1.0, as shown in K. Under lower heating conditions (L, M), the intensity was decreased progressively (K > L > M). Other protocols using pH 6.0 or 10.0 gave poor results, similar to a lack of pretreatment (T). Diaminobenzidine (DAB) was used as the chromogen, with hematoxylin counterstaining. Original magnification 100×. Scale bar = 50 μm. Reprinted with permission from Reference 90.

MONOCLONAL Ki-67 ANTIBODY AND VARIANTS

The optimal diagnostic reagent to detect cycling cells would be an antibody that can identify proteins specifically restricted to the various phases of the cell cycle and that does not require fresh tissue preincubation. Candidate proteins with these characteristics that have been identified include the Ki-67-defined antigen (detected by antibodies MIB-1, Ki-S5, Ki-S1, and polyclonal Ki-67), proliferating cell nuclear antigen (PCNA/cyclin), and DNA topoisomerase II-α. A number of other antibodies have been developed including those to the M1 subunit of ribonucleotide reductase, p105, PAA, and C_5F_{10}, the latter identifying cells in the M-phase of the cell cycle; these are mostly not immunoreactive in fixed tissue and have not been extensively used (14). In situ hybridization for localization of histone H3 and/or H4 m RNA is a more recent technique to study the S-phase of dividing cells, but this is not an immunohistochemical procedure.

The Ki-67 monoclonal antibody was generated to a Hodgkin's disease cell line and was determined to identify a nuclear antigen present only in proliferating cells (11). The antigen recognized by Ki-67 is a 345- to 395-kDa nonhistone protein complex that is susceptible to protease treatment (12). The gene encoding the Ki-67 protein is localized to chromosome 10 and organized into 15 exons. The center of the gene is formed by an extraordinary 6845-bp exon containing 16 successively repeated homologous segments of 366 bp, known as the Ki-67 repeats, each containing a highly conserved new motif of 66 bp, the Ki-67 motif. The Ki-67 antigen appears to play a pivotal role in maintaining cell proliferation, as Ki-67 protein antisense oligonucleotides significantly inhibit the uptake of radioactive thymidine in human tumor cell lines in a dose-dependent manner (9). This protein complex is expressed during all non-G_0 phases of the cycle and is thus a useful marker for all cycling cells. The limitation of the Ki-67 monoclonal antibody was that it could only be used on fresh frozen tissue sections, as the antigen was susceptible to most forms of fixation and tissue processing.

A large number of studies have validated the efficacy and sensitivity of this reagent by comparing the proliferation index of Ki-67 immunostaining with that obtained by titriated thymidine uptake and BrdU labeling. Furthermore, many studies have validated the usefulness of Ki-67 as a prognostic determinant in a variety of malignant tumors including those of the breast, prostate, peripheral nerve sheath, epidermis, cartilage, esophagus, liver, and ovary (5,15,55,58,81).

Several alternative antibodies to the Ki-67 antigen are now available that are immunoreactive in routinely fixed paraffin-embedded sections, namely, MIB-1, Ki-S1, Ki-S5, and polyclonal Ki-67 (44). These antibodies appear to be suitable substitutes for the monoclonal antibody Ki-67 in assessment of tumor cell proliferative index (39), are obviating the need for fresh frozen tissue. Several MIB antibodies are available commercially, but MIB-1 is the antibody of choice for the assessment of cell proliferation antigens in paraffin sections. These reagents have now been widely employed for the assessment of the proliferative index of a variety of malignant tumors.

PROLIFERATING CELL NUCLEAR ANTIGEN

PCNA, a 36-kDa nonhistone nuclear protein, was first described independently by two groups of investigators and represents a component of the DNA polymerase-delta (4). An antibody was described in the sera of selected patients with systemic lupus

183

erythematosus that reacted with a nuclear antigen in proliferating cells (51). The sera did not react with the nuclei of renal tubular or hepatic parenchymal cells but did react with the lymphocytes of lymphoid follicles. However, normal peripheral lymphocytes were not labeled, and 20% of the cells became positive on mitogenic stimulation with phytohemagglutinin. Bravo and Celis (3) employed high-resolution two-dimensional gel electrophoresis to screen for proteins whose rate of synthesis increased substantially in proliferating, compared with resting cells. They found a protein, called cyclin, in small amounts in normal or nondividing cells; it was synthesized by normal proliferating cells, with levels being strikingly increased in the S-phase. While initially thought to be the same as PCNA, it is now clearly established that PCNA and cyclin are two different proteins.

There are at least two forms of PCNA, one associated with the replicon structure and the other more loosely associated with the cell nucleus. Although both are retained following formalin fixation, alcoholic fixatives such as methacarn only preserve the former (4). The level of PCNA has been shown to correlate with cellular proliferation (specifically with DNA synthesis), rising during late G_1 and peaking during S-phase, and declining during G_2 and M-phases. In tumors, there is good correlation between PCNA expression and the S-phase fraction, as determined by flow cytometry. Earlier work with anti-PCNA auto-antisera suggested that PCNA positivity correlated with mitotic activity and tumor grade (59). PCNA has since been widely used to study the proliferative index of tumors. It appears to correlate with mitotic activity and tumor grade and parallels the results of flow cytometric determination of S-phase (10).

Several caveats apply when using anti-PCNA antibodies to assess cell proliferation in tissue sections. It has been observed that in malignant cell lines such as HeLa, PCNA levels increase during S-phase but do not remain at zero during the other phases of the cell cycle. Furthermore, it seems that relative amounts of PCNA differ in different tumor cell types and that the relationship of immunohistochemically stainable PCNA to the phase of the cell cycle varies with the cell type (14). One explanation for this finding is that it reflects a "loss of control" of PCNA expression in neoplastic transformation. While it has been established that different components of the antigen are preserved by formalin compared with alcohol-based fixatives, a greater limiting factor is the extreme sensitivity of the antigen to formalin fixation. Immunohistochemical demonstration of the antigen progressively diminishes with increasing durations of fixation. As such, the interpretation of PCNA values should be done with a great deal of caution, especially as the fixation process is difficult to standardize between laboratories and even within the same laboratory (38). Furthermore, there are variations between antibody clones (50), with marked differences in sensitivity between two common commercial clones, PC10 and 19A2. The former produces much stronger staining intensity and labels a significantly larger proportion of tumor cells (38). Nevertheless, there is a demonstrable correlation between PC10 and 19A2 counts with those obtained with Ki-67. However, the two anti-PCNA antibodies produce much higher counts (39), thought to be due to the long half-life of PCNA, which has been shown to be about 20 hours (84). Noncycling cells may thus display stainable PCNA. Weakly stained cells show poor correlation with the S-phase, and only strongly stained cells should be counted when employing anti-PCNA antibodies.

Despite these important limitations and the lack of standardization, anti-PCNA antibodies continue to be used extensively in the determination of tumor proliferative indices, raising serious questions concerning the validity of reported results and interpretations.

184

DNA TOPOISOMERASE II-α

Topoisomerase II (Topo II) is a eukaryotic homodimeric nuclear enzyme that exists in two isoforms in human cells, the 170-kDa form (Topo II-α) and the 180-kDa form (Topo II-β). Topo II-α is a key enzyme in DNA metabolism, with important roles in DNA replication and chromosome partitioning during cell division; the function of Topo II-β is poorly understood (80) but is probably not related to mitotic function (16). Topo II-α has been shown to be a marker of cell proliferation in both normal (18,82) and neoplastic tissue, its expression correlating with MIB-1 counts (46). Topo II-α has been studied in a variety of malignant tumors including carcinomas of the breast (46, 78), urinary bladder (52), salivary gland (19), ovary (20,73), and lung (24), as well as melanocytic nevi and malignant melanoma (47,57), and malignant lymphoma (1,17). This proliferation marker has also been employed in the study of human gastric disorders (20,83) and for the distinction of adrenocortical adenomas and carcinomas (21).

Interestingly, chemotherapeutic agents targeted against Topo II interfere with its DNA cleavage-rejoining action, trapping Topo II-α enzyme with DNA in a noncleavable complex. This results in the accumulation of stabilized double-stranded DNA breaks, which are lethal to the cell at the G_2M-phase of the cell cycle (54). In vitro studies indicate that sensitivity to Topo II-inhibiting drugs is dependent on the expression level of the Topo II-α gene in target cells. These observations have resulted in the labeling of this enzyme as a marker of drug sensitivity. For example, high levels of Topo II-α expression correlate with sensitivity to doxorubicin treatment in invasive breast carcinoma, particularly in the presence of amplification of the c-*erb*B-2 gene (46).

Ki-S1 antibody has been shown to be identical with Topo II-α (2); Ki-S1 stained a protein in immunoblots of *Saccharomyces cerevisiae* expressing human topo II-α. The demonstration of this enzyme in fixed embedded sections requires pretreatment using heat-induced AR with one of several solutions including citrate buffer (pH 6.0), EDTA (pH 8.0), or Tris-buffered saline (pH 7.6) (22–24, 46).

ANTIGEN RETRIEVAL METHODS FOR PROLIFERATION MARKERS

Fixatives

Certain antigens, particularly cell surface antigens that are expressed weakly in fresh frozen tissue, may be completely lost during routine tissue processing and embedding. Leong and Gilham (34) clearly demonstrated that tissues fixed in formaldehyde displayed a distinct and progressive loss of many tissue antigens, frequently proportional to the duration of exposure to the fixative. To circumvent this, a variety of alternative fixatives have been employed. The alcohol-based reagents such as ethanol, Carnoy's solution, and methacarn appear to optimize the immunostaining of intermediate filament proteins; heavy metal fixatives such as B5 and Zenker's solution are preferred for intranuclear antigens; Bouin's solution is used for neuropeptides and biogenic amines; and periodate-lysine-paraformaldehyde oxidizes carbohydrate moieties and stabilizes lipids and proteins as well as some membrane proteins (27). In addition, special methods of tissue processing such as freeze drying (53), freeze substitution with low-temperature plastics, and the acetone-methyl benzoate-xylene procedure (60) have been advocated for the preservation of labile tissue antigens. All these methods have met with varying success, but at the expense of good cytomorphologic preservation (27). The extent of protein denaturation, which results from the action of fixative, is not critically important for morphologic preservation; however, it is significant in immunolabeling. The risk of antigenic denaturation is particularly high with fixatives containing acid substances, because these cause destruction of the tertiary and quaternary structures of cellular proteins. Thus, when formalin is used, it should be carefully buffered, since oxidation to formic acid occurs when it stands. No single fixative appears to be universally ideal for all antigens, and different mordants seem to afford varying levels of preservation for different antigens.

Microwave irradiation has been successfully employed as the primary mode of tissue fixation in the routine diagnostic laboratory, accelerating the fixation process and producing excellent quality sections and cytomorphology (25,30,31,68) and accelerating immunolabeling (35). Importantly, tissues fixed by irradiating in normal saline and processed through graded alcohols and xylene before paraffin embedding clearly displayed better preservation of cellular antigens compared with those fixed in 10% buffered formalin for durations as short as 8 hours (28,33,34). Subsequent work established that this method of physical fixation with microwaves produced good preservation of nuclear antigens including the proliferative markers MIB-1, Ki-S1, Ki-S5, and polyclonal Ki-67 (36,39).

Proteolytic Digestion

For a variety of reasons, 10% formalin has remained the most widely used routine fixative, despite its deleterious effects on antigen preservation. Proteolytic digestion was a popular AR method for formalin-fixed tissues, although it was quite clear that its efficacy varied according to the antigen tested. While enhancing some antigens, enzyme pretreatment had deleterious effects on others (33,34). The formaldehydes are thought to induce fixation through their property of forming cross-links between proteins, thereby forming a gel that retains cellular constituents in their in vivo relationships to each other. Soluble proteins are fixed to structural proteins and rendered insoluble, so that the entire structure is given some mechanical strength, allowing it to withstand the rigors of subsequent processing. The cross-linkage of protein occurs mostly between the basic amino acid lysine molecules, although other groups such as imino, amido, peptide, guanidyl, hydroxyl, carboxyl, sulphydryl, and aromatic rings may also be involved. Only the exterior lysine residues react, accounting for 40% to 60% of the total lysine residues. It is thought that the cross-linkage of protein residues caused by formaldehyde, a property valued for its fixative action, may mask antigenic sites of interest, making their detection difficult. Proteolytic predigestion breaks these masking cross-linkages, in turn enhancing immunostaining. While effective for a number of antigens including the intermediate filament proteins, proteolytic digestion on its own imparts little benefit to the immunolabeling of cell proliferation markers.

Heat-Induced Antigen Retrieval

The introduction of heat (microwave)-induced AR by Shi et al. (61) represented a major breakthrough in the immunostaining of formalin-fixed, paraffin-embedded tissue sections. These authors heated paraffin-embedded sections in the presence of heavy metal solutions, such as lead thiocyanate and zinc sulphate, up to temperatures of 100°C to unmask a wide variety of antigens for immunohistology. It was subsequently shown that microwave irradiation of deparaffinized and rehydrated tissue sections in 10 mmol citrate buffer at pH 6.0 produced, with few exceptions, increased intensity and extent of immunostaining (8,13,36,37).

Heat-induced AR made it possible to optimize immunolabeling in fixed tissue sections (36,37) and cytologic preparations (29,69), making immunohistology a reproducible and indispensible adjunct to diagnostic pathology (27,32,41,74). The adoption of citrate buffer as the AR solution eliminated the need to employ heavy metal solutions, which, when heated, generate toxic fumes. While we are far from fully understanding the actions of AR techniques on protein preservation, some important observations have emerged in recent years. It has been demonstrated that heat-induced AR is dependent on several factors, namely, the nature of the retrieval solution, osmolarity, pH, temperature, and time (63,75). Several of these factors have been investigated in relation to the immunolabeling of cell proliferation markers.

Combined Proteolytic Digestion and Heat-Induced Antigen Retrieval

Most antibodies to cell proliferation markers are significantly enhanced by heat-induced AR (44,75). Immunostaining with the MIB-1 antibody is weak without heat-induced AR. However, immunostaining can be further enhanced when heat-induced AR is combined with proteolytic digestion, the enzymatic treatment being applied before the heat-induced AR procedure (39). We found that treatment with trypsin type II, 0.25 mg/mL for 3 minutes at 37°C, produced optimal staining. The same enzyme was effective for the staining of Ki-S1 but was not required for Ki-S5 or polyclonal Ki-67 (39). It has similarly been demonstrated that the effects of heat-induced AR can be further boosted by proteolytic digestion, in a number of selected antigens (36,37). Interestingly, many of these antigens, such as the cytokeratins, benefit from enzymatic digestion applied after heat-induced AR, in contrast to the sequence for MIB-1 and Ki-S.

Temperature

The application of microwaves to produce AR was a major milestone in immunohistochemistry and spawned the development of a variety of methods to generate heat for AR. These have included the use of pressure cookers, steam generated by domestic steamers and other devices, autoclaves, water baths, and plastic pressure cookers in microwave ovens (reviewed in References 64 and 65). These devices were employed to generate heat, which is thought to be the agent responsible for AR. However, the recent demonstration that ultrasound could be employed to produce equally effective AR (56) lent credence to our concept that molecular kinetics may play a role in AR (41,45,72).

When heat is employed, optimal results of AR generally correlate with the product of heating temperatures and duration. Shi et al (63), using archival paraffin-embedded material for retrieval of MIB-1, PCNA (PC10), and a number of other antigens, demonstrated that the lower the temperature of heating used for AR, the longer the time required to reach the same intensity of AR immunostaining compared with that obtained by higher temperature heating. Some authors have claimed that pressure cooking or the combination of microwave heating and pressure cooking gives the most optimal results over a wide range of antigens (49,76). The pressure cooker allows generation of temperatures above boiling point, so-called superheating. A recently developed ultrarapid microwave (MicroMed URM; Milestone, Sorisole, Bergamo, Italy) that produces accurate and constant superheating by microwaves (79) was employed for AR of MIB-1 (70). Exquisite localization of the Ki-67 protein was demonstrated (70,79) to the nucleolus, nucleoplasm, nuclear membrane, and chromosomes of melanoma cells, corresponding to each phase of the cell cycle. This exquisitely sensitive immunolabeling was not possible with heat generated by microwaves alone, suggesting that controlled superheating may provide the optimal AR method.

pH

While the chemical composition of the retrieval solution may have an influence on its efficacy, no single chemical has been identified to be essential or best for the process (40). Currently, several AR solutions have been used to achieve satisfactory results of AR-immunohistochemistry for archival paraffin sections (6,13,36,37,42,48, 66,70,75). In contrast, Shi et al. (62) clearly demonstrated that the pH of the buffer might be critical to the antigen being detected. Their studies of a number of antigens indicated that AR immunoreactivity fell into three essential groups. In one group [L26, proliferating cell nuclear antigen (PCNA), AE1, epithelial membrane antigen (EMA), and neuron-specific enolase (NSE)], there was no significant change in immunoreactivity through pH values ranging from 1.0 to 10.0. A second group (MIB-1 and estrogen receptor) displayed a dramatic decrease in immunostaining at pH values of 3.0 to 6.0 (depending on the type of buffer). Strong immunostaining was seen at pH values above and below this critical range. The third group (MT1 and HMB45) showed gradually increasing intensities of staining with increasing pH and weak staining with buffers of pH values 1.0 to 2.0.

CONCLUSION

The proliferative index of tumors has been demonstrated to be an important biologic determinant. The development of antibodies specific to proteins found in proliferating cells offers a powerful alternative to previous methods of assessment, which were both cumbersome and laborious (as with thymidine labeling) or inaccurate and not standardized (as with mitosis counting). Several antibodies have been generated to the Ki-67 protein which is found in all cycling cells. The demonstration of DNA topoisomerase II-α (MIB-5) has also been shown to be a marker of cell proliferation. This nuclear enzyme appears to be the target of doxorubicin and may thus be a marker of drug sensitivity. While these markers are immunoreactive in paraffin sections, they all require some form of AR for their optimal demonstration. The most effective method, as with most other antigens in fixed, embedded tissue sections, is heat-induced AR. The mechanisms of AR are incompletely understood. While several buffers serve adequately as retrieval solutions, the pH of the solution is critical for its efficacy. The temperature generated and the duration of heating are other important factors.

The factors affecting AR of cell proliferation markers are no different from those for other tissue antigens. Optimal AR is achieved with the correct pH, which, in the case of cell proliferation markers, is alkaline. Superheating appears to provide optimal AR, especially for MIB-1, provided the temperature can be accurately delivered and maintained in a constant manner, as with the new MicroMed URM instrument. When employing an antibody to a new proliferation marker, it is imperative that adequate in-house testing be conducted to determine the optimal AR solution and its optimal pH.

REFERENCES

1. **Bauman, M.E., J.A. Holden, K.A. Brown, W.G. Harker, and S.L. Perkins.** 1997. Differential immunohisto-chemical staining for DNA topoisomerase II alpha and beta in human tissues and for DNA topoisomerase II beta in non-Hodgkin's lymphomas. Mod. Pathol. *10*:168-175.

2. **Boege, F., A. Andersen, S. Jensen, R. Zeidler, and H. Kreipe.** 1996. Proliferation-associated nuclear antigen Ki-S1 is identical with topoisomerase II alpha: delineation of a carboxyl-terminal epitope with peptide antibodies. Am. J. Pathol. *146*:1302-1308.

3. **Bravo, R. and J.E. Celis.** 1980. A search for differential polypeptide synthesis throughout the cell cycle of HeLa cells. J. Cell Biol. *84*:795-798.

4. **Bravo, R. and H. Macdonald-Bravo.** 1987. Existence of two populations of cyclin/proliferating cell nuclear antigen during the cell cycle: association with DNA replication sites. J. Cell Biol. *105*:1549-1554.

5. **Brown, D.C. and K.C. Gatter.** 1990. Monoclonal antibody Ki-67: its use in histopathology. Histopathology *17*:489-503.

6. **Cattoretti, G., M.H. Becker, and G. Key.** 1992. Monoclonal antibodies against recombinant parts of the Ki-67 antigen (MIB1 and MIB3) detect proliferating cells in microwave-processed formalin-fixed paraffin sections. J. Pathol. *168*:357-363.

7. **Coon, J.S., A.L. Landay, and R.S. Weinstein.** 1987. Biology of disease: advances in flow cytometry for diagnostic pathology. Lab. Invest. *57*:453-478.

8. **Cuevas, E.C., A.C. Bateman, B.S. Wilkins, and P.A. Johnson.** 1994. Microwave antigen retrieval immunohisto-chemistry: a study of 80 antibodies. J. Clin. Pathol. *47*:448-452.

9. **Duchrow, M., C. Schluter, and G. Key.** 1995. Cell proliferation-associated nuclear antigen defined by antibody Ki-67, a new kind of cell cycle-maintaining proteins. Arch. Immunol. Ther. Exp. *43*:117-121.

10. **Garcia, R.L., M.D. Coltrera, and A.M. Gown.** 1989. Analysis of proliferative grade using anti-PCNA/cyclin monoclonal antibodies in fixed, embedded tissues: comparison with flow cytometric analysis. J. Pathol. *134*:733-739.

11. **Gerdes, J., H. Lemke, and H. Baisch.** 1984. Cell cycle analysis of a cell proliferation-associated human nuclear antigen defined by the monoclonal antibody Ki-67. J. Immunol. *133*:1710-1715.

12. **Gerdes, J., L. Li, and D.D. Schlueter.** 1991. Immunohistochemical and mo;ecular biologic characterization of the cell proliferation-associated antigen that is defined by the monoclonal antibody Ki-67. Am. J. Pathol. *138*:867-873.

13. **Gown, A.M., N. de Wever, and H. Battifora.** 1993. Microwave-based antigenic unmasking. A revolutionary new technique for routine immunohistochemistry. Appl. Immunohistochem. *1*:256-266.

14. **Gown, A.M. and A.S.-Y. Leong.** 1993. Immunohistochemistry of solid tumors: poorly differentiated round cell and spindle cell tumors II, p. 73-108. *In* A.S.-Y. Leong (Ed.), Applied Immunohistochemistry for the Surgical Pathologist. Edward Arnold, London.

15. **Grigioni, W.F., M. Fiorentino, and A. D'Errico.** 1995. Overexpression of c-met pro-oncogene product and raised Ki-67 index in hepatocellular carcinomas with respect to benign liver conditions. Hepatology *21*:1543-1546.

16. **Grue, P., A. Grasser, M. Schested, P.B. Jensen, A. Uhse, T. Straub, W. Ness, and F. Boege.** 1998. Essential mitotic functions of DNA topoisomerase II-alpha are not adopted by topoisomerase II beta in human H69 cells. J. Biol. Chem. *273*:3360-3366.

17. **Guinee, D.G., Jr., S.L. Perkins, W.D. Travis, J.A. Holden, S.R. Tripp, and M.N. Koss.** 1998. Proliferation and cellular phenotype in lymphomatoid granulomatosis: implications of a higher proliferation index in B cells. Am. J. Surg. Pathol. *23*:1093-1110.

18. **Heck, M.M.S. and W.C. Earnshaw.** 1986. Topoisomerase II: a specific marker for cell proliferation. J. Cell Biol. *103*:2569-2581.

19. **Hirabayshi, S.** 1999. Immunohistochemical detection of DNA to[poisomerase type II alpha and Ki-67 in adenoid cytstic carcinoma and pleomorphic adenoma of the salivary gland. J. Oral Pathol. Med. *28*:131-136.

20. **Holden, J.A.** 1997. Immunohistochemical localization of DNA topoisomerase II in human gastric disorders. Am. J. Pathol. *151*:313.

21. **Iino, K., H. Sasano, N. Yabuki, Y. Oki, A. Kikuchi, T. Yoshimi, and H. Nagura.** 1997. DNA topoisomerase II alpha and Ki-67 in human adrenocortical neoplasms: a possible marker of differentiation between adenomas and carcinomas. Mod. Pathol. *10*:901-907.

22. **Jarvinen, T.A.H., K. Holli, T. Kuukasjarvi, and J.J. Isola.** 1998. Predictive value of topoisomerase II alpha and other prognostic factors for epirubicin chemotherapy in advanced breast cancer. Br. J. Cancer *77*:2267-2273.

23. **Kellner, U., H.-J. Heidebrecht, P. Rudolph, H. Biersack, F. Buck, T. Dakowski, H.-H. Wacker, M. Domanowski, A. Seidel, O. Westergaard, and R. Parwaresch.** 1997. Detection of human topoisomerase IIα in cell lines and tissues: characterization of five novel monoclonal antibodies. J. Histochem. Cytochem. *45*:251-263.

24. **Kreisholt, J., M. Sorensen, P.B. Jensen, B.S. Nielsen, C.B. Andersen, and M. Sehested.** 1998. Immunohisto-chemical detection of DNA topoisomerase II aplha, P-glycoprotein and multidrug resistance protein (MRP) in small cell and non-small cell lung cancer. Br. J. Cancer *77*:1469-1473.

25. **Leong, A.S.-Y.** 1988. Applications of microwave irradiation in histopathology. Pathol. Annu. *23*:213-234.

26. **Leong, A.S.-Y.** 1992. Leading article: new vistas in the histopathological assessment of cancer. Med. J. Aust. *157*:699-701.

27. **Leong, A.S.-Y.** 1993. Immunohistochemistry – theoretical and practical aspects, p. 1-22. *In* A.S.-Y. Leong (Ed.), Diagnostic Immunohistochemistry for the Surgical Pathologist. Edward Arnold, London.

189

28. **Leong, A.S.-Y.** 1994. Microwave technology for morphological analysis. Cell Vision *1*:278-288.
29. **Leong, A.S.-Y.** 1996. Microwave technology in immunohistology – the past twelve years. J. Cell Pathol. *1*:99-108.
30. **Leong, A.S.-Y., M.E. Daymon, and J. Milios.** 1985. Microwave irradiation as a form of fixation for light and electron microscopy. J. Pathol. *146*:313-321.
31. **Leong, A.S.-Y. and C.G. Duncis.** 1986. A method of rapid fixation of large biopsy specimens using microwave irradiation. Pathology *18*:222-225.
32. **Leong, A.S.-Y. and J. Wright.** 1987. The contributions of immunohistochemical staining in tumor diagnosis. Histopathology *11*:1295-1305.
33. **Leong, A.S.-Y., J. Milios, and C.G. Duncis.** 1988. Antigen preservation in microwave-irradiated tissues: a comparison with formaldehyde fixation. J. Pathol. *156*:275-282.
34. **Leong, A.S.-Y. and P.N. Gilham.** 1989. The effects of progressive formaldehyde fixation on the preservation of tissue antigens. Pathology *21*:266-271.
35. **Leong, A.S.-Y. and J. Milios.** 1990. Accelerated immunohistochemical staining by microwaves. J. Pathol. *161*:327-334.
36. **Leong, A.S.-Y. and J. Milios.** 1993. An assessment of the efficacy of the microwave antigen-retrieval procedure on a range of tissue antigens. Appl. Immunohistochem. *1*:267-274.
37. **Leong, A.S.-Y. and J. Milios.** 1993. Comparison of antibodies to estrogen and progesterone receptor and the influence of microwave-antigen retrieval. Appl. Immunohistochem. *1*:282-288.
38. **Leong, A.S.-Y., J. Milios, and S.K. Tang.** 1993. Is immunolocalization of proliferating cell nuclear antigen (PCNA) in paraffin sections a valid index of cell proliferation? Appl. Immunohistochem. *1*:127-135.
39. **Leong, A.S.-Y., S. Vinyuvat, C. Suthipintawong, and J. Milios.** 1995. A comparative study of cell proliferation markers in breast carcinomas. J. Clin. Pathol. Mol. Pathol. *48*:M83-M87.
40. **Leong, A.S.-Y., J. Milios, and F.J.W.-M. Leong.** 1996. Epitope retrieval with microwaves. A comparison of citrate buffer and EDTA with three commercial retrieval solutions. Appl. Immunohistochem. *4*:201-207.
41. **Leong, A.S.-Y. and F.J.W.-M. Leong.** 1997. Applications and protocols of microwave technology for morphological analysis, p. 69-90. *In* J. Gu (Ed.), Analytical Morphology: Theory, Applications and Protocols. Eaton Publishing, Natick, MA.
42. **Leong, A.S.-Y., M.R. Wick, and P.E. Swanson.** 1997. Immunohistology and Electron Microscopy of Anaplastic and Pleomorphic Tumors, p. 7-31. Cambridge University Press, Cambridge, England.
43. **Leong, A.S.-Y. and F.J.W.-M. Leong.** 1998. What we need to know about cancer genes. Diagn. Cytopathol. *18*:33-40.
44. **Leong, A.S.-Y., K. Cooper, and F.J.W.-M. Leong.** 1999. A manual of diagnostic antibodies for immunohistology, p. 223-224; 285-287. Greenwich Medical Media, London.
45. **Leong, A.S.-Y. and R. Sormunen.** 1999. Microwave procedures for electron microscopy and resin-embedded sections. Micron *29*:397-409.
46. **Lynch, B.J., D.G. Guinee, and J.A. Holden.** 1997. Human DNA topoisomerase II alpha: a new marker of cell proliferation in invasive breast cancer. Hum. Pathol. *28*:1180-1188.
47. **Lynch, N.B.L., G. Komaromy-Hiller, I.R. Bronstein, and J.A. Holden.** 1998. Expression of DNA topoisomerase I, DNA topoisomerase II alpha and p 53 in metastatic malignant melanoma. Hum. Pathol. *29*:1240-1245.
48. **Merz, H., O. Rickers, S. Schrimel, K. Orscheschek, and A.C. Feller.** 1993. Constant detection of surface and cytoplasmic immunoglobulin heavy and light chain expression in formalin-fixed and paraffin-embedded materials. J. Pathol. *170*:257-264.
49. **Miller, R.T. and C. Estran.** 1995. Heat-induced epitope retrieval with a pressure cooker – suggestions for optimal use. Appl. Immunohistochem. *3*:190-193.
50. **Mintze, K., N. Macon, K.E. Gould, and G.E. Sandusky.** 1995. Optimization of proliferating cell nuclear antigen (PCNA) immunohistochemical staining: a comparison of methods using three commercial antibodies, various fixation times, and antigen retrieval solution. J. Histotechnol. *18*:25-30.
51. **Miyachi, K., M.J. Fritzler, and E.M. Tan.** 1987. Autoantibody to a nuclear antigen in proliferating cells. J. Immunol. *121*:2228-2234.
52. **Monnin, K.A., I.B. Bronstein, D.K. Gaffney, and J.A. Holden.** 1999. Elevations of DNA topoisomerase I in transitional cell carcinoma of the urinary bladder; correlation with DNA topoisomerase II-alpha and p53 expression. Hum. Pathol. *30*:384-391.
53. **Murray, G.L. and S.W.B. Ewen.** 1991. A novel method for optimal biopsy specimen preservation for histochemical and immunohistochemical analysis. Am. J. Clin. Pathol. *95*:131-136.
54. **Nitiss, J.L. and W.T. Beck.** 1996. Antitopoisomerase drug action and resistance. Eur. J. Cancer *32A*:958-966.
55. **Polkowski, W., J.J. van Lanschot, F.J. Ten Kate, J.P. Baak, G.N. Tytgat, H. Obertop, W.J. Voorn, and G.J. Offerhaus.** 1995. The value of p53 and Ki-67 as markers for tumor progression in the Barrett's dysplasia-carcinoma sequence. Surg. Oncol. *4*:163-171.
56. **Portiansky, E.L. and E.J. Gimeno.** 1996. A new epitope retrieval method for the detection of structural cytokeratins in the bovine prostatic tissue. Appl. Immunohistochem. *4*:208-214.
57. **Randolph, P., M. Tronnier, and R. Menzel, et al.** 1998. Enhanced expression of Ki-67, Topoisomerase II alpha, PCNA, p53 and p21[WAF/Cip1] reflecting proliferation and repair activity in UV-irradiated melanocytic nevi. Hum. Pathol. *29*:1480-1487.
58. **Raymond, W.A. and A.S.-Y. Leong.** 1998. The relationship between growth fractions and oestrogen receptors in

human breast carcinoma, as determined by immunohistochemical staining. J. Pathol. *158*:203-211.

59.**Robbins, B.A., D. de la Vega, and K. Ogata.** 1987. Immunohistochemical detection of proliferating cell nuclear antigen in solid human malignancies. Arch. Pathol. Lab. Med. *111*:841-845.

60.**Sato, Y., K. Muukai, S. Furuya, T. Kayema, and S. Hirohashi.** 1992. The AMEX method: a multipurpose tissue processing and paraffin embedding method. Extraction of protein and application to immunoblotting. Am. J. Pathol. *140*:775-779.

61.**Shi, S., M.E. Key, and K.L. Kalra.** 1991. Antigen retrieval in formalin-fixed, paraffin-embedded tissues: an enhancement method for immunohistochemical staining based on microwave oven heating of tissue sections. J. Histochem. Cytochem. *39*:741-748.

62.**Shi, S.-R., B. Chaiwun, L. Young, R.J. Cote, and C.R. Taylor.** 1993. Antiogen retrieval technique utilizing citrate buffer or urea solution for immunohistochemical demonstration of androgen receptor in formalin fixed paraffin sections. J. Histochem. Cytochem. *41*:1599-1604.

63.**Shi, S.-R., S.A. Imam, L. Young, R.J. Cote, and C.R. Taylor.** 1995. Antigen retrieval immunohistochemistry under the influence of pH using monoclonal antibodies. J. Histochem. Cytochem. *43*:193-201.

64.**Shi, S.-R., R.J. Cote, and C.R. Taylor.**1997. Antigen retrieval immunohistochemistry: past, present and future. J. Histochem. Cytochem. *45*:327-343.

65.**Shi, S.-R., R.J. Cote, L. Young, and C.R. Taylor.** 1997. Antigen retrieval immunohistochemistry: practice and development. J. Histotechnol. *20*:145-154.

66.**Shin, H.J.C., D.M. Shin, and Y.Y. Ro.** 1994. Optimization of proliferating nuclear antigen immunohistochemical staining by microwave heating in zinc sulphate solution. Mod. Pathol. *7*:242-248.

67.**Siitonen, S.M., O.-P. Kallioniemi, and J.J. Isola.** 1993. Proliferating cell nuclear antigen immunochemistry using monoclonal antibody 19A2 and anew antigen retrieval technique has prognostic impact in archival paraffin-embedded node-negative breast cancer. Am. J. Pathol. *142*:1081-1089.

68.**Sormunen, R.T. and A.S.-Y. Leong.** 1998. Antigen retrieval for fixed acrylic resin embedded sections for light and electron microscopic examination. Appl. Immunohistochem. *6*:234-240.

69.**Suthipintawong, C., A.S.-Y. Leong, and S. Vinyuvat.** 1996. Immunostaining of cell preparations: a comparative evaluation of common fixatives and protocols. Diagn. Cytopathol. *15*:167-174.

70.**Suurmeijer, A.H.J. and M.E. Boon.** Pretreatment in a high pressure microwave processor for MIB-1 immunostaining of cytological smears and paraffin tissue sections to visualize the various phases of the mitotic cycle. J. Histochem. Cytochem. (In press).

71.**Takagi, S., M.L. McFadden, and R.E. Humphreys.** 1993. Detection of 5-bromo-2-deoxyuridine (BrdUrd) incorporation with mononuclear anti-BrdUrd antibody after dexoyribonuclease treatment. Cytometry *14*:640-648.

72.**Takes, P.A., J. Kohrs, R. Krug, and S. Kewley.** 1989. Microwave technology in immunohistochemistry: application to avidin-biotin staining of diverse antigens. J. Histotechnol. *12*:95-98.

73.**Tanoguchi, K., H. Sasano, N. Yabuki, A. Kikuchi, K. Ito, S. Sato, and A. Yajima.** 1998. Immunohistochemical and two-parameter flow cytometric studies of DNA topoisomerase II alpha in human epithelial ovarian carcinoma and germ cell tumor. Mod. Pathol. *11*:186-193.

74.**Taylor, C.R. and R.J. Cote.** 1994. Immunomicroscopy: A Diagnostic Tool for the Surgical Pathologist, WB Saunders, Philadelphia.

75.**Taylor, C.R., S.-R. Shi, B. Chaiwun, and L. Young.** 1994. Strategies for improving the immunohistochemical staining of various intranuclear prognostic markers in formalin-paraffin sections: androgen receptor, estrogen receptor, progesterone receptor, p53, proliferating cell nuclear antigen, and Ki-67 antigen revealed by antigen retrieval techniques. Hum. Pathol. *25*:263-270.

76.**Taylor, C.R., S.-R. Shi, and R.J. Cote.** 1996. Antigen retrieval for immunohistochemistry. Status and need for greater standardization. Appl. Immunohistochem. *4*:144-146.

77.**Tischler, A.S.** 1995. Triple immunohistochemical staining for bromodeoxyuridine and catecholamine biosynthetic enzymes using microwave antigen retrieval. J. Histochem. Cytochem. *43*:1-4.

78.**Turley, H., M. Comley, S. Houlbrook, N. Nozaki, A. Kikuchi, I.D. Hickson, K. Gatler, and A.L. Harris.** 1997. The distribution and expression of the two isoforms of DNA topoisomerase II in normal and neoplastic human tissues. Br. J. Cancer. *75*:1340-1346.

79.**Visinoni, F., J. Milios, A.S.-Y. Leong, M.E. Boon, and L.P. Kok.** 1998. Ultra rapid microwave accelerated tissue processing—description of a new tissue processor. J. Histotechnol. *21*:219-224.

80.**Wang, J.C.** 1996. DNA topoisomerases. Annu. Rev. Biochem. *65*:635-692.

81.**Wintzer, H.O., I. Zipfel, and E. Schulte-Monting.** 1991. Ki-67 immunostaining in breast tumors and its relationship to prognosis. Cancer *67*:421-428.

82.**Woessner, R.D., M.R. Mattern, and C.K. Mirabelli, et al.** 1991. Proliferation and cell cycle-dependent differences in expression of the 170 kilodalton and 180-kilodalton forms of topoisomerase II in NIH-3T3 cells. Cell Growth Differ. *2*:209-214.

83.**Yabuki, N., H. Sasano, and K. Kato, et al.** 1996. Immunohistochemical study of DNA topoisomerase II in human gastric disorders. Am. J. Pathol. *149*:997-1007.

84.**Yu, C.C.-W., E.A. Dublin, R.S. Camplejohn, and D.A. Levison.** 1995. Optimization of immunohistochemical staining of proliferating cells in breast carcinoma using antibodies to proliferating cell nuclear antigen and the Ki-67 antigen. Ann. Cell. Pathol. *9*:45-52.

Ki-67 Antigen Retrieval in Tissues and Cells

12

Albert J.H. Suurmeijer[1] and Mathilde E. Boon[2]

1Department of Pathology and Laboratory Medicine, University Hospital Groningen, Groningen, and 2Cytology and Pathology Laboratory, Leiden, The Netherlands

INTRODUCTION

The description in the literature of a new technique or a major development in an existing method used in biology and medicine often drives scientific advances. Important developments in immunohistochemistry (IHC) are the introduction of the monoclonal antibody (mAb) technique, several immunolabeling methods, and the antigen retrieval (AR) technique. These advances allow the specific and sensitive detection of a large number of antigens in routinely processed tissue. In surgical pathology, AR is responsible for less false-negative immunostaining, which translates into increased diagnostic accuracy and improved patient care. AR increases the sensitivity of IHC in routinely processed tissue to such an extent that many of the IHC findings reported before the advent of AR, e.g., in certain tumors, are now considered to be of little value. Shi et al. (35) first described the AR method in 1991. These authors revolutionized the field of IHC, showing that high-temperature microwave (MW) heating of tissue sections in an aqueous solution had a beneficial rather than deleterious effect on tissue antigenicity and immunostaining results. It was rather surprising that the exposure of formaldehyde-fixed tissue sections to temperatures well above 60°C did not induce destruction of tissue antigens and deterioration of tissue morphology. Now we know, from experiments in which purified proteins are exposed to high temperatures, that formaldehyde fixation has some protective effect on the primary and secondary protein structure (26). It seems that AR recovers the tertiary and quaternary structure of the tissue antigen by breaking at least some of the steric barriers induced by formaldehyde cross-linking.

Antigen Retrieval Techniques
Edited by Shan-Rong Shi, Jiang Gu, and Clive R. Taylor
©2000 Eaton Publishing, Natick, MA

Table 1. The Original Standard Microwave-Antigen Retrieval Method for Paraffin-Embedded Tissue

1. Paraffin sections (4 μm) are picked up on tissue slides coated with a good tissue adhesive. Best results are obtained with 3-aminopropyltriethoxysilane and poly-L-lysine (Sigma, St. Louis, MO, USA). The slides are placed in rectangular plastic (Mellendahl-type) staining jars containing about 75 mL AR solution. These jars can contain up to 16 slides.

2. Jars are covered with loose-fitting caps and heated in the center of a household microwave oven with an output of at least 700 W, until boiling occurs. To prevent boiling over and excessive evaporation at higher power levels, irradiation of at least two jars at the same time is advised. One jar can serve as a water load. The retrieval solution is kept boiling for two cycles of 5 minutes. Between these boiling cycles, the amount of retrieval solution evaporated can be replenished. The time interval between the boiling cycles is at least 1 minute.

3. After heating, the staining jars are removed from the oven and allowed to cool for at least 15 minutes.

4. Slides are rinsed in distilled water twice and in phosphate-buffered saline for 5 minutes.

5. Proceed with immunohistochemical staining.

The original MW method of Shi et al. (shown in Table 1) has been modified and optimized by Shi et al. (36–38) and others (7,8,44–47). These additional studies have revealed that the product of heating time and temperature, as well as the pH and composition of the buffer solution, are important factors determining AR-IHC outcome (36,37,47). Moreover, high-temperature heating sources other than the conventional household MW oven have been tested, such as pressure cookers (28,48) and wet autoclaves (12,17,40,48). With these pieces of equipment, tissue sections are typically heated at temperatures above 100°C for 2 to 20 minutes, so-called superheating. Another approach is the heating of tissue sections at lower temperatures for a longer period, e.g., at 70°C overnight in a conventional laboratory oven (20,25).

These studies were all designed to develop a standard AR method to be used in histopathology with many diagnostically useful antigens (38). Although significant progress has been made with all these adjustments, there still remain some antigens that require refined manipulation of AR or protease treatment (7). In this chapter, we provide the reader with important information on the many variables determining AR results. We show how optimal AR results can be obtained by refined manipulation of these retrieval conditions, focusing on Ki-67 staining with the mAb MIB-1 in formaldehyde-fixed tissue and ethanol-fixed cells. This knowledge should allow the reader to adapt AR in an optimal way, using any other antibody. We use the term antigen retrieval (AR) for Shi's original MW method, for modified MW, and for alternative heating methods, even though the synonym heat-induced epitope retrieval (HIER) is also recommended.

Ki-67 IMMUNOSTAINING IN TISSUES AND CELLS

The protein pKi-67 was discovered by chance during the preparation of mAbs with nuclear extracts of Hodgkin cells (14). The mAb Ki-67 recognizes this nuclear protein pKi-67, which is expressed in all active phases of the cell cycle, the G_1, S-, G_2, and M-cell cycle phases, and not in quiescent cells in the G_0 phase. Thus, mAbs reactive with Ki-67 can be used as selective markers of cell proliferation, for instance in oncology research (16). The original mAb Ki-67 could be applied only with cryostat sections or cell preparations and not with formaldehyde-fixed and paraffin-embedded tissue, hampering retrospective studies of archive material in pathology laboratories (14).

Gene technology has demonstrated the existence of two mRNA species and two isoforms of pKi-67. The shortest of the cDNA isoforms lacks exon 7. The central exon 13 of pKi-67 cDNA has 16 tandemly repeated 366-bp elements. These repeats encode for the epitope recognized by mAb Ki-67 (34). Using recombinant DNA technology, a new series of paraffin-grade mAbs has been developed, the MIB series (6). These mAbs were raised against a peptide containing one of the Ki-67 repeats. At present, one of these mAbs, MIB-1, is widely used for cell and tissue research, in particular for the estimation of cell proliferation and prognosis in different tumor types. Comparative IHC studies have shown that the proliferating tissue compartment stained with MIB-1 is equivalent to that seen with Ki-67.

The exact function of the nuclear protein recognized by Ki-67 and MIB-1 is still unknown. Nevertheless, in flow cytometric studies there is accumulating evidence that pKi-67 binds to DNA. During the S-phase of the cell cycle, when DNA replication takes place, the amount of pKi-67 increases and reaches a maximum in the M-phase (21). Moreover, with DNAse pretreatment of cells, Ki-67 immunolabeling becomes negative, whereas RNAse treatment has no influence (33).

Interestingly, in buffer solution, double-stranded DNA appears to modulate the three-dimensional conformation of pKi-67, and this altered structure has stronger affinity for the mAbs Ki-67 and MIB-1 (24). Finally, with fluorescence in situ hybridization, Ki-67 colocalizes with centomeric, telomeric, and satellite III DNA, which is heterochromatic in nature (4).

Several cell kinetic studies have shown that the nuclear distribution of pKi-67 is related to the cell cycle (3,11,18,49) and compatible with a chromatin-associated function (41). For instance, Du Manoir et al. (11) have found that Ki-67 immunostaining is related to DNA content and nuclear size. In their analysis of the diploid human mammary cancer cell line MCF-7, it appears that cells follow two different pathways when going through the 2c compartment (G_1). In about 10% of cells, the amount of pKi-67 remains constant, the Ki-67 stable pathway, and these cells typically show a speckled nuclear staining pattern. In a large number of cells, however, there is a postmitotic decrease in the amount of pKi-67, the Ki-67 decrease pathway, and these cells have either small nuclei with nucleoplasmic staining or intermediate-sized nuclei showing nucleolar staining. The larger nuclei in the G_0 phase are negative. During the DNA replication (S) phase, the amount of pKi-67 increases progressively in intermediate-sized nuclei. Here, nuclear enlargement is accompanied by both nucleolar staining and increased nucleoplasmic staining. During the mitotic phase, pKi-67 covers the surface of chromosomes, which is most apparent in metaphase spreads of cell monolayers.

It is possible to obtain these staining patterns described in cell cultures in cell samples of fine needle aspirations or cervical smears, as well as in routinely processed tissue sections. Actually, we have recently used these qualitative features in addition to quantative data of MIB-1 IHC to optimize AR with a newly marketed high-pressure MW processor (ultrarapid microwave processor [URM]; MicroMed, Sorisole, Bergamo, Italy).

Ki-67 MICROWAVE-ANTIGEN RETRIEVAL IN FORMALDEHYDE-FIXED TISSUE

Microwave Heating and Microwave-Antigen Retrieval

To achieve reproducible effects with MW-AR methods, data on size, shape, and volume of the load, dilution and ionic strength of the AR solution, place of the load in the oven, and, in particular, temperature control are essential. In the original (standard) MW-AR method of Shi et al. (Reference 35 and Table 1) two boiling cycles of 5 minutes are applied. With three 50-mL cylindrical Coplin jars in an MW oven of 700 W power the boiling point (100°C) is reached in 140 to 145 seconds. Thus, net boiling time is less than 8 minutes. This is also observed with two 75-mL rectangular Hellendahl staining jars. However, it is well appreciated that the heating performance of different microwaves at a certain power level may vary considerably due to hot spots, in particular with different shapes of containers and small volumes, even when they are placed in the center of the MW cavity. These inconsistencies result in variations in the efficiency of MW-AR. To obtain some kind of standardization, the calibration method of Tacha and Chen (46) can be used. With their modification of the standard MW method, slides are brought to boiling temperature and subsequently kept boiling at a lower power setting for the remainder of the AR heating period, using the formula $S = 250/P \times 10$, where S is the power setting and P is the highest output power of MW oven. Here, the net power P of the MW used can be determined with the simple procedure given in the *Microwave Cookbook for Microscopists* by Kok and Boon (19).

With regard to heating time, several publications have indicated that optimal Ki-67 immunostaining requires controlled boiling for more than 10 minutes in citrate buffer of pH 6.0 (1,27,30,50). Moreover, it is known that the efficacy of Ki-67 retrieval is influenced by formaldehyde fixation, in particular fixation time (1,30). In tissue fixed in neutral buffered formalin for 48 hours, for instance, a heating time of at least 14 minutes should be applied (30). Prolonged MW heating does not have a detrimental effect on Ki-67 antigenicity. Routine fixation in surgical pathology often implies that the length of formaldehyde fixation may vary from a few hours to several days. In the experience of most investigators, 20 minutes of heat exposure for AR provides a good safeguard. During the cooling phase of 15 minutes, the temperature of the buffer solution decreases to about 50°C. Actually, the sections are left standing in hot buffer solution for a few minutes, which may explain the experience of some authors that AR is less effective if this cooling step is omitted after 10 minutes of MW heating.

Composition and pH of the Buffer Solution

A major drawback of Shi's original MW method was the use of toxic lead thiocyanate. In the early days of AR, Cattoretti et al. (7) and Suurmeijer and Boon (45) tested other metal salts and buffer solutions and found that the results with aluminum chloride, urea, and citrate buffer were superior to those obtained with lead thiocyanate (8). In their extensive study, Cattoretti et al. (7) reported that 110 of 255 antibodies (43%) showed increased immunoreactivity with MW-AR. For 25 of these antibodies reported to work only with frozen sections, MW heating completely restored reactivity with paraffin-embedded tissue. One of these antibodies was MIB-1. With 53 antibodies, immunoreactivity was strongly enhanced, and in 32 cases, the antigens unmasked by MW heating could also be detected with protease digestion, although

MW-AR gave superior results, particularly in specimens fixed for more than 18 hours.

These authors recognized that the molarity of the retrieval solution was an important factor. It appeared that some antigens, e.g., most intermediate filament proteins, depend on strong denaturation conditions (heating in high molar solutions like 6 mol/L urea and 0.3 mol/L aluminum chloride), whereas other antigens need fine-tuning in molarity and salt composition. For instance, MIB-1 staining is strong after 15 minutes of AR in 0.3 mol/L aluminum chloride but completely negative when 0.01 mol/L aluminum chloride is used (44). On the other hand, immunoreactivity for α-smooth muscle actin (1A4), desmin (D33), Ber-Ep4, and low-molecular-weight cytokeratins (Cam 5.2) is optimal with 0.01 mol/L aluminum chloride and comparable to IHC after trypsin digestion (44). The excellent immunostaining results Cattoretti et al. (7) obtained with 0.01 mol/L citrate buffer, pH 6.0, for a broad range of antigens were confirmed by other groups (5,9,15,23,50), and in the following years their modification was adopted in the scientific community as an efficient AR method. Actually, most of the IHC studies found in the literature today use citrate buffer.

Major progress was made in the field of AR in 1995, when Shi et al. (36) noted the importance of the pH value of the buffer solution in addition to high-temperature heating. They compared different buffer solutions with pH values ranging from 1.0 to 10.0 using the standard AR method and evaluated mAbs to cytoplasmic antigens [AE1, HMB-45, neuron-specific enolase (NSE)], nuclear antigens [MIB-1, proliferating cell nuclear antigen (PCNA), estrogen receptor (ER)], and cell surface antigens [MT1, L26, epithelial membrane antigen (EMA)] on formalin-fixed and paraffin-embedded tissue.

Three pH-influenced AR immunostaining patterns were found: a type A pattern (for AE1, NSE, PCNA, L26, and EMA) with excellent retrieval throughout the pH range; a type B pattern (for MIB-1 and ER) with strong immunostaining at very low pH and at neutral to high pH, and a strong decrease in staining intensity at pH 3.0 to 6.0; and a type C pattern (for HMB-45 and MT1) with increasing staining intensity with increasing pH but weak staining at low pH. For these antibodies, the advantage of a buffer solution of high pH value is evident. Furthermore, it appeared that the chemical composition of the buffer solution was less important than the pH value. The Tris-HCl buffer was preferred because it does not need the addition of NaOH to obtain a high pH value. Moreover, in some cases weak false-positive nuclear staining was noted using MIB-1 after low-pH AR. With Tris-HCl buffer, pH 9.0, however, excellent and specific immunostaining is seen with good morphologic detail and a clean background. Using this AR solution, Evers et al. (13) obtained good IHC staining results with five antibodies [parvalbumin, calbindin, microtubule-associated protein (MAP)-2, MAP-5, and SMI-32] in vibratome sections of human brain fixed in formaldehyde for as long as 10 months.

The comparative study by Pileri et al. (31) showed that the application of 1 mmol/L EDTA-NaOH solution, pH 8.0, as AR solution for MIB-1 staining is the most efficient and better than Tris-HCl buffer, pH 9.0, and citrate buffer, pH 6.0, when 20 slides were MW heated in 200 mL buffer solution for three cycles of 5 minutes each. In the next paragraph, we elaborate on other heating methods by which good results can also be obtained with Tris-HCl buffer, pH 9.0, and citrate buffer, pH 6.0. We stress again that temperature control is of major importance, because the effectiveness of AR is a function of time and temperature.

Other Heating Sources

The MW-AR methods are based on MW heating of tissue sections for 10 minutes, with boiling at 100°C for less than 8 minutes. So-called superheating at temperatures higher than 100°C is possible with hydrated autoclaving (12,17,40,48), with pressure cooking (28,48), and by combining microwaving and pressure cooking (48). The use of these alternative heating sources eliminates the need to adjust the volume of the AR solution. Larger volumes can be used that are apt to give a more even heating pattern with greater numbers of slides in a single batch. The autoclave and pressure cooker have the inconvenience of the additional time and handling required for warming up the AR solution. However, in the experience of many laboratories, these superheating methods are bound to give better AR results, in particular with large numbers of slides, compared with MW-AR (48).

Shin et al. (40) first used an autoclave for tau immunostaining in Alzheimer's disease. Inspired by this paper, Emanuals et al. (12) applied the autoclave for AR-IHC with MIB-1. With their method, tissue sections are immersed in distilled water and heated at 115°C or 121°C for 2 cycles of 17 minutes each, with one cycle consisting of 2 minutes of warming plus 5 minutes heating and 10 minutes of cooling. Thus, the total time needed to achieve strong MIB-1 staining by hydrate autoclaving is comparable to the time needed with MW-AR. Autoclaving in Tris-HCl buffer, pH 9.5, with 5% urea at 120°C for 10 minutes is superior to MW heating for 20 minutes (5 min × 4) in the same AR solution (48).

A household pressure cooker is, of course, more readily available than an autoclave and a much cheaper alternative. In the pressure cooker method described by Miller et al. (28), 3 L of citrate buffer, pH 6.0, are brought to boiling, and AR heating begins when full pressure is reached. MIB-1 immunostaining results were found to be superior with a 2-minute pressure cooker heating time (immunoscore 5+) compared with 30-minute MW heating (immunoscore 4+). With one run in the pressure cooker, up to 100 slides can be treated. With this amount it is possible to save 90 minutes, if the pressure cooker is used as opposed to the MW. It is also possible to combine microwaving and pressure cooking. A plastic pressure cooker is available (Nordicware, Minneapolis, MN, USA) for use with a conventional MW. Here, 600 mL distilled water is used for AR with three staining jars, each containing 24 slides. Comparing different heating methods, Taylor et al. (48) found better MIB-1 staining with MW plus pressure cooker (immunoscore 4+) compared with MW alone (immunoscore 3+).

Recently, a new high-pressure MW processor has come on the market, the ultrarapid microwave (URM; MicroMed). This apparatus allows controlled superheating under high pressure in the MW. It has a maximum power output of 1000 W. Time, temperature, and pressure can be adjusted using a touch screen personal computer. MW power and pressure are regulated through sophisticated software. The jar with the AR solution is placed in a glass dome and during microwaving, the apparatus controls and adjusts the pressure in this glass dome as a function of the temperature measured in the AR solution by a fiberoptic sensor. Under these circumstances the AR solution can be heated at constant temperatures higher than 100°C.

We have tested the URM for AR efficiency in formalin-fixed tissue. The test battery approach suggested by Shi et al. (38) helps one to establish an optimum for a particular antibody. Our test battery included four different temperatures (90°, 95°, 100°, and 115°C), four different heating periods (2.5, 5, 10, and 20 min), and three pH values (Tris buffer of pH 2.0, citrate buffer of pH 6.0, and Tris buffer of pH 9.0). The slides were heated in a plastic staining jar with 250 mL AR solution. The panel of antibodies included MIB-1 (Ki-67) from Immunotech (Marseille, France), KL-1 (cytokeratins), V9 (vimentin), L26 (CD20), UCHL-1 (CD45RO), and QBEND

(CD34), all purchased from DAKO (Glostrup, Denmark). The results of this study demonstrate again that for each antibody the perfect match of AR solution (pH), temperature, and heating time must be established. By refined manipulation of these three factors, optimal IHC staining results can be determined for each antibody.

Optimal MIB staining was seen under the following conditions: 2.5 to 20 minutes in Tris buffer, pH 2.0, at 100°C or 10 to 20 minutes in citrate buffer, pH 6.0, at 115°C. The results with citrate buffer, pH 6.0, at 100°C and with Tris buffer, pH 9.0, at 115°C were suboptimal. For the other five antibodies, 20 minutes of AR in citrate buffer, pH 6.0, or Tris buffer, pH 9.0, at 115°C was the most efficient. With Tris buffer of pH 2.0 at 115°C, tissue morphology became very poor, and nuclear counterstaining with hematoxylin became very pale. Thus, for our small antibody panel, heating at 115°C in citrate buffer, pH 6.0, for 20 minutes proved to be the best general choice. In the histologic sections, the MIB-1 nuclear staining index proved to be highly reproducible.

Compared with the other devices, the main advantage of the URM is good control of the main factors determining AR outcome, such as time, temperature, and pH. Thus, the URM could well be used to standardize AR. However, its high price will probably limit its use by many laboratories.

Another good strategy for AR is low-temperature heating overnight in an appropriate AR solution using a conventional laboratory oven. This approach was, among others (16,24), studied by Koopal et al. (20) for 16 antibodies. MIB-1 was tested extensively. With overnight heating (for approximately 15 h) at 80°C, optimal MIB-1 staining was obtained with both citrate buffer of pH 6.0 and Tris buffer of pH 9.0. With 11 of the other 15 antibodies, however, Tris buffer of pH 9.0 yielded the most consistent results, and citrate buffer of pH 6.0 proved less effective, which is in contrast with the results seen with superheating, in which citrate buffer of pH 6.0 is, in general, the best choice. The nuclear antigens (Ki-67, ER, PR, p53, and Rb) did not survive low-temperature overnight heating in citrate buffer of pH 1.0, and tissue morphology was severely damaged, in contrast to MW heating in the same AR solution for 10 minutes. On the other hand, tissue morphology obtained by low-temperature heating overnight in Tris buffer of pH 9.0 is excellent and, in general, better than that seen with MW-AR in the same AR solution.

From a practical viewpoint, the simplicity of Koopal's modification is appealing, in particular for laboratories faced with increasing workloads and on a working schedule permitting overnight low-temperature heating. A large number of slides can be placed in AR solution at the end of the working day and heated overnight, with IHC applied the next morning. The consistent heat effect obtained with Koopal's method makes it useful for standardization, just like the superheating variants. With this alternative heating method, optimal retrieval conditions for a particular antibody can be determined by varying the pH and/or the composition of the retrieval solution, in addition to heating intensity.

Influence of Formaldehyde Fixation

The studies outlined in the previous paragraphs all aimed at optimization and standardization of AR in order to find a method that works with many antibodies used for diagnosis or research in pathology. Needless to say, the results of IHC staining are not only dependent on the potential of AR, but also on histotechnique, especially on formaldehyde fixation parameters (see review by Larsson in Reference 22).

The chemistry of formaldehyde fixation is complex and not fully understood. The reaction of formaldehyde with amino acid groups of proteins is maximal at alkaline pH. However, the formation of secondary cross-links has an acidic pH optimum. Apart from pH, formaldehyde fixation by formation of cross-links also depends on temperature and, in particular, on fixation time. It is remarkable that these three factors also determine the outcome of AR. This reinforces the concept that most of the reactions of formaldehyde with proteins are unstable and reversible by AR protocols. Heating of formaldehyde-fixed tissue in a low- or high-pH buffer solution induces hydrolysis, which may hypothetically result in breakage of some of formaldehyde-induced cross-links and/or partial cleavage of tissue proteins near cross-links. The kinetics of hydrolysis are influenced by the intensity of heating, that is, the product of temperature and heating time, as well as the molarity and pH of the buffer solution. However, although reversal of formaldehyde fixation may be an important mechanism, there is also evidence that other molecular mechanisms must be invoked in AR (see below). Nevertheless, for many antigens, formaldehyde fixation causes a time-related loss of immunoreactivity. It is well appreciated that completion of formaldehyde fixation, meaning extensive cross-linking, takes at least several days. For this reason, it is conceivable that AR is most successful in tissue specimens that are not overfixed. In fact, data on MIB-1 retrieval support this assumption.

It appears that, with the MW citrate method, the degree of AR is proportional to the duration or intensity of heating and is related to duration of formaldehyde fixation (30). Using MW-AR with citrate buffer of pH 6.0, quantitative MIB-1 immunostaining is suboptimal if tissue is fixed for longer than 24 hours (1,30). However, the various AR modifications described earlier seem to have stronger AR potential and can be applied with archival paraffin-embedded tissues that are routinely fixed in formalin from less than 24 hours to a couple of days. Using citrate buffer, pressure cooker AR yields better results compared with MW-AR (28). With EDTA buffer, equivalent good results are seen with both MW and pressure cooker, even in tissue fixed for up to 1 week (31). The same result can be obtained with low-temperature heating overnight in Tris buffer of pH 9.0 (20). For routinely fixed histological specimens, we generally obtain the best results using pressure cooker AR with EDTA buffer.

In daily pathology practice, formaldehyde fixation is not standardized, which is mainly due to variations in specimen size and fixation time. Variations in fixation time can be responsible for discordant IHC staining results between different laboratories using routine formalin fixation. Nowadays, the rigorously optimized AR techniques may overcome this negative influence of prolonged formaldehyde fixation on IHC staining in many cases. However, the detrimental effect of formaldehyde fixation on tissue antigenicity can also be prevented by starting with optimal formaldehyde fixation when the tissue is received in the laboratory. For this purpose, microwaves can also be applied.

The benefits of this approach were recently described by Ruijter et al. (32). In their study whole prostates were injected with formalin, so that the fixative is present within the tissue as the temperature is increased by MW irradiation. Here, MW irradiation is thought to stimulate the diffusion and chemical reaction of the fixative. Whatever the precise mechanism, both histology and IHC (e.g., for E-cadherin) were very good in the whole-mount tissue sections of these prostates. The lesson to be remembered from this observation is that AR is nothing more than damage control. We try to undo a negative effect that we could have prevented initially. Unfortunately, at present, little attention is paid to optimization of formaldehyde fixation, even though it is at least as important for IHC as optimization of AR.

Ki-67 ANTIGEN RETRIEVAL IN CYTOLOGIC SPECIMENS

In cytology, immunostaining of cytologic preparations can provide important additional diagnostic information. Optimization of cytotechnique is of major importance for adequate immunostaining in cytology [immunocytochemistry (ICC)]. Dalquen et al. (10) mention the following prerequisites for optimal ICC: *(i)* cell sampling and fixation should be easy to handle for the clinician who sends the specimen to the cytology laboratory; *(ii)* nonspecific background staining, often a problem in samples rich in blood and protein, should not occur; *(iii)* ideally, the ICC technique should be applicable to all kinds of cytologic material, including both fixed and air-dried smears that have been stored for some days; and *(iv)* cellular and nuclear details should not be destroyed by the ICC technique, so that immunostained cells can still be differentiated by their morphology.

In routine cytology practice, specimens are either unfixed, air-dried, and stained with the Giemsa technique or ethanol-fixed and stained with the Papanicolaou (Pap) technique.

Some studies have been performed to obtain a universal ICC method to be used with air-dried cytologic smears. Analogous to IHC, ICC strongly depends on type and duration of fixation. To meet the requirements for specific ICC staining in cytology, Suthipintawong et al. (42) tested 23 fixation protocols for air-dried smears, involving acetone, acetone/methanol, acetone/formalin, glutaraldehyde, ethanol, methanol, and formal saline. Fixation in 0.1% formal saline (also known as van der Griendt's fluid) overnight at room temperature, followed by 10 minutes of fixation in 100% ethanol and MW-AR in citrate buffer of pH 6.0 produced the most consistent and optimal preservation of immunoreactivity with 18 diagnostically useful antibodies. Moreover, background staining was removed, allowing proper evaluation of immunostaining.

These authors also published a more simplified protocol that is very effective and practical for immunostaining of pKi-67 with MIB-1 (43). With this modification, freshly made smears are air-dried for 20 minutes to 14 hours at room temperature, before immersion in 10% buffered formalin for 2 to 14 hours. Immunostaining follows MW-AR in citrate buffer of pH 6.0. Importantly, this study revealed that MIB-1 counts in the cytologic smears strongly correlated with MIB-1 counts in corresponding tissue sections. The fact that the air-dried smears may be left at room temperature for at least 14 hours is very advantageous, because the need for ICC in cytodiagnosis is often unanticipated and only evident after cytologic specimens have been prepared and examined routinely. Moreover, the formalin-fixed smears can be kept at room temperature for at least 1 week without loss of MIB-1 immunoreactivity.

With AR protocols, de novo MIB-1 immunostaining can also be obtained in ethanol-fixed cell smears, as shown by Boon et al. (2) for routinely processed Pap smears. For AR-IHC, the coverslips of previously stained smears can be removed with xylene and the slides rehydrated through ethanols. Destaining of the Pap smear is achieved with MW-AR in citrate buffer. The merits of this MIB-1 immunostaining in cervical cytology are described in Chapter 3.

We have recently applied the MicroMed URM for MIB-1 AR-IHC of ethanol-fixed cytologic smears, using the optimal protocol for tissue sections: superheating at 115°C in citrate buffer of pH 6.0 for 10 minutes. In the cytologic smears, we were able to see the different nuclear cell cycle-related staining patterns described by Du Manoir et al. (11). Figure 1 illustrates three different MIB-1 staining patterns found in a smear with melanoma cells. Figure 1a shows perinucleolar staining in G_1 phase,

Figure 1b shows perinuclear and nucleoplasmic staining in S-phase, and Figure 1c shows surface staining of chromosomes in metaphase. It is striking that the morphology of the nuclei of the tumor cells is well preserved with high-pressure MW superheating, despite the high temperature of 115°C. In the IHC stainings, the association of Ki-67 with nucleoli, chromatin, and chromosomes is still easily discerned. No denaturing and boiling effect of nuclei is seen. It appears that the constant temperature during MW heating under pressure in the URM is responsible for both good morphology and consistent MIB-1 immunostaining results.

Surprisingly, in studies with quantitative immunostaining with MIB-1, little or no attention has been paid to these differential, cell cycle-related Ki-67 staining patterns. One wonders what is meant by the MIB-1 index used in many reports. It appears that only weak, moderate, and strong nuclear MIB-1 staining is included in MIB-1 counts and indices, and that the perinuclear (late G_1) staining pattern is disregarded. We observed that under suboptimal conditions only nuclei with a large amount of Ki-67 protein stain positive and only late S-G_2 and M-phase staining patterns are seen. We stress that only optimally stained cytologic smears and histologic sections should be used for quantitation.

BACKGROUND CHEMISTRY

The mode of action of AR in routinely processed tissue is not fully understood. Tissue sent to the pathology laboratory for histologic examination routinely undergoes fixation in neutral buffered formalin, dehydration in ascending ethanol concentrations, clearing in xylene, and embedding in paraffin. Completion of formaldehyde fixation takes at least several days. However, routine formalin fixation often lasts less than 1 day, which implies that ill-understood changes related to ethanol dehydration and embedding may also contribute to loss of tissue antigenicity, in addition to the detrimental effects of formaldehyde fixation. On the molecular level, the following mechanisms of AR have been considered: *(i)* rupture of protein cross-linkages induced by formaldehyde fixation, *(ii)* rehydration and renaturation of proteins, and *(iii)* removal of divalent metal complexes.

The first hypothesis is supported by chemical data on the reversibility of formaldehyde-induced protein cross-linkages by heat and acid or alkaline hydrolysis (22). Formaldehyde fixation can alter the three-dimensional structure of the epitope by the formation of different cross-links, including those between the epitope and unrelated proteins or those between the epitope and DNA. It might well be that blocking proteins are modified or dissolved and extracted by AR, freeing the epitope. Moreover, DNA may be modified by heat and extremes of pH. Under these denaturing conditions, it is conceivable that DNA unfolds and refolds. In this way, renatured double-

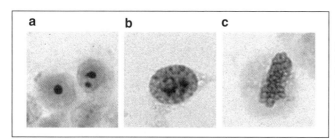

Figure 1. MIB-1 immunostaining in melanoma cells in different phases of the cell cycle (see text for further details). (a) Perinucleolar staining in the G_1 phase. (b) Perinuclear and nucleoplasmic staining in the S-phase. (c) Surface staining of chromosomes in metaphase.

stranded DNA may influence the conformation of the Ki-67 epitope and its antigenicity (24). Theoretically, a similar mechanism may be involved in AR of other DNA binding nuclear proteins.

In general, AR has no enhancing effect on immunoreactivity in ethanol-fixed tissues or cells (35,42), with one exception: immunostaining with MIB-1 in methacarn or ethanol-fixed tissues or cells benefits from AR (2,15). Methacarn and ethanol are coagulative fixatives that induce denaturation of proteins by dehydration. Here, rehydration and renaturation of the pKi-67 and the epitope recognized by MIB-1 may be responsible for the recovery of immunoreactivity. On the other hand it can be assumed that AR restores the conformation of the pKi-67 epitope by modification of DNA or nearby proteins, as discussed above.

The third mechanism was proposed by Morgan et al. (29), who studied the effect of calcium chloride and EDTA-mediated calcium chelation at different pH levels on AR for MIB-1 immunostaining in formaldehyde-fixed tissue. These authors found that calcium ions strongly inhibit AR at high pH values but have no effect at very low pH. Moreover, calcium chloride inhibits AR with chaotropic denaturing agents, such as guanidine HCl and urea, whereas it has no effect on AR with aluminum chloride. However, Shi et al. (39) recently showed by IHC that calcium modifies Ki-67 protein conformation before and independent of formalin fixation; they concluded that calcium does not necessarily play a role in AR.

We conclude that current literature data strongly support the notion that breakage of formaldehyde-induced cross-links with restoration of the three-dimensional architecture of the epitope plays a key role in AR.

REFERENCES

1. **Benini, E., S. Rao, M.G. Daidone, S. Pilotti, and R. Silvestrini.** 1997. Immunoreactivity to MIB-1 in breast cancer: methodological assessment and comparison with other proliferation indices. Cell Prolif. *30*:107-115.
2. **Boon, M.E., E.D. Kleinschmidt-Guy, and N.E. Ouwerkerk.** 1994. PAPNET for analysis of proliferating (MIB-1 positive) cell populations in cervical smears. Eur. J. Morphol. *32*:78-85.
3. **Braun, N., T. Papadopoulos, and H.K. Muller-Hermelink.** 1988. Cell cycle dependent distribution of the proliferation-associated Ki-67 antigen in human embryonic lung cells. Virchows Arch. B Cell Pathol. *56*:25-33.
4. **Bridger, J.M., I.R. Kill, and P. Lichter.** 1998. Association of pKi-67 with satellite DNA of the human genome in early G1 cells. Chromosome Res. *6*:13-24.
5. **Brown, R.W. and R. Chirala.** 1995. Utility of microwave-citrate antigen retrieval in diagnostic immunohistochemistry. Mod. Pathol. *8*:515-520.
6. **Cattoretti, G., M.H. Becker, G. Key, M. Duchrow, C. Schluter, J. Galle, and J. Gerdes.** 1992. Monoclonal antibodies against recombinant parts of the Ki-67 antigen (MIB 1 and MIB 3) detect proliferating cells in microwave-processed formalin-fixed paraffin sections. J. Pathol. *168*:357-363.
7. **Cattoretti, G., S. Pileri, C. Parravicini, M.H.G. Becker, S. Poggi, C. Bifulco, G. Key, L. D'Amato, E. Sabattini, E. Feudale, et al.** 1993. Antigen unmasking on formalin-fixed, paraffin embedded tissue sections. J. Pathol. *171*:83-98.
8. **Cattoretti, G. and A.J.H. Suurmeijer.** 1995. Antigen unmasking on formalin-fixed paraffin-embedded tissues using microwaves: a review. Adv. Anat. Pathol. *2*:2-9.
9. **Cuevas, E.C., A.C. Bareman, B.S. Wilking, P.A. Johnson, H. Williams, A.H.S. Lee, D.B. Jones, and D.H. Wright.** 1994. Microwave antigen retrieval in immunocytochemistry: a study of 80 antibodies. J. Clin. Pathol. *47*:448-452.
10. **Dalquen, P., G. Sauter, R. Epper, B. Kleiber, G. Feichter, and F. Gudat.** 1993. Immunocytochemistry in diagnostic cytology. Recent Res. Cancer Res. *133*:47-80.
11. **Du Manoir, S., P. Guillaud, E. Camus, D. Seigneurin, and G. Brugal.** 1991. Ki-67 labeling in postmitotic cells defines different Ki-67 pathways within the 2c compartment. Cytometry *12*:455-463.
12. **Emanuels, A., H. Hollema, and J. Koudstaal.** 1994. Autoclave heating: an alternative method for microwaving? Eur. J. Morphol *32*(2–4 suppl):337-340.
13. **Evers, P., H.B.M. Uylings, and A.J.H. Suurmeijer.** 1998. Antigen retrieval in formaldehyde-fixed human brain tissue. Methods: Companion Methods Enzymol. *15*:133-140.

14. **Gerdes, J., U. Schwab, H. Lemke, and H. Stein.** 1983. Production of a mouse monoclonal antibody reactive with a human nuclear antigen associated with cell proliferation. Int. J. Cancer *31*:13-20.
15. **Gown, A.M., N. de Wever, and H. Battifora.** 1993. Microwave-based antigen unmasking. A revolutionary new technique for routinely immunohistochemistry. Appl. Immunohistochem. *1*:256-266.
16. **Hofstadter, F.** 1995. Cell proliferation assessment in oncology. Virchows Arch. *427*:323-341.
17. **Igarashi, H., H. Sugimura, K. Maruyama, Y. Kitayama, I. Otha, M. Suzuki, M. Tanaka, Y. Dobashi, and I. Kino.** 1994. Alteration of immunoreactivity by hydrated autoclaving, microwave treatment, and simple heating of paraffin-embedded tissue sections. APMIS *102*:295-307.
18. **Isola, J., H. Helin, and O.-P. Kalloniemi.** 1990. Immunoelectron-microscopic localization of a proliferation-associated antigen Ki-67 in MCF-7 cells. Histochem. J. *22*:498-506.
19. **Kok, L.P. and M.E. Boon.** 1992. Microwave Cookbook for Microscopists: Art and Science of Visualization, p. 63-64. Coulomb Press Leyden, Leiden, The Netherlands.
20. **Koopal, S.A., M. Iglesias Coma, A.T.M.G. Tiebosch, and A.J.H. Suurmeijer.** 1998. Low temperature heating overnight in Tris-HCl buffer pH 9 is a good alternative for antigen retrieval in formalin-fixed paraffin-embedded tissue. Appl. Immunohistochem. *6*:228-233.
21. **Landberg, G., E.M. Tan, and G. Roos.** 1990. Flow cytometric multiparameter analysis of proliferating cell nuclear antigen/cyclin and Ki-67 antigen: a new view of the cell cycle. Exp. Cell Res. *187*:111-118.
22. **Larsson, L.I.** 1993. Tissue preparation methods for light microscopic immunohistochemistry. Appl. Immunohistochem. *1*:2-6.
23. **Leong, A.S.Y. and J. Milios.** 1993. An assessment of the efficacy of the microwave antigen retrieval procedure on a range of tissue antigens. Appl. Immunohistochem. *1*:267-274.
24. **Lopez, F., F. Belloc, F. Lacombe, P. Dumain, J. Reiffers, P. Bernard, and M.R. Boisseau.** 1994. The labelling of proliferating cells by Ki-67 and MIB-1 antibodies depends on the binding of a nuclear protein to the DNA. Exp. Cell Res. *210*:145-153.
25. **Man, Y. and F.A. Tavassoli.** 1996. A simple epitope retrieval method without the use of microwave oven or enzyme digestion. Appl. Immunohistochem. *4*:139-141.
26. **Mason, J.T. and J.T. O'Leary.** 1991. Effects of formaldehyde fixation on protein secondary structure: a calorimetric and infrared spectroscopic investigation. J. Histochem. Cytochem. *39*:225-229.
27. **McCormick, D., H. Chong, C. Hobbs, C. Datta, and P.A. Hall.** 1993. Detection of Ki-67 antigen in fixed and wax-embedded sections with the monoclonal antibody MIB1. Histopathology *22*:355-360.
28. **Miller, K., J. Auld, E. Jessup, A. Rhodes, and M. Ashton-Key.** 1995. Antigen unmasking in formalin-fixed routinely processed paraffin-wax-embedded sections by pressure cooking: a comparison with microwave oven heating and traditional methods. Adv. Anat. Pathol. 2:60-64.
29. **Morgan, J.M., H. Navabi, and B. Jasani.** 1997. Role of calcium chelation in high-temperature antigen retrieval at different pH values. J. Pathol. *182*:233-237.
30. **Munakata, S. and J.B. Hendricks.** 1993. Effect of fixation time and microwave oven heating on retrieval of the Ki-67 antigen from paraffin-embedded tissue. J. Histochem. Cytochem. *41*:1241-1246.
31. **Pileri, S.A., G. Roncador, C. Ceccarelli, M. Piccioli, A. Briskomatis, E. Sabbatini, S. Ascani, D. Santani, P.P. Piccaluga, O. Leone, et al.** 1997. Antigen retrieval techniques in immunohistochemistry: comparison of different methods. J. Pathol. *183*:116-123.
32. **Ruijter, E.T., G.J. Miller, T.W. Aalders, C.A. van der Kaa, J.A. Schalken, F.M. Debruyne, and M.E. Boon.** 1997. Rapid microwave-stimulated fixation of entire prostatectomy specimens. J. Pathol. *183*:369-375.
33. **Sasaki, K., T. Murakami, M. Kawasaki, and M. Takahashi.** 1987. The cell cycle associated change of the Ki-67 reactive nuclear antigen expression. J. Cell. Physiol. *133*:579-584.
34. **Schluter, C., M. Duchrow, C. Wohlenberg, M.H. Becker, G. Key, H.D. Flad, and J. Gerdes.** 1993. The cell proliferation-associated antigen of antibody Ki-67: a very large, ubiquitous nuclear protein with numerous repeated elements, rpresenting a new kind of cell-cycle-maintaining proteins. J. Cell Biol. *123*:513-522.
35. **Shi, S.-R., M.E. Key, and K.L. Kalra.** 1991. Antigen retrieval in formalin-fixed, paraffin-embedded tissues: an enhancement method for immunohistochemical staining based on microwave oven heating of tissue sections. J. Histochem. Cytochem. *39*:741-748.
36. **Shi, S.-R., S.A. Imam, L. Young, R.J. Cote, and C.R. Taylor.** 1995. Antigen retrieval immunohistochemistry under the influence of pH using monoclonal antibodies. J. Histochem. Cytochem. *43*:193-201.
37. **Shi, S.-R., R.J. Cote, L. Young, A.S. Imam, and C.R. Taylor.** 1996. Use of pH 9.5 Tris-HCl buffer containing 5% urea for antigen retrieval immunohistochemistry. Biotech. Histochem. *71*:190-196.
38. **Shi, S.-R., R.J. Cote, and C.R. Taylor.** 1997. Antigen retrieval immunohistochemistry: past, present, and future. J. Histochem. Cytochem. *45*:327-343.
39. **Shi, S.-R., R.J. Cote, D. Hawes, S. Thu, Y. Shi, L.L. Young, and C.R. Taylor.** 1999. Calcium-induced modification of protein conformation demonstrated by immunohistochemistry. What is the signal? J. Histochem. Cytochem. *47*:463-470.
40. **Shin, R.-W., T. Iwaki, T. Kitamoto, and J. Tateishi.** 1991. Hydrated autoclave pretreatment enhances tau immunoreactivity in formalin-fixed normal and Alzheimer's disease brain tissues. Lab. Invest. *64*:693-702.
41. **Starborg, M., K. Gell, E. Brundell, and C. Hoog.** 1996. The murine Ki-67 cell proliferation antigen accumulates in the nucleolar and heterochromatic regions of interphase cells and at the periphery of chromosomes in a process

essential for cell cycle progression. J. Cell Sci. *109*:143-153.

42. **Suthipintawong, C., A.S. Leong, and S. Vinyuvat.** 1996. Immunostaining of cell preparations: a comparative evaluation of common fixatives and protocols. Diagn. Cytopathol. *15*:167-174.

43. **Suthipintawong, C., A.S. Leong, K.-W. Chan, and S. Vinyuvat.** 1997. Immunostaining of estrogen receptor, progesterone receptor, MIB1 antigen, and c-erb-2 oncoprotein in cytologic specimens: a simplified method with formalin fixation. Diagn. Cytopathol. *17*:127-133.

44. **Suurmeijer, A.J.H.** 1994. Optimizing immunohistochemistry in diagnostic tumor pathology with antigen retrieval. Eur. J. Morphol. *32*(2–4 suppl):325-330.

45. **Suurmeijer, A.J.H. and M.E. Boon.** 1993. Optimizing keratin and vimentin retrieval in formalin-fixed, paraffin-embedded tissue with the use of heat and metal salts. Appl. Immunohistochem. *1*:143-148.

46. **Tacha, D.E. and T. Chen.** 1994. A modified antigen retrieval method. A calibration technique for microwave ovens. J. Histotechnol. *17*:365-366.

47. **Taylor, C.R., S.-R. Shi, B. Chaiwun, L. Young, S.A. Imam, and R.J. Cote.** 1994. Strategy for improving the immunohistochemical staining of various intranuclear prognostic markers in formalin-paraffin sections: androgen receptor, estrogen receptor, progesterone recepter, p53 protein, proliferating cell nuclear antigen, and Ki-67 antigen revealed by antigen retrieval technique. Hum. Pathol. 25:263-270.

48. **Taylor, C.R., S.-R. Shi, C. Chen, L. Young, C. Yang, and R.J. Cote.** 1996. Comparative study of antigen retrieval heating methods—microwave, microwave and pressure cooker, autoclave and steamer. Biotech. Histochem. *71*:263-270.

49. **Van Dierendonck, J.H., R. Keijzer, C.J.H. van de Velde, and C.J. Cornelisse.** 1989. Nuclear distribution of the Ki-67 antigen during the cell cycle: comparison with the growth fraction in human breast cancer cells. Cancer Res. *49*:2999-3006.

50. **Von Wasielewski, R., M. Werner, M. Nolte, L. Wilkens, and A. Georgii.** 1994. Effects of antigen retrieval by microwave heating in formalin-fixed tissue sections on a broad panel of antibodies. Histochemistry *102*:165-172.

Immunohistochemical Detection of Tumor Suppressor Genes Using Antigen Retrieval Technique

13

Debra Hawes, Richard J. Cote, Shan-Rong Shi, and Clive R. Taylor

Department of Pathology, University of Southern California Keck School of Medicine, Los Angeles, CA, USA

INTRODUCTION

Neoplasia has been defined as a disorder in proliferation characterized by uncontrolled cell division regulation (7). Therefore, an understanding of the factors that regulate the cell cycle is important to the understanding of tumor development and progression. During the past several years, a great deal of information has been generated dealing with the factors that govern the cell cycle of nucleated cells (8). Among these are the so-called tumor suppressor genes; the most well known are the retinoblastoma (Rb) protein, *p53, p27, p21, p16*, and *PTEN/MMAC*. The existence of tumor suppressor genes (also known as antioncogenes) was first suggested by Knudson in 1971 (33), who explained the epidemiology of retinoblastoma by postulating multiple hits (double deletion) of both alleles of a recessive *Rb* gene that normally acts to inhibit the formation of tumors. The primary characteristics of tumor suppressor genes are that *(i)* they encode normal cellular products involved in growth control, and *(ii)* since the abnormality is recessive, both the alleles must be inactivated for loss of function (i.e., loss of tumor suppression) to occur. This is in contrast to the abnormalities described for oncogenes (positive growth factors), which are dominant, and thus require mutation in only one allele.

Several putative tumor suppressor genes have been identified, including the *Rb* gene, *p53, DCC* (deleted in colon cancer), the Wilms' tumor gene, and the neurofibromatosis type I gene (*NF1*) (33,45). *NM23* may also be an example of a tumor suppressor gene (35). The two best characterized are the *Rb* and the *p53* genes; the gene products for both have been identified and studied by immunohistochemical methods. Both *p53* and *Rb* gene products are thought to be involved in growth control

Antigen Retrieval Techniques
Edited by Shan-Rong Shi, Jiang Gu, and Clive R. Taylor
©2000 Eaton Publishing, Natick, MA

through regulation of transcription; wild-type p53 protein has been shown specifically to activate transcription, which may then lead to production of products that control cell growth (17). Both are nuclear phosphoproteins, and there is evidence that phosphorylation inactivates the Rb protein. In addition, a variety of viral oncoproteins, including SV40 T antigen, e1A from adenovirus, and E6 from human papilloma virus, bind to and neutralize Rb and/or p53 proteins. More recently, a cellular oncoprotein (MDM2) has been described, which binds to and may neutralize p53 protein (49).

GENES

Rb

The *Rb* gene is located on chromosome 13q14 and spans a region of more than 200 000 bases, including 27 exons. The protein has a molecular weight of 105 000 Da, and a number of antibodies have been developed that recognize specific parts of this protein (71). The *Rb* gene is the only tumor suppressor for which there is direct clinical evidence of suppression of tumor formation. Alterations in this gene have been described in a number of human tumors, including retinoblastoma, osteosarcoma, other sarcomas, leukemias, lymphomas, and certain carcinomas, including those derived from breast, lung, prostate, bladder, kidney, and testes (9,26,53). Gene alterations also have been associated with advanced tumor grade and stage in a variety of tumors (9). In the case of breast carcinoma, alterations of the *Rb* gene have been associated with other signs of progression, such as loss of hormone receptor expression. Furthermore, there is growing evidence that gene alterations may identify primary tumors that are at higher risk of developing metastases (14).

It is now clear that genetic alterations in the *Rb* gene correlate with loss of expression of Rb protein as determined by immunohistochemical methods (71). In fact, it has been suggested that immunohistochemical analysis of Rb protein may detect *Rb* gene inactivation more rapidly, specifically, and reliably than direct screening of DNA for gene abnormalities (2). Assessment of *Rb* gene loss by immunohistochemistry (IHC) is based on loss of detectable nuclear staining for Rb protein. This is in contrast to the immunohistochemical staining pattern seen in tumors with altered *p53*, in which staining is increased due to accumulation of mutant protein. Interestingly, we have recently found that not only loss of Rb expression, but Rb overexpression is also indicative of a poor prognosis in patients with demonstrated bladder cancer (10). This finding is based on immunohistochemical analysis of 185 patients with transitional cell carcinoma of the bladder who underwent radical cystectomy. This presents the interesting notion that a nonfunctional Rb protein may exist in tumor cells. Preliminary studies of these cases using the Western blotting technique showed that most of the Rb protein in these high-expressing tumors was in the phosphorylated form (Chatterjee et al., unpublished data).

p53

The p53 protein was originally described as a nuclear protein (MW, 53 000 Da) expressed in methylcholanthrene-induced mouse sarcomas, but not in normal mouse cells (13). Originally thought to be a cellular oncoprotein specifically expressed by tumor cells, it is now included in the tumor suppressor family. The p53 protein is expressed by all normal cells, but the half-life of the wild-type (normal) protein is so short (6–30 min) that it does not accumulate to levels high enough to be detected by standard immunohistochemical techniques; mutant p53 protein, by contrast, has an extended half-life, accumulates, and is readily detectable in the cell nucleus; hence mutation is indicated by positive staining.

The *p53* gene is located on chromosome 17p13.1. Alterations of the *p53* gene, identified by cytogenetic, molecular, and immunohistochemical methods, are extremely common in human cancer and have been described in bladder, colon, lung, breast, and other carcinomas, as well as astrocytomas, leukemias, sarcomas, and mesotheliomas (11,15,16,44,67). Loss of *p53* suppressor function usually results from complete loss of one allele associated with a point mutation in the second allele; the mutant *p53* gene continues to be expressed but lacks the regulatory activity of the wild-type *p53*. Mutant p53 protein has several important properties: it can bind to and neutralize residual wild-type p53 proteins (i.e., it has "antisuppressor" or oncogenic effects), and it is a metabolically stable protein, with a long half-life (hence accumulation and detection).

There is increasing evidence that the immunohistochemical detection of p53 protein in the nucleus identifies cells that have mutations in the *p53* gene (16). However, a small percentage of tumors having *p53* mutations do not show detectable p53 nuclear accumulation by IHC, for reasons that are unclear.

Data suggest that the immunohistochemical analysis of p53 may not only be more sensitive than molecular methods in detecting *p53* gene alterations but that IHC may detect important alterations in *p53* function that do not involve mutations at the gene level (16). In addition, when p53 nuclear reactivity is detected by IHC, significant heterogeneity in the staining pattern (percentage of reactive tumor cell nuclei) is observed, even within the same tumor type. While some of the variation may be due to differences in fixation, there is now evidence that this may be due to a property of the mutant p53 protein (16). The heterogeneity in the staining pattern is apparently due (at least in part) to different sites of mutation, resulting in differing half-lives for the expressed proteins.

Another possible mechanism of heterogeneous staining is that some cells in a tumor may have a mutant *p53* gene, while others do not. While this mechanism has been suggested for some tumors (particularly astrocytomas), it may be uncommon, as p53 is apparently an early event in most of the common tumors, such as breast, prostate, and bladder carcinoma (16).

Because of the importance of *p53* alterations in human cancer and the ease of detecting p53 mutations by molecular or immunohistochemical techniques, p53 alterations have been the focus of intense examination. As with *Rb* alterations, *p53* alterations are associated with tumors of high histologic grade and tumors with a high proliferative index (again suggesting a relationship between tumor suppressor genes and control of cell growth). In the case of breast tumors, *p53* alterations are associated with loss of hormone receptor expression and hormone-independent tumor growth (as are *Rb* alterations), again suggesting that tumors that lose normal growth controls may do so because they become independent of normal growth regulators (5,14). There is growing evidence that, at least for some types of tumors, *p53* alterations identify patients with shorter disease-free interval and poorer overall survival (16,23,34). In the case of breast and bladder carcinoma, the association between p53 alterations and prognosis appears strongest in the earliest stage tumors, thus emphasizing the potential value of *p53* examination in assessing the future behavior of the tumor. It appears that in many tumors, p53 alterations are an early event in tumorigenesis and can be detected in in situ carcinomas (in the case of breast and bladder cancer) (5,15,16,69), or even in dysplastic lesions (in prostate and colon carcinoma). Thus, tumors that are at highest risk for progression may be identified even prior to becoming invasive.

One final concern relates to the possible instability of p53 in cut sections. Some investigators have reported loss of p53 staining in stored cut paraffin-embedded sections (30). We have confirmed this finding. However, the problem can be remedied by the use of appropriate antigen retrieval methods (see below), again emphasizing the importance of optimizing and standardizing the total stain procedure (60,67,68).

CYCLIN-DEPENDENT KINASE INHIBITORS

The cyclin-dependent kinase (cdk) inhibitors are a family of negative cell cycle regulators. Their primary mechanism of functioning appears to be through the formation of stable complexes with cdk proteins. These complexes inactivate the catalytically operative units. Among most the well known and clinically relevant are the p21, p27, and p16.

p21

p21, a member of the WAF/CIP/KIP family of cdk inhibitors, is probably the best characterized of the cdk inhibitors. It appears that the rate of *p21* gene aberrations is very low and that the main mechanism of inactivation may rest at the level of expression, since its transcription is directly activated by p53, and *p53* gene mutations are predominant events in cancer (8), although there is growing evidence for a p53-independent pathway (24,54). It acts as a regulator of epithelial carcinogenesis and differentiation and is thought to play an important role in tumor suppression by regulating cell cycle progression, DNA replication, and DNA repair (20). The protein expression of *p21* has been studied in a variety of tumor types including breast (54), gastric (29), ovary (1), colorectal (62), and bladder carcinomas (65,72). The loss of protein expression assessed by immunohistochemical methods has been associated with a higher grade of tumor and a worse prognosis.

p27

Analysis of genes and proteins involved in cell cycle regulation has yielded important prognostic and treatment information in many tumor systems. Recently, cell cycle inhibitors have been demonstrated to play a potentially important role in tumor progression (64). One of these, the cyclin-kinase inhibitor *p27*[kip1] (also known as *p27*), is a member of the cip/kip family of cdk inhibitors (50). It is involved in regulation of the cell cycle at the G_1/S transition, ultimately through inhibition of Rb protein phosphorylation (7). Mutations in the human *p27* gene appear to be rare (18,51). However, loss of *p27* expression has been shown to be associated with colon, breast, and prostate cancer progression (6,12,39,52). It is interesting that this loss of *p27* expression appears to be due to an increased proteasome-mediated protein degradation and to altered *p27* gene transcription or p27 mRNA stability (39). This demonstrates that p27 analysis must take place at the level of the protein. Thus, immunohistochemical methods for detecting p27, such as those described here, have the potential to become the tool of choice for determining p27 status (12).

p16

The p16 protein was first identified in association with cdk4, in DNA virus-transformed cells. It was found that the usual cyclin D-cdk4 complex was largely replaced by a p16-cdk4 complex preventing cell division (70). Numerous studies have found the presence of abnormal p16 protein in a variety of tumor types including melanomas, gliomas, esophageal, pancreatic, lung, and bladder carcinomas as well as in certain types of lymphoma (4,25,27,28,31,32,42,47,48,56,57). Numerous studies have demonstrated that immunohistochemical expression of Rb and p16 are inversely correlated in a variety of tumors (22,46,55). Recent work using immunohistochemical and molecular methods in our laboratory has supported this finding.

Obviously, application of antigen retrieval (AR)-IHC for the detection of tumor suppressor genes, as well as other markers on archival formalin-fixed, paraffin-embedded tissue sections, has provided a valuable approach to the study of the pathways of cell growth and death, which is, of course, a key factor in the understanding of cancer progression.

PTEN/MMAC1/TEP-1

PTEN, which stands for phosphatase and tensin homolog deleted on chromosome 10, is a relatively new candidate tumor suppressor gene. It is also known as *MMAC1* (mutation in many advanced carcinomas) and *TEP-1* (TGF-β-regulated and epithelial cell-enriched phosphastase). Protein tyrosine phosphatases have been shown to act as either positive or negative regulators during signal transduction, cell cycle progression, and cellular transformation. One hypothesis concerning the mechanism by which *PTEN* acts as a tumor suppressor is that it antagonizes protein tyrosine kinase (21). Somatic mutations of *PTEN* have been identified in glioma, breast, and prostate tumor cell lines (3,37,63). It has also been identified as the gene predisposing to Cowden disease (3,38). Frequent inactivation of the *PTEN* gene has also been found in primary prostate cancer (3). However, it is difficult to identify physiologic protein substrates (43). It has been suggested that overexpression of PTEN may negatively regulate cellular adhesion and cell mobility through PTEN-mediated dephosphorylation of focal adhesion kinase (FAK) (66). More recent studies have noted that PTEN may function as a lipid phosphatase for phosphatidylinositol 3,4,5-triphosphate (PIP3) (40). Subsequent studies have confirmed this finding and demonstrated that the major consequence of loss of PTEN function is deregulation of the phosphoinositide (PI) 3-kinase/Akt pathway, which is oncogenic in several tumor models (19,36). PTEN functions as a negative regulator of this pathway by dephosphorylating PIP_3 and decreasing activated Akt.

Immunohistochemical study of PTEN using AR techniques in archival paraffin-embedded tissue sections has already been documented (41). This research group found that loss of PTEN protein is correlated with a poor prognosis in prostate cancer. Our group has optimized an AR protocol for the detection of PTEN protein in archival paraffin-embedded sections and has demonstrated that PTEN is expressed in the cytoplasm and with much lower intensity of immunostaining in prostate cancer cells than in normal glands. Our results support the hypothesis that PTEN plays an important role in the initiation and progression of prostate cancer (unpublished data).

ANTIGEN RETRIEVAL TECHNIQUE FOR IHC DETECTION OF TUMOR SUPPRESSOR GENES

The high-temperature heating AR technique is used for IHC detection of all tumor suppressor genes that have been discussed in this chapter. In our experience, AR is a simple and effective method of pretreating tissue to optimize immunostaining results

Table 1. Primary Antibodies

Antibody	Clone/Cat. No.	Source	Concentration[a] (µg/mL)
p53	1801/OP09-200UG	Oncogene, Cambridge, MA, USA	5
p53	DO7/Code#M7001	DAKO, Carpinteria, CA, USA	1
p21	WAF1 (Ab-1)/OP64-100UG	Oncogene	5
p27	DCS-72.F6/MS-256-P	NeoMarker, Union City, CA, USA	4
p16	/13251A	PharMingen, San Diego, CA, USA	5
Rb	G3-245/14001A	PharMingen	5
Rb	PAb RB-WL-1	Ref. 59	0.6
PTEN	PAb	Zymed, South San Francisco, CA, USA	5

[a]Concentration is used for overnight incubation of the primary antibody at room temperature, detected by using the ABC system (Vector Laboratories, Burlingame, CA, USA).

of p53, p21, p16, p27, Rb, and PTEN on routinely formalin-fixed, paraffin-embedded tissue sections. The major technical issues are summarized as follows:

1. The test battery approach based on two major factors that influence the effectiveness of AR-IHC is helpful to establish an optimal protocol for each marker of interest (see Appendix for details).

2. Fresh tissue sections may be used to confirm the immunostaining results obtained by archival paraffin-embedded tissue section cut from the same tumor in order to avoid any false staining patterns resulting from AR treatment, as exemplified by our application of the optimal AR protocols for Rb and thrombospondin (58,59).

3. A test model system using cell lines may be applied to establish optimal protocols similar to the use of fresh tissue sections discussed above. In addition, it may allow for quantitative IHC results, which are reported as the percentage of cells present that are positive. Cell lines may also be processed in the same way as routinely formalin-fixed, paraffin-embedded tissue sections to establish optimal protocols for these tissues. Our laboratory has successfully applied various cell line model systems from cytospin smears (fixed in formalin or acetone, or unfixed), centrifuged cell pellets embedded in an embedding medium such as OCT compound (Tissue-Tek®; Sakura Fintek, Torrance, CA, USA) (used as frozen tissue section), and routinely processed cell pellets embedded in paraffin (as routine paraffin section), for IHC study of most antibodies to tumor suppressor genes.

4. Most nuclear markers (i.e., p53, Rb, p16) tend to have a stronger intensity when the tissue sections are heated in AR solutions with lower pH values (59,60).

5. Previously cut and stored paraffin-embedded tissue sections have been shown to display a reduced intensity of immunostaining for p27 and p53 over a period of time. This has been especially problematic for p27 (12). The reduced immunoreactivity for p53 found in stored tissue samples may be restored by using an optimized AR protocol. We have found that satisfactory immunostaining results for p27 in stored paraffin-embedded sections can be achieved by combining an optimal AR protocol and an enhanced detection system such as a PowerVision™ (ImmunoVision, Daly City, CA, USA) two-step detection reagent (61).

Table 2. Summary of Antigen Retrieval Protocols

Antibody	Heating Temperature °C	Heating Time (min)	AR Solution	AR Solution pH	Notes
Rb	90	10	Acetic buffer	1–2	Ref. 59[a]
Rb	120	10	Tris-HCl buffer	10	Ref. 59[a]
p53	100	10	Citrate buffer	6	Low pH solution may achieve stronger staining (60)
p21	100	10	Citrate buffer	6	
p16	95	5	Tris-HCl buffer	1–2	—[b]
p27	100	10	Citrate buffer	6	—[c]
PTEN	100	10	Citrate buffer	6	

[a]Both protocols are optimal for Rb immunostaining.

[b]In our laboratory, this lower temperature is controlled by using a microwave oven (around 1000 W), setting at high power for 1 min, and then changing to 40% power setting for 5 min.

[c]For stored paraffin sections, a combined use of an optimal AR protocol (EDTA-NaOH solution of pH 8.0) with a two-step PowerVision™ detection system may achieve a satisfactory result of IHC for p27 (61).

ANTIGEN RETRIEVAL PROTOCOLS

Materials and Reagents

- Refer to the Appendix for details concerning basic equipment and materials for AR-IHC.
- A cryostat for cutting frozen tissue sections, as well as equipment for performing cell culture, cell centrifuge, and cytospin.
- Primary antibodies to tumor suppressor genes listed in Table 1.

Procedures

Refer to the Appendix for AR protocols in detail. Different optimal AR protocols are summarized in Table 2.

REFERENCES

1. **Barboule, N., V. Baldin, S.J. Ozan, S. Vidal, and A. Valette.** 1998. Increased level of p21 in human ovarian tumors is associated with increased expression of cdk2, cyclin A and PCNA. Int. J. Cancer. *76*:891-896.
2. **Borg, A., Q.-A. Zhang, P. Alm, H. Olsson, and G. Sellberg.** 1992. The retinoblastoma gene in breast cancer, allele loss is not correlated with loss of gene protein expression. Cancer Res. *52*:2991-2994.
3. **Cairns, P., K. Okami, S. Halachmi, N. Halachmi, M. Esteller, J.G. Herman, J. Jen, W.B. Isaacs, G.S. Bova, and D. Sidransky.** 1997. Frequent inactivation of PTEN/MMAC1 in primary prostate cancer. Cancer Res. *57*:4997-5000.

4. **Caldas, C., S.A. Hahn, L.T. da Costa, M.S. Redston, M. Schutte, A.B. Seymour, C.L. Weinstein, R.H. Hruban, C.J. Yeo, and S.E. Kern.** 1994. Frequent somatic mutations and homozygous deletions of the p16 (MTS1) gene in pancreatic adenocarcinoma [published erratum appears in Nat. Genet. 1994 Dec; 8(4):410]. Nat. Genet. *8*:27-32.

5. **Cattoretti, G., S. Andreola, C. Clemente, L. DAmato, and F. Rilke.** 1988. Vimentin and p53 expression on epidermal growth factor receptor-positive, oestrogen receptor-negative breast carcinomas. Br. J. Cancer *57*:353-357.

6. **Catzavelos, C., N. Bhattacharya, Y.C. Ung, J.A. Wilson, L. Roncari, C. Sandhu, P. Shaw, H. Yeger, L. Morava-Protzner, L. Kapusta, et al.** 1997. Decreased levels of the cell-cycle inhibitor p27^{Kip1} protein: prognostic implications in primary breast cancer. Nat. Med. *3*:227-230.

7. **Cordon-Cardo, C.** 1995. Mutation of cell-cycle regulators. Biological and clinical implications for human neoplasia. Am. J. Pathol. *147*:545-560.

8. **Cordon-Cardo, C. and V.E. Reuter.** 1997. Alterations of tumor suppressor genes in bladder cancer. Semin. Diagn. Pathol. *14*:123-132.

9. **Cordon-Cardo, C., D. Wartinger, D. Petrylak, G. Dalbagni, W.R. Fair, Z. Fuks, and V.E. Reute.** 1992. Altered expression of the retinoblastoma gene product: prognostic indicator in bladder cancer. J. Natl. Cancer Inst. *84*:1251-1256.

10. **Cote, R.J., M.D. Dunn, S.J. Chatterjee, J.P. Stein, S.R. Shi, Q.C. Tran, S.X. Hu, H.J. Xu, S. Groshen, C.R. Taylor et al.** 1998. Elevated and absent pRb expression is associated with bladder cancer progression and has cooperative effects with p53. Cancer Res. *58*:1090-1094.

11. **Cote, R.J., S.C. Jhanwar, S. Novick, and A. Pillicer.** 1991. Genetic alterations of the p53 gene are a feature of malignant mesotheliomas. Cancer Res. *51*:5410-5416.

12. **Cote, R.J., Y. Shi, S. Groshen, A.-C. Feng, C. Cordon-Cardo, D. Skinner, and G. Lieskovsky.** 1998. Association of p27Kip1 levels with recurrence and survival in patients with stage C prostate carcinoma. J. Natl. Cancer Inst. *90*:916-920.

13. **DeLeo, A.B., G. Jay, E. Appella, G.C. Dubois, L.W. Law, and L.J. Old.** 1979. Detection of a transformation-related antigen in chemically induced sarcomas and other transformed cells of the mouse. Proc. Natl. Acad. Sci. USA *76*:2420-2424.

14. **Drobnjak, M., R.J. Cote, A.D. Saad, T. Drudis, Z. Fuks, and C. Cordon-Cardo.** 1993. p53 and Rb alterations in primary breast carcinoma: correlation with hormone receptor expression and lymph node metastases. Int. J. Oncol. *2*:173-178.

15. **Esrig, D., D. Elmajian, S. Groshen, J.A. Freeman, J.P. Stein, S.C. Chen, P.W. Nichols, D.G. Skinner, P.A. Jones, and R.J. Cote.** 1994. Accumulation of nuclear p53 and tumor progression in bladder cancer. N. Engl. J. Med. *331*:1259-1264.

16. **Esrig, D., C.H. Spruck, P.W. Nichols, B. Chaiwun, K. Steven, S. Groshen, S.C. Chen, D.G. Skinner, P.A. Jones, and R.J. Cote.** 1993. p53 nuclear protein accumulation correlates with mutations in the p53 gene tumor grade and stage in bladder cancer. Am. J. Pathol. *142*:1389-1397.

17. **Farmer, G., J. Bargonetti, H. Zhu, P. Friedman, R. Prywes, and C. Prives.** 1992. Wild-type p53 activates transcription in vitro. Nature *358*:83-86.

18. **Ferrando, A.A., M. Balbin, A.M. Pendas, F. Vizoso, G. Velasco, and C. Lopez-Otin.** 1996. Mutational analysis of the human cyclin-dependent kinase inhibitor p27kip1 in primary breast carcinomas. Hum. Genet. *97*:91-94.

19. **Funari, F., H.J. Huang, and W.K. Cavenee.** 1998. The phosphoinositol phosphatase activity of PTEN mediates a serum-sensitive G1 growth arrest in glioma cells. Cancer Res. *58*:5002-5008.

20. **Funk, J.O., M.A. McShea, E. Espling, J.-T. Eppel, and D.A. Galloway.** 1999. p21CIP1 acts as a positive regulator of cyclin B through carboxy-terminal association with a novel protein, CARB. J. Invest. Dermatol. *113*:431.

21. **Furnari, F., H. Lin, H.-J. Su Huang, and W.K. Cavenee.** 1997. Growth suppression of glioma cells by PTEN requires a functional phosphatase catalytic domain. Proc. Natl. Acad. Sci. USA *94*:12479-12484.

22. **Gerdts, J., K.M. Fong, P.V. Zimmerman, R. Maynard, and J.D. Minna.** 1999. Correlation of abnormal RB, p16ink4a, and p53 expression with 3p loss of heterozygosity, other genetic abnormalities, and clinical features in 103 primary non-small cell lung cancer. Clin. Cancer Res. *5*:791-800.

23. **Hamada, H., Y. Ogawa, H. Seguchi, M. Terashima, A. Nishioka, T. Inomata, S. Yoshida, S. Kishsimoto, and H. Saito.** 1995. Immunohistochemical study of p53 expression in cancer tissues from patients undergoing radiation therapy. Histol. Histopathol. *10*:611-617.

24. **Hayama, H., A. Iavarone, and S.A. Reeves.** 1998. Regulation of the cdk inhibitor p21 gene during cell cycle progression is under the control of transcription factor E2F. Oncogene *16*:1513-1523.

25. **Hebert, J., J.M. Cayuela, J. Berkeley, and F. Sigaux.** 1994. Candidate tumor-suppressor genes MTS1 (p16INK4A) and MTS2 (p15INK4B) display frequent homozygous deletions in primary cells from T- but not from B-cell lineage acute lymphoblastic leukemias [see comments]. Blood *84*:4038-4044.

26. **Horowitz, J.M., S.H. Park, E. Bogenmann, J.C. Cheng, D.W. Yandell, F.J. Kaye, J.D. Minna, T.P. Dryja, and R.A. Weinberg.** 1990. Frequent inactivation of the retinoblastoma anti-oncogene is restricted to a subset of human tumor cells. Proc. Natl. Acad. Sci. USA *87*:2775-2779.

27. **Hunter, T. and J. Pines.** 1994. Cyclins and cancer. II: cyclin D and CDK inhibitors come of age [see comments]. Cell *79*:573-582.

28. **Hussussian, C.J., J.P. Struewing, A.M. Goldstein, P.A. Higgins, D.S. Ally, M.D. Sheahan, W.H. Clark, Jr.,**

M.A. Tucker, and N.C. Dracopoli. 1994. Germline p16 mutations in familial melanoma [see comments]. Nat. Genet. *8*:15-21.

29. Ikeguchi, M., H. Saito, K. Katano, S. Tsujitani, M. Maeta, and N. Kaibara. 1998. Expression of p53 and p21 are independent prognostic factors in patients with serosal invasion by gastric carcinoma. Dig. Dis. Sci. *43*:964-970.

30. Jacob, T.W., J.E. Prioleau, J.E. Stillman, and S.J. Schnitt. 1996. Loss of tumor marker-immunostaining intensity on stored paraffin slides of breast cancer. J. Natl. Cancer Inst. *88*:1054-1059.

31. Jen, J., J.W. Harper, S.H. Bigner, D.D. Bigner, N. Papadopoulos, S. Markowitz, J.K. Willson, K.W. Kinzler, and B. Vogelstein. 1994. Deletion of p16 and p15 genes in brain tumors. Cancer Res. *54*:6353-6358.

32. Kamb, A., D. Shattuck-Eidens, R. Eeles, Q. Liu, N.A. Gruis, W. Ding, C. Hussey, T. Tran, Y. Miki, and J. Weaver-Feldhaus. 1994. Analysis of the p16 gene (CDKN2) as a candidate for the chromosome 9p melanoma susceptibility locus. Nat. Genet. *8*:23-26.

33. Knudson, A.G., Jr. 1971. Mutation and cancer: statistical study of retinoblastoma. Proc. Natl. Acad. Sci. USA *68*:820-823.

34. Lazaris, A., G.E. Theodorpoulos, P. Anastassopoiulos, L. Nakapoulou, D. Panoussopoulos, and K. Pamadimitrious. 1995. Prognostic significance of p53 and c-erbB-2 immunohistochemical evaluation in colorectal adenocarcinoma. Histol. Histopathol. *10*:661-668.

35. Leone, A., O.W. McBride, A. Weston, M.G. Wang, P. Angland, C.S. Cropp, J.R. Goepel, and R. Lidereau. 1991. Somatic allelic deletion of nm23 in human cancer. Cancer Res. *51*:2490.

36. Li, D. and H. Sun. 1998. PTEN/MMAC1/TEP1 suppresses the tumorigenicity and induces G1 cell cycle arrest in human glioblastoma cells. Proc. Natl. Acad. Sci. USA *95*:15406-15411.

37. Li, J., C. Yen, D. Liaw, K. Podsypanina, S. Bose, S.I. Wang, J. Puc, C. Miliaresis, L. Rogers, R. McCombie, et al. 1997. PTEN, a putative protein tyrosine phosphatase gene mutated in human brain, breast, and prostate cancer. Science *275*:1943-1947.

38. Liaw, D., D.J. Marsh, J. Li, P.L.M. Dahia, S.I. Wang, Z. Zheng, S. Bose, K.M. Call, H.C. Tsou, M. Peacock et al. 1997. Germline mutations of PTEN gene in Cowden disease, an inherited breast and thyroid cancer syndrome. Nat. Genet. *16*:64-67.

39. Loda, M., B. Cukor, S.W. Tam, P. Lavin, M. Fiorentino, G.F. Draetta, J. M. Jessup, and M. Pagano. 1997. Increased proteasome-dependent degradation of the cyclin-dependent kinase inhibitor p27 in aggressive colorectal carcinomas. Nat. Med. *3*:231-234.

40. Maehama, T. and J.E. Dixon. 1998. The tumor suppressor, PTEN/MMAC1, dephosphorylates the lipid second messenger, phosphatidylinoditol 3,4,5-triphosphate. J. Biol. Chem. *273*:13375-13378.

41. McMenamin, M., P. Soung, S. Perera, I. Kaplan, M. Loda, and W.R. Sellers. 1999. Loss of PTEN expression in paraffin-embedded primary prostate cancer correlates with high Gleason score and advanced stage. Cancer Res. *59*:4291-4296.

42. Mori, T., K. Miura, T. Aoki, T. Nishihira, S. Mori, and Y. Nakamura. 1994. Frequent somatic mutation of the MTS1/CDK4I (multiple tumor suppressor/cyclin-dependent kinase 4 inhibitor) gene in esophageal squamous cell carcinoma. Cancer Res. *54*:3396-3397.

43. Myers, M., J.P. Stolarov, C. Eng, J. Li, S.I. Wang, and M.H. Wigler. 1997. PTEN, the tumor suppressor from human chromosome 10q23, is a dual-specificity phosphatase. Proc. Natl. Acad. Sci. USA *94*:9052-9057.

44. Nigro, J.M., S.J. Baker, A.C. Preisinger, J.M. Jessup, R. Hostetter, K. Cleary, S.H. Bigner, N. Davidson, S. Baylin, and P. Devilee. 1989. Mutations in the p53 gene occur in diverse human tumor types. Nature 342:705-708.

45. Nowell, P.C. and C. Croce. 1986. Chromosomes genes and cancer. Am. J. Pathol. *125*:7-16.

46. Okami, K., A.I. Reed, P. Cairns, W.M. Koch, W.H. Westra, S. Wehage, J. Jen, and D. Sidransky. 1999. Cyclin D1 amplification is independent of p16 inactivation in head and neck squamous cell carcinoma. Oncogene *18*:3541-3545.

47. Okamoto, A., D.J. Demetrick, E.A. Spillare, K. Hagiwara, S.P. Hussain, W.P. Bennett, K. Forrester, B. Gerwin, M. Serrano, and D.H. Beach. 1994. Mutations and altered expression of p16INK4 in human cancer. Proc. Natl. Acad. Sci. USA *91*:11045-11049.

48. Okuda, T., S.A. Shurtleff, M.B. Valentine, S.C. Raimondi, D.R. Head, F. Behm, A.M. Curcio-Brint, Q. Liu, C.H. Pui, C.J. Sherr, et al. 1995. Frequent deletion of p16INK4a/MTS1 and p15INK4b/MTS2 in pediatric acute lymphoblastic leukemia. Blood 85:2321-2330.

49. Oliner, J.D., K.W. Kinzler, P.S. Meltzer, D.L. George, and B. Vogelstein. 1992. Amplification of a gene encoding a p53-associated protein in human sarcomas [see comments]. Nature *358*:80-83.

50. Polyak, K., M.H. Lee, H. Erdjument-Bromage, A. Koff, J.M. Roberts, P. Tempst, and J. Massague. 1994. Cloning of p27Kip1, a cyclin-dependent kinase inhibitor and a potential mediator of extracellular antimitogenic signals. Cell *78*:59-66.

51. Ponce-Castaneda, M.V., M.H. Lee, E. Latres, K. Polyak, L. Lacombe, K. Montgomery, S. Mathew, K. Krauter, J. Sheinfeld, J. Massague, and C. Cordon-Cardo. 1995. p27Kip1: chromosomal mapping to 12p12-12p13.1 and absence of mutations in human tumors. Cancer Res. *55*:1211-1214.

52. Porter, P., K.E. Malone, P.J. Heagerty, G.M. Alexander, L.A. Gatti, E.J. Firpo, J.R. Daling, and J.M. Roberts. 1997. Expression of cell-cycle regulators p27Kip1 and cyclin E, alone or in combination, correlate with survival in young breast cancer patients. Nat. Med. *3*:222-225.

215

53. Reissmann, P.T., M.A. Simon, W.-H. Lee, and D.J. Slamon. 1989. Studies of retinoblastoma gene in sarcomas. Oncogene *4*:839-843.

54. Rey, M.J., P.L. Fernandez, P. Jares, M. Munoz, A. Nadal, N. Peiro, I. Nayach, C. Mallofre, J. Muntan, E. Campo, et al. 1998. p21WAFa/Cip1 is associated with cyclin D1CCND1 expression and tubular differentiation but is independent of p53 overexpression in human breast carcinoma. J. Pathol. *184*:265-271.

55. Sartor, M., F. Elamin, J. Gaken, S. Warnkulasuriya, M. Partridge, N. Thakker, N.W. Johnson, and M. Tavassoli. 1999. Role of p16/MTS1, cyclin D1 and RB in primary oral cancer and oral cancer cell lines. Br. J. Cancer *80*:79-86.

56. Schmidt, E.E., K. Ichimura, G. Reifenberger, and V.P. Collins. 1994. CDKN2 (p16/MTS1) gene deletion or CDK4 amplification occurs in the majority of glioblastomas. Cancer Res. *54*:6321-6324.

57. Sherr, C.J. and J.M. Roberts. 1995. Inhibitors of mammalian G1 cyclin-dependent kinases. Genes Dev. *9*:1149-1163.

58. Shi, S.-R., R.J. Cote, and C.R. Taylor. 1997. Antigen retrieval immunohistochemistry: past, present, and future. J. Histochem. Cytochem. *45*:327-343.

59. Shi, S.-R., R.J. Cote, C. Yang, C. Chen, H.-J. Xu, W.F. Benedict, and C.R. Taylor. 1996. Development of an optimal protocol for antigen retrieval: A 'test battery' approach exemplified with reference to the staining of retinoblastoma protein (pRB) in formalin-fixed paraffin sections. J. Pathol. *179*:347-352.

60. Shi, S.-R., R.J. Cote, L. Young, B. Chaiwun, Y. Shi, D. Hawes, T. Chen, and C.R. Taylor. 1998. Standardization of immunohistochemistry based on antigen retrieval technique for routine formalin-fixed tissue sections. Appl. Immunohistochem. *6*:89-96.

61. Shi, S.-R., J. Guo, R.J. Cote, L.L. Young, D. Hawes, Y. Shi, S. Thu, and C.R. Taylor. 1999. Sensitivity and detection efficiency of a novel two-step detection system (PowerVision) for immunohistochemistry. Appl. Immunohistochem. Mol. Morphol. *7*:201-208.

62. Sinicrope, F.A., G. Roddey, M. Lemoine, S. Ruan, L.C. Stephens, M.L. Frazier, Y. Shen, and W. Zhang. 1998. Loss of p21/WAF1/Cip1 protein expression accompanies progression of sporadic colorectal neoplasms but not hereditary nonpolyposis colorectal cancers. Clin. Cancer Res. *45*:1251-1261.

63. Steck, P.A., M.A. Pershouse, S.A. Jasser, W.K. Yung, H. Lin, A.H. Ligon, L.A. Langford, M.L. Baumgard, T. Hattier, T. Davis, et al. 1997. Identification of a candidate tumor suppressor gene MMAC1, at chromosome 10q23 that is mutated in multiple advanced cancers. Nat. Genet. *15*:356-362.

64. Steeg, P.S. and J. Abrams. 1997. Cancer prognostics: past, present and p27. Nat. Med. *3*:152-154.

65. Stein, J.P., D.A. Ginsberg, G.D. Grossfeld, S.J. Chatterjee, D. Esrig, M.G. Dickinson, S. Groshen, C.R. Taylor, P.A. Jones, D.G. Skinner, and R.J. Cote. 1998. Effect of p21WAF/CIP1 expression on tumor progression in bladder cancer. J. Natl. Cancer Inst. *90*:1072-1079.

66. Tamura, M., J. Gu, K. Matsumoto, S.-I. Aota, R. Parsons, and K.M. Yamada. 1998. Inhibition of cell migration, spreading, and focal adhesions by tumor suppressor PTEN. Science *280*:1614-1617.

67. Taylor, C.R. and R.J. Cote. 1994. Immunomicroscopy. A diagnostic tool for the surgical pathologist, 2nd ed., Ch. 4. W.B. Saunders, Philadelphia.

68. Taylor, C.R., S.-R. Shi, and R.J. Cote. 1996. Antigen retrieval for immunohistochemistry. Status and need for greater standardization. Appl. Immunohistochem. *4*:144-166.

69. Walker, R.A., S.J. Dearing, D.P. Lane, and J.M Varley. 1991. Expression of p53 protein in infiltrating and in situ breast carcinomas. J. Pathol. *165*:203-211.

70. Xiong, Y., H. Zhang, and D. Beach. 1993. Subunit rearrangement of the cyclin-dependent kinases is associated with cellular transformation. Genes Dev. *7*:1572-1583.

71. Xu, H.-J., S.-X. Hu, P.-T. Cagle, G.E. Moore, and W.F. Benedict. 1991. Absence of retinoblastoma protein expression in primary non-small cell lung carcinomas. Cancer Res. *51*:2735-2739.

72. Yamashita, M., S. Hodges, D. Johnston, C. Bogdan, and W. F. Benedict. 1999. Loss of p21/WAF1/CIP1 expression is an important predictor of aggressive behavior in urinary bladder cancer. J. Urol. *161*:151.

Section IV

Standardization and Combination of the Antigen Retrieval Technique

Combination of Antigen Retrieval Techniques and Signal Amplification of Immunohistochemistry In Situ Hybridization and FISH Techniques

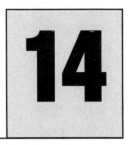

Hartmut Merz, Katharina Ottesen, Wibke Meyer, Anke Mueller, Yanming Zhang, and Alfred Christian Feller

Department of Pathology, Medical University of Luebeck, Luebeck, Germany

INTRODUCTION

Since the introduction of monoclonal antibodies, immunohistochemistry has become an important tool in research and surgical pathology. Immunohistochemistry is a well-established and widely used method for detecting cellular antigens in daily diagnostic work and for research purposes. It allows defined antigens to be visualized in situ on cryostat and paraffin sections (15,25,34,77). One of its disadvantages is that many of the well-characterized antigens cannot be detected in formalin-fixed tissue with the available immunohistochemical techniques (45,46). Immunohistochemical evaluation of frozen material has its limitations, because the morphology is not well preserved, and fresh frozen material also is frequently not available.

The most widely used fixative in routine histopathology is formaldehyde, which has become the gold standard for morphologic tissue preservation. Aldehyde fixation of proteins is a method that preserves the overall cellular and/or tissue architecture well, but the mechanisms of its chemical reactivity are still not understood completely (17). It was believed that the fixation process irreversibly destroys most cellular antigens, but recent developments in immunohistochemistry have suggested that complex aldehyde-linked protein aggregates are formed in which primary and secondary protein structures may be preserved, while the tertiary or quaternary

Antigen Retrieval Techniques
Edited by Shan-Rong Shi, Jiang Gu, and Clive R. Taylor
©2000 Eaton Publishing, Natick, MA

protein structures are altered by extensive cross-linking. Although the molecular mechanism underlying tissue fixation is not well understood, it has become clear that available immunoreactive antigenic epitopes are progressively lost during the fixation process. This is accomplished by a time-dependent increase in protein-protein and/or nucleic acid cross-linking.

Cross-linking is a special form of chemical modification that can be defined as a process involving the joining of two molecular components by covalent bonds achieved by the use of the cross-linking reagent formalin (63,76). Tissue fixation can be divided into a two-step procedure: the primary reaction is defined by the additional reaction of the amine and an aldehyde (e.g., formalin) or ketone (e.g., acetone), $R-NH_2 + HCHO \rightarrow R-NH-CH_2OH$, followed by a secondary condensation reaction: $R-NH-CH_2OH + H_2N-CO-R' \rightarrow R-NH-CH_2-NH-CO-R' + H_2O$ (63). Both aldehyde and ketone are carbonyl compounds that can react with amino groups of proteins to form Schiff bases. Formalin fixation is a complicated process that is difficult to predict and that depends on a variety of conditions (e.g., time, concentration of fixatives, pH, and additives such as buffers, salts, etc.) and may lead to a variety of protein alterations (18–20), which increase during the time of tissue fixation.

Antibodies recognize specific epitopes localized in a particular spatial configuration within the protein molecule and the amino acid sequence. These structures might be linear but in many instances are discontinuous, because the antigenic determinants are composed of residues from different parts of the amino acid sequence recognizing a two- or three-dimensional structure (3,6). Formalin fixation may induce a change in protein conformation, or, with greater likelihood, a change in accessibility of the residues encoding the antigenic epitope, thus masking the tissue antigenicity.

In other words, the use of cross-linking fixatives is usually responsible for the non-reactivity of many antibodies. Therefore, formalin-sensitive antigens/antigenic epitopes might not be irreversibly destroyed during the fixation process, but the accessibility of antigenic epitopes is suggested to be limited by steric barriers caused by the aldehyde. If the three-dimensional conformation is modified by the cross-linking process, an optimal retrieval system might give access to the antigenic epitopes, thereby reversing such hindrances by antigen retrieval (AR) techniqes (35,41,45,46,57,59).

Recent results in routine immunohistochemistry have offered some support for the above-mentioned hypothesis. While monoclonal anti-immunoglobulin antibodies frequently functioned inadequately in formalin-fixed tissues, polyclonal anti-immunoglobulin antibodies were shown to produce reproducible staining results; however, the results were dependent on the conditions of the fixation process of tissues. Moreover, staining sensitivity could be improved by using enzyme-mediated tissue digestion and by controlling the fixation process (45).

Taking this into account, it appeared possible that most cellular antigens might not be irreversibly destroyed, but only masked and may therefore be accessible to AR techniques.

A variety of hidden antigens can be retrieved and/or the sensitivity of the immunohistochemical methods can be increased by pretreating the fixed tissue in various ways, e.g., with detergent treatment, by protease digestion, or by microwave heating.

The introduction of high-temperature heating AR techniques has significantly enhanced the sensitivity of immunohistochemistry in formalin-fixed, paraffin-embedded tissue. The use of different AR solutions, as well as different AR conditions with or without the combination of protease digestion, leads to a tremendous increase in sensitivity without loss of specificity; the results may be comparable to or even better than those achieved using fresh frozen material, with the added advantage of well-preserved morphology (45).

The sensitivity of these methods depends on the optimization of both AR and staining techniques.

Although some antigens may be retrieved under appropriate AR conditions, there may still be many antigens for which available antigenic epitopes are still too sparse to be visualized after formalin fixation. This has been observed for a large number of leukocyte differentiation antigens and for antigens expressed at very low levels such as cytokines, cytokine receptors, or cell cycle regulating proteins.

In the past, a number of attempts have been made to overcome these obstacles, including the introduction of new reagents recognizing formalin-resistant epitopes, attempts to retrieve formalin-fixed antigenic sites for initially nonreactive antibodies, and efforts to achieve signal amplification with an acceptable signal-to-noise ratio (35, 41,45,46,57–59). Our reliable approach to resolve this dilemma is the combination of an optimized AR system and a recently described powerful immunohistochemical staining protocol introducing a biotinyl-tyramine amplification step, in which signal amplification is accomplished by covalent deposition of biotin molecules (46).

While AR pretreatment resulted in moderately improved immunostaining, biotinylated tyramine enhancement proved to be the most efficient step, although it is not sufficient for many antigens when used without pretreatment steps. The combination of an AR step with the biotinylated tyramine enhancement step may result in a 100- to 10 000-fold boost in sensitivity.

With this approach, many defined antigens can be reproducibly detected in formalin-fixed, paraffin-embedded tissues, and the sensitivity of the method is tremendously enhanced. Moreover, it also allows many previously unreactive or unsatisfactorily reactive antigens to be detected, yielding a sensitivity in formalin-fixed, paraffin embedded tissues comparable to or even better than that achieved in cryostat sections, without resulting in a loss of specificity, provided the conditions are controlled appropriately.

COMPARISON OF DIFFERENT ANTIGEN RETRIEVAL STEPS

Several AR steps have been suggested to improve the staining intensity. Until recently, attempts to unmask antigenic sites have been based on section pretreatment with proteinases, involving trypsin, proteinase K, pronase E, pepsin, or others; the accepted mode of action of these enzymes is digestion of proteins and the release of appropriate epitopes for immunstaining. However, it is not clear whether there is a true liberalization of fixative-caused bonds or whether the partial tissue digestion is responsible for an increase in antibody penetration and binding; it is possible that both factors may be relevant. As these enzymes also digest proteins/antigenic epitopes, which are native, e.g., not cross-linked, it is conceivable that a loss in immunoreactivity may result after prolonged tissue digestion.

Heat-induced AR methods are based on biochemical studies of the chemical reaction between protein and formalin by Fraenkel-Conrat and co-workers (18–20) in the 1940s; these studies indicated that hydrolysis of cross-linkages between formalin and protein is limited by certain amino acid side chains, such as imidazol and indol, but that these cross-linkages can be reversed by high-temperature heating (120°C) or strong alkaline treatment. This observation formed the basis for the development of AR techniques in 1991 by Shi et al. (57), who should receive credit for being the first to describe the use of a microwave oven to deliver energy for AR. Microwaves had previously been used only for application of small amounts of energy to hasten fixation and staining.

Superheating of tissue sections at high energy levels, in contradiction to the established doctrine, improved immunoreactivity for a wide range of antigens. Indeed, it soon became clear that some antigens formerly inaccessible in formalin-fixed tissues could be efficiently detected after heat-induced AR.

Heating is thought to transport energy to the protein-protein or protein-nucleic acid cross-links, which results in their partial disruption or breakdown and release for subsequent staining. However, the way heat is applied does not seem to be very important; improvement in immunohistochemistry was reported for heating with the microwave, pressure or autoclave cooker, or a simple water bath. The method of choice will depend either on the available equipment or on the experience of the individual user/researcher (63).

One common problem with this new technique is focal superheating (which occurs in liquids heated in the microwave oven after excessive boiling or after prolonged heating at elevated energy levels), overboiling, and buffer evaporation. This may explain inconsistencies from staining to staining, foci of little or no staining, significantly altered morphology such as the phenomenon of "nuclear melting," especially when larger batches of slides were stained (24,42,60). Another pitfall may be the reduction in intensity of staining due to placing the slides at different locations in the oven, thereby moving them away from the point of microwave focus. Some of these obstacles can be overcome by using a pressure cooker. This technique is both an economical and practical alternative for the routine laboratory (50).

To demonstrate the clinical significance of AR-based immunohistochemistry (AR-IHC), it is necessary to compare the intensity of AR-IHC with that obtained by routine IHC (without AR) of frozen and paraffin sections and to study the correlations among the different methods. The preferable result of any AR method is the unmasking of all hidden epitopes, irrespective of the degree of fixation or AR method. However, as we have learned from fixation experiments, overfixation cannot be readily overcome by simply adjusting AR. Nevertheless, the critical factor in unmasking epitopes might be the relationship between the degree of fixation and the period of time for which the slides are exposed to high temperature with or without pressure. It has been suggested that the higher the temperature, the shorter the time in which maximum AR is obtained. This was elegantly demonstrated by Shi et al. (61). Moreover, the use of a test battery for optimization of AR for new antibodies has been suggested: different buffer solutions with varying pHs in combination with various pretreatments (e.g., autoclave/pressure cooker, microwave, or water bath) were used to define the optimal conditions for maximum intensity of immunostaining (61).

Materials and Reagents

In our laboratory we usually perform a similar, although somewhat different, approach in defining the best pretreatment for individual antibodies. We also performed a test battery (Table 1) using either citrate buffer (10 mmol/L) at pH 6.0, EDTA (10 mmol/L) at pH 8.0, or Tris HCl/urea (100 mmol/L/5%) at pH 9.5; all solutions were brought to a boil in a conventional microwave oven (600 W, operating at a frequency of 2.45 GHz with five power level settings) using full power (600 W); after boiling temperature was reached, the power setting was reduced to level 2, with a maximum power of 240 W. Coplin jars were filled with buffer, and silica-glass beads

Table 1. Test Battery for Defining the Best Pretreatment

Microwave-buffer/enzyme	Source[a]	Concentration	pH	Time	Temperature (°C)
Citrate	Sigma	10 mmol/L	6.0	3 × 5 min	~100°
EDTA	Sigma	10 mmol/L	8.0	3 × 5 min	~100°
Tris-HCl/urea	Sigma	100 mmol/L/5%	9.5	3 × 5 min	~100°
Trypsin	Sigma	0.1%	7.5	5 min	~37°
Proteinase K	Roche Molecular Biochemicals	20, 50, or 100 µg/mL	7.5	5 min	~37°
Microwave + enzyme		As above	As above	3 × 5 min + 5 min	~100° + ~37°

[a]Sigma-Aldrich, Deisenhofen, Germany; Roche Molecular Biochemicals, Mannheim, Germany

(Roth, Heidelberg, Germany) were added to prevent overboiling and jar breakage. Jars were covered with loose-fitting plastic lids and heated.

Since the temperature during microwave treatment can be influenced by the volume and number of jars, both parameters were always kept constant, with the jars in the identical position in the microwave oven. After every 5 minutes of treatment, the Coplin jars were filled up with buffer to prevent dry microwave heating. After heating, slides were immediately rinsed in distilled water and subsequently transferred to phosphate-buffered saline (PBS). Moreover, we pretreat additional slides with proteases, usually trypsin (0.1% solution for 5 minutes at 37°C) and proteinase K (20, 50, and 100 µg/mL for 5 minutes at 37°C) and use one untreated slide as a control. Finally, we use a combination of heating and proteolysis, using the best mode of microwave heating (as implied by the results of the above-mentioned preliminary microwave experiments) and a subsequent proteolytic treatment. For individual antibodies (e.g., immunoglobulins or steroid hormone receptors), this combination may increase the intensity of staining without resulting in loss of sensitivity.

However, the prolonged use of high concentrations of urea (4 or 6 mol/L) or metal salts (saturated solution of lead isothiocyanate or manganese or magnesium chloride) in AR buffers (in our laboratory as well as others in the early days of microwave-based AR), with or without additional proteolytic treatment, may lead to poor morphologic results, as these reagents are able to solubilize proteins via reversible denaturation of secondary and higher structures. Formalin-fixed tissue may show some resistance to such treatment, although ultimately high molar concentrations of denaturing solutions in conjunction with microwave/heat treatment will also lead to destruction of the morphology. Increasing treatment time or concentrations of buffer solutions (like urea) will lead to enhancement of staining intensity but will also result in poorer morphologic preservation. Therefore, a compromise has to be chosen to achieve good staining results as well as a reasonably preserved morphology.

Such a test battery can be used for rapid screening or establishing optimal protocols for new antibodies, resulting in working protocols for routine analysis of any antibody to be used. We also believe that optimal retrieval conditions will be found and that a standardized and validized protocol for immunostaining can be established; this will also allow comparison of results among different laboratories and may provide a basis for defining the clinical significance of defined patterns or levels of antigen expression.

PITFALLS, ARTIFACTS, AND GENERAL COMMENTS

Although data continue to accumulate, a universal AR solution has not yet been found. High pH Tris-HCl/urea (62,71), EDTA (16,27,52,59), or citrate solutions (5,43,59,70) may be convenient, as described above, but these solutions are not beneficial for all antibodies. There are still antibodies that need no pretreatment, and there are antibodies that may benefit from proteolytic tissue pretreatment only. However, recent reviews have described a good number of antibodies (for which clone numbers and sources are available) including the optimized retrieval conditions (36,50,57). In summary, it may be possible to obtain equivalent intensities of staining with several different AR solutions, if the pH value of the AR solution and the heating conditions are optimized.

Another disadvantage is that some solutions may produce high background staining or false-negative results for some antibodies (androgen receptor, cyclin D1, etc.), when they are heated to very high temperatures using an autoclave or pressure cooker (Reference 71 and authors' observations).

False nuclear positivity is sometimes found in focal areas, particularly in the peripheral regions of the tissue section, but the intensity of the false positivity is frequently much weaker than that produced by specific binding of antibodies (4,47,60).

One potential cause of increased background staining after AR heating may be the unmasking of endogenous biotin, which is also sometimes found in frozen tissue sections (55). This effect can be avoided by use of a routine blocking procedure with avidin followed by a saturating concentration of D-biotin. It is important to keep in mind that any background staining that may be found in frozen tissue sections can also be found in the microwave-heated archival paraffin sections, because the paraffin sections having undergone AR treatment may have the same or even higher sensitivity than the frozen sections. However, these problems are seldomly significant in AR-IHC.

After AR heating in solution with a low pH (1.0–2.0), the hematoxylin counterstain will often be weak, even if the hematoxylin staining time was extended; the nuclei may additionally show granular disruption or nuclear melting under higher magnification. Vigorous heating in buffers with a high pH (9.0–10.0) may result in extensive tissue loss in a few instances. [This frequently occurs when using the autoclave or pressure cooker (19)].

The standardization of immunohistochemistry depends on three major factors: first, the fixation process (including size of the tissue, fixative used and its concentration, use of buffer ingredients, and time of fixation); second, tissue processing and pretreatment; and third, the immunohistochemical procedure. It will be difficult to standardize all these parameters, but some can be standardized at one's own institution at least. Many studies concerning formalin fixation of tissues have shown that the influence of formalin on tissue antigenicity is dependent on the total time of fixation (7,17). Therefore, the duration of fixation (e.g., 24 h for routine material and 4 h for biopsies in 4% buffered formaldehyde may be acceptable and reproducible parameters) should be standardized, as can be achieved by tissue processing performed in automatic or semi-automatic tissue processors. One of the most important factors influencing immunohistochemistry is the standardization of the staining process itself. This important issue involves three areas: antibodies and reagents, technical procedures, and interpretation (70). The AR technique can be used to help standardize immunohistochemistry on archival paraffin sections (69,70,74). Several studies have suggested that increased heating may reverse the effects of longer fixation (49).

THE ImmunoMax METHOD: CATALYZED REPORTER DEPOSITION/TYRAMINE AMPLIFICATION

The introduction of new methods allowed a revolutionary ongoing development in diagnostic pathology. The challenges of modern pathology are both numerous and complex and require special knowledge not only of macro- and microscopy but also of recently developed techniques including immunohistochemistry and molecular pathology. Since the introduction of immunofluorescence techniques in 1941 by Coons et al. (13), immunohistochemistry has become an important method of providing objective and standardized diagnostics. Modern immunohistochemical techniques are based on sandwich techniques such as horseradish peroxidase (HRP)-conjugated anti-HRP antibody complex (PAP)-(68), alkaline phosphatase (AP)-conjugated anti-AP antibody complex (APAAP) (14), or avidin-biotin complex (ABC) (26) techniques using bridging antibodies for signal increase. However, these methods, although effective, still suffer from low sensitivity in detecting many important antigens when used in formalin-fixed and paraffin-embedded tissues (46).

It has been reported by others and ourselves that the retrieval of a variety of hidden antigens in formalin-fixed tissues (using chaotropic substances or heavy metal salts in combination with microwave treatment) still left a significant number of antigens that could not be detected even after enforced AR in formalin-fixed, paraffin-embedded tissues (45,57). One reliable approach to circumvent these limitations could be a signal amplification technique, which should allow the signal to be enhanced above a critical threshold so that it can then be visualized.

Based on these observations and stimulated by reports (1,9–11) according to which a 30- to 200-fold signal amplification was achieved by covalent deposition of biotin reporter molecules, we combined and modified the retrieval and amplification steps and ended up with a new maximized immunohistochemical staining protocol, which we have termed the ImmunoMax method (46) and which is now established as the tyramine enhancement or catalyzed reporter deposition technique. This method enhances the sensitivity of the reaction 100- to 10 000-fold compared with conventional immunohistochemical reactions. Antigens previously thought to be nonreactive or insufficiently detectable in formalin-fixed, paraffin-embedded tissues can now be detected.

Materials and Reagents

Primary antibodies were either from DAKO (Hamburg, Germany) or Dianova (Hamburg, Germany); secondary bridging antibodies were either biotinylated rabbit anti-mouse or biotinylated mouse anti-rabbit antibodies (Dianova and DAKO, respectively). The ABC complexes were from DAKO (but Vector-reagents from Böhringer-Ingelheim, Ingelheim, Germany may be used with no difference). Diaminobenzidine (DAB; Sigma-Aldrich, Deisenhofen, Germany) was used as a substrate for HRP, and naphthol AS-BI phosphate (Sigma) and new fuchsin (Chroma, Köngen, Germany) was used for AP.

Preparation of Biotinyl-Tyramine

NHS-LC biotin (Pierce via Bender und Hobein, München, Germany) and tyramine hydrochloride (Sigma) were used. Tyramine hydrochloride was prepared as a 290 µmol/L stock solution (50 mg/L). One milliliter of this solution was added to 39 mL of a solution containing 100 mg of NHS-LC biotin in borate buffer (100 mmol/L, pH > 8.0, usually 8.5; Sigma) resulting in molarities of 7.25 for tyramine hydrochloride and 7 µmol/L for NHS-LC biotin. The solution was agitated overnight with light protection, passed through a 45-µm sterile filter, and stored frozen at –70°C indefinitely. Each sample of biotinyl-tyramine stock has to be tested individually for sensitivity of enhancement (dilutions from 1:25 to 1:250 in 50 mmol/L Tris/100 mmol/L NaCl, pH 8.0). *Note*: Tyramide Signal Amplification™ (TSA) has been patented. Products are available from NEN (Boston, MA, USA) and DAKO (the Catalyzed Signal Amplification [CSA]-system).

AR and enzyme digestion were used as noted above, or they may be performed for convenience according to individual laboratory standards.

General Discussion

A comparison of the tyramine-based enhancement method on formalin-fixed, paraffin embedded tissues and the standard ABC method was made. (Either formalin-fixed, paraffin-embedded or frozen tissues were used. The latter is supposed to be the gold standard of maximum sensitivity.) The results obtained were analyzed, and the increase in sensitivity achieved with additional pretreatments or biotinylated tyramine enhancement was measured by further diluting the primary antibodies. This results in a semiquantitative measurement of signal intensities and staining patterns for the individual technical steps and the recognition of additive or supraadditve effects on the overall staining results as a means of dilution of the primary antibody.

Extensive aldehyde cross-linking camouflages the overwhelming number of antibody binding sites. If pretreatment steps (proteases, microwave, chaotropic substances) allow the retrieval of a varying number of these antibody binding sites, a system that strongly amplifies standard immunohistochemical procedures should allow the detection of these (few) partly demasked antigens.

The bridging techniques (e.g., APAAP and ABC methods), although optimized, still suffer from problems with background staining when used repeatedly or in higher concentrations. It was therefore desirable to find a way to increase the available number of enzyme or reporter molecules in the vicinity of the antigen. In terms of chemically defined molecular interactions, it is clear that only a covalent linkage will result in stable, background-free interaction. This was achieved by modifying a biotin-based amplification procedure (9–11) at the antigenic binding site, which resulted in strong enhancement of the subsequent immunohistochemical staining method (1).

In our procedure, this enhancement is critically dependent on the deposition of biotinylated tyramine on the tissue by the catalytic action of HRP, which liberates free radicals by oxidizing H_2O_2. It is thought that radicalized biotinylated tyramine will be covalently attached to electron-rich moieties (tyrosine, phenylalanine, tryptophane, or others), e.g., to many protein molecules at the site of HRP activity. Then the covalently bound biotin molecules themselves act as binding sites and may further be detected with enzyme-labeled streptavidin-biotin complexes or with enzyme-labeled streptavidin. Therefore, the biotin molecule itself acts as a "new" secondary, covalently bound antigen at the site of the primary antigen (around the peroxidase activity), e.g., on a variety of different neighboring proteins. In principle, the biotinyl-tyramine will react with another biotinyl-tyramine molecule to catalyze the dimerization of the compounds; however, the concentrations of reporter molecules used in the procedure are low (and titrated in preliminary experiments) so that dimerization will be less likely to occur. The radicalized tyramine reporter molecule will interact with electron-rich moieties in the direct vicinity of the enzyme, especially at the site of antigen to be detected. It is of interest that dimerized molecules are no longer reactive and thus do not take further part in the staining process; they are readily washed away after finishing the enhancement step. Moreover, as mentioned above, the reaction takes place only in the closest vicinity of the HRP enzyme, causing no significant background problems. Because diffusion artifacts are few and false, nonspecific binding will not occur. One of the factors, which is efficient in reducing nonspecific binding, may be the ongoing biotinylation of the enzyme itself via biotinylated tyramine, which soon results in loss of enzyme activity, thus stopping the catalyzing activity and further deposition of biotinylated tyramine. The method is summarized in Figure 1.

Peroxidase has to be introduced into the system for the tyramine-reporter amplification step. The amplification step then takes place by radicalization of tyramine reporter, which is then covalently bound to other electron-rich moieties (e.g., other tyramine molecules) around the peroxidase activity. This is shown schematically in Figure 1, a and b. Figure 1c shows a schematic comparison with the ABC method.

A single biotinylated tyramine enhancement step allows primary antibodies to be used at a dilution up to 500 times higher than the dilution used in the standard ABC technique. This was demonstrated for several antibodies. Furthermore, the signal can be enhanced to a level comparable to or sometimes even better than the signal obtained on cryostat sections, when optimized AR steps are included. Moreover, many antibodies can be strongly and reproducibly detected with the same tissue distribution they show on cryostat sections but with well-preserved morphology and without background staining. The addition of a single biotinylated tyramine enhancement step requires only 30 to 45 minutes more working time, which is not much compared with the whole procedure of tissue processing, pretreatment, and staining.

However, one has to be aware of possible artifacts and pitfalls. In some experiments we observed a paradoxically low signal or no signal at all when the tyramine enhancement method was used in combination with high antibody concentrations (e.g., concentrations that would be good or optimal for conventional ABC staining). We suspect that this may be due to the so-called Bigbee effect, as demonstrated by Bigbee et al. (8) for multistep immunohistochemical reactions, in which primary, secondary, and tertiary reagents were not well tuned.

We have also seen that the enhancement was weaker than expected for various antibodies. As we have learned from our experiments, this is frequently the case with antigens that are highly sensitive to formalin fixation and with antigens that cannot be easily retrieved by any of the AR techniques. We try to circumvent this problem by using several antibodies for the same antigen; these antibodies recognize different epitopes of the molecule, for example, of seven different commercially available CD5 antibodies, only two work with acceptable efficiency, only one of which is highly consistent and reproducible, while it is still dependent on the fixation time and AR pretreatment of the tissue. Frequently background problems occur when the reaction is weak, e.g., when the antigen is sensitive to fixation and alternatives to the employed antibody are not available. In these instances, focal false-positive stainings are observed; they may be nuclear stainings or dots evenly or randomly distributed over the slide.

It has also been demonstrated that AR steps may allow the partial retrieval of some hidden antigens. Each antigen should therefore be tested with a variety of AR methods or even with a combination of the AR techniques mentioned above. When using overfixed tissues, the AR steps and/or dilutions of primary antibodies have to be optimized and titrated; much higher concentrations of enzyme or antibodies may be needed to achieve the same degree of AR.

Furthermore, the biotin molecules may be amplified by biotin-bridging antibodies at steps 5 or 7 of the protocol (flow chart, Table 2). As expected, the enhancement effect was stronger when the bridging antibody was used after the deposition of biotinylated tyramine (data not shown). This supports the hypothesis that covalently bound molecules stabilize the system, resulting in a better signal-to-noise ratio. Such a step may not only increase the overall staining results as much as 20-fold, but may also be beneficial for steric reasons and helpful in the balance of background staining.

The same degree of amplification could be observed with a second round of biotin-

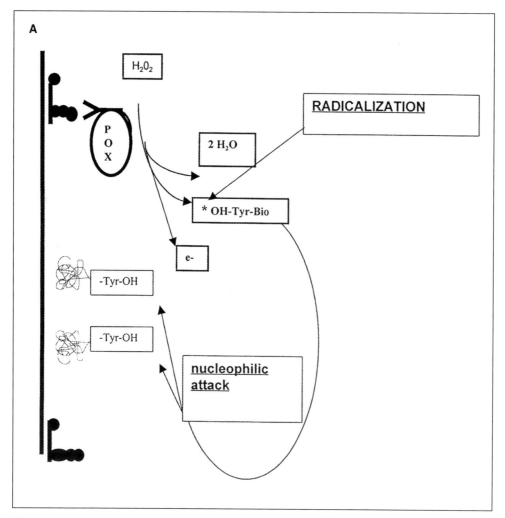

Figure 1. The ImmunoMax technique. (A) Amplification.

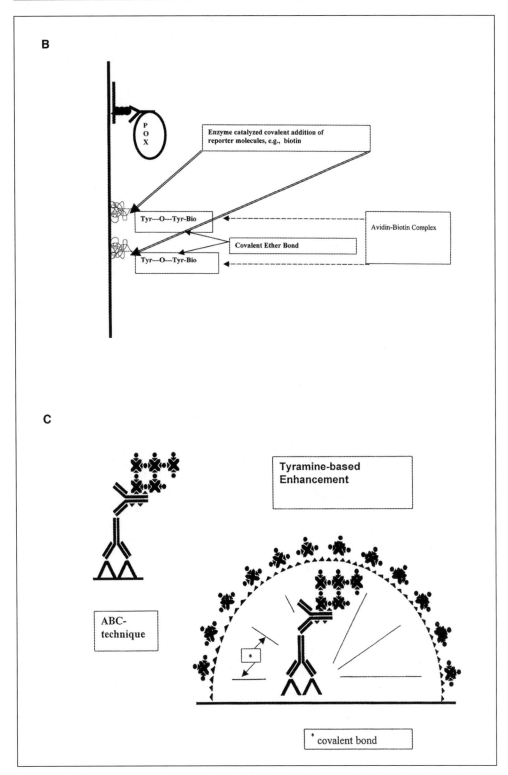

Figure 1 (continued). The ImmunoMax technique. (B) Tyramine-reporter deposition. (C) Comparison with the ABC method.

Table 2. Flow Chart of the Tyramine-Enhancement Technique (ImmunoMax Method) Compared with the Avidin-Biotin Complex (ABC) Method

Step	Method	
	ABC	ImmunoMax
1	—	Antigen retrieval steps
2	H_2O_2 blocking, rabbit/mouse or other normal serum	H_2O_2 blocking, rabbit/mouse or other normal serum
3	Primary antibody	Primary antibody
4	Secondary biotinylated rabbit anti-mouse or mouse anti-rabbit or any other species-specific secondary reagent necessary for the detection of the primary antibody	
5	—	Optional: antibiotin-bridging antibody and additional quaterny reagents necessary to end up with peroxidase enzyme (proceed with step 7)
6	—	ABC-peroxidase + H_2O_2 + biotinylated tyramine
7	—	Optional: as in step 5
8	—	Optional: ABC-peroxidase + H_2O_2 + biotinylated tyramine
9	ABC-peroxidase/alkaline phosphatase	
10	Color development	Color development

ylated tyramine deposition, although these additional enhancement steps may not really be necessary in routine diagnostic staining, except for the detection of antigens with low expression and/or for methodologic reasons (e.g., in situ hybridization; see below).

With the tyramine enhancement technique, it may thus be possible to dilute the primary antibody down to $1:1 \times 106$ (10 000-fold—compared with dilutions used for conventional ABC, as we have shown for CD30, UCHL1, and other antigens). If this is calculated, taking into account the amount of antibody molecules used per slide and the expected amount of antigen molecules per cell and cells per slide, it could mean that as few as 100 to 1000 antibody molecules can be detected. The detection limit for conventional ABC or APAAP techniques is thought to be at least 10 to 100 times higher. These results demonstrate the power of such an enhancement technique, which attains a level of sensitivity superior to all known detection levels at the protein level and which can only be achieved or overcome at the DNA/RNA level with the polymerase chain reaction (PCR) technique (48). Finally, we have observed that many previously nonreactive antibodies functioned in well-fixed paraffin sections when using this technique. Some examples of the potency of the technique are shown in Figures 2 to 4.

THE InsituMax TECHNIQUE

The InsituMax technique involves AR and tyramine-based enhancement of immunohistochemical detection of nonradioactively labeled nucleic acids in in situ hybridization experiments.

The regulation of gene expression is of fundamental importance for the understanding of normal and disregulated cell biology. Since the introduction of in situ hybridization histochemistry, such questions can be addressed at the single cell level, combining both molecular and cytologic information. DNA and RNA in situ hybridization are recognized to be of potential diagnostic value within a pathologic setting, such as the detection of chromosomal aberrations, the localization of viruses [Epstein-Barr virus (EBV), human papillomavirus, human immunodeficiency virus, cytomegalovirus, etc.], bacteria (mycobacteria and others), and cellular gene products, which may be involved in the pathogenesis of certain diseases (21,53,54).

The two principal systems in in situ hybridization histochemistry are radioactive and nonradioactive techniques. The former include the disadvantages of using hazardous materials, special equipment, and long exposure times; the latter sometimes suffer from poor morphology and, more importantly, low sensitivity, especially when single-copy genes, short sequences, or genes expressed with low abundance are involved (12,21,56).

Although some DNA and RNA molecules can be detected under appropriate conditions, there may still be many proper probes and/or reliable in situ hybridization histochemistry conditions are not available. Furthermore, gene expression of interest is frequently too sparse to be visualized, as observed, e.g., for sparsely expressed genes, such as cytokines. Another disadvantage of the method is the need for experience, careful experimental design, and high-quality material and reagents.

One reliable approach toward resolving this dilemma is the use of a combination of

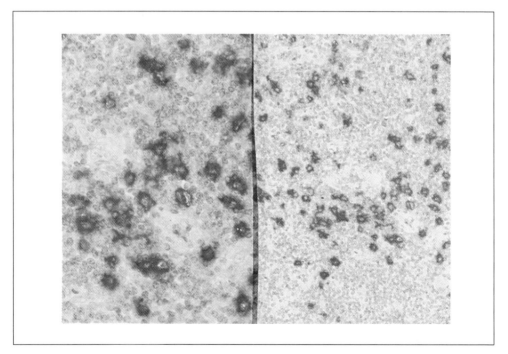

Figure 2. CD30 is demonstrated in both panels using AR (citrate buffer for 15 min), HRS4 antibody (kind gift of Prof. Pfreundschuh, Hamburg, Germany), and TSA. HRS4 was used at 1/100th of the dilution used in the conventional ABC technique. Typically, CD30-positive blasts were seen in a case of florid Epstein-Barr virus infection. **(See color plate A8).**

an optimized tissue pretreatment (29,32,39,54,64,67,72,75), an optimized probe preparation, simplified hybridization strategy system, and a powerful immunohistochemical detection protocol introducing a tyramine enhancement-based amplification step, in which signal amplification is accomplished by covalent deposition of a high number of reporter molecules, as shown above for the ImmunoMax method (30,46,56,73,75).

For this purpose cryostat and paraffin sections were hybridized to digoxigenin-, biotin-, or fluorescein isothiocyanate (FITC)-labeled oligonucletide probes, washed, and then detected either with the ABC technique or, for comparison, with the tyramine-enhancement method, resulting in a new maximized in situ hybridization histochemistry staining protocol, which we accordingly termed the InsituMax Method.

Similar to protein antigens it was believed that the fixation process irreversibly destroys cellular DNA/RNA molecules, but recent developments in immunohistochemistry (see above) have suggested that the accessibility of cellular targets may be limited by steric barriers caused by the aldehyde. Such hindrances may be partially reversed by retrieval techniques (e.g., microwave-based retrieval, protease digestion, or a combination of both strategies) (12,29,32,39,54,64,67,72,75).

Each step in tissue treatment is important: the fixation and tissue processing, AR, probe labeling, and detection. Optimization of all steps is necessary to achieve good and reproducible results.

AR is the basis for susceptibility of the detection procedure (29,32,39,54,64,67, 72,75). The principles used to achieve availability of nucleic acids for hybridization are identical to those used for immunohistochemistry. We use the microwave-based technique with citric acid or urea followed by a short and optimized proteolytic step,

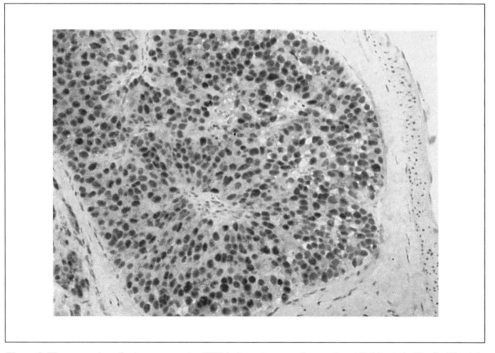

Figure 3. The expression of estrogen receptor (ER) in breast cancer tissue using AR (citrate buffer for 30 min), the anti-ER-Ab (DAKO), and TSA. Anti-ER-Ab was used at 1/10th of the dilution used in the conventional ABC technique. The strong nuclear staining of ER is highlighted in this intraductal carcinoma. (See color plate A9).

which should on the one hand allow better probe penetration and on the other hand destroy residual nucleases. The AR step is of critical importance, since no or little pretreatment may result in false-negative staining, as will overtreatment of tissue slides (no or little accessibility of the target and washing out of target, respectively)

The labeling of the probe is another important point to consider. The success of probe labeling has to be monitored, and only those probes, which have incorporated enough label for detection should be used. It will be shown later how this can be accomplished. However, optimal probe labeling resulted only in moderately improved in situ staining, and the reporter molecule (either digoxygenin, biotin, or FITC) enhancement step proved to be more efficient, although the latter is sometimes not sufficient for genes expressed in low abundance. For this purpose we sometimes use additional bridging steps. The combination of optimized AR, improved probe labeling with monitoring of its efficiency, and the enhancement step of hybridized reporter molecules resulted in a tremendous boost in sensitivity without a loss of specificity.

Using this protocol, genes can be reproducibly detected in cryostat and formalin-fixed, paraffin-embedded tissues. On the one hand, the sensitivity of the method is extremely enhanced, and on the other hand, morphology is well preserved when compared with other in situ hybridzation protocols. Moreover, rare gene transcripts that were previously insufficiently or very rarely detectable in formalin-fixed, paraffin-embedded tissues, but for which more sensitive methods [such as PCR or reverse-transcribed (RT)-PCR] have shown the presence of the gene products, can now also be visualized in defined cellular compartments, as shown for interleukin-6 (Il-6) in Figures 5 and 6).

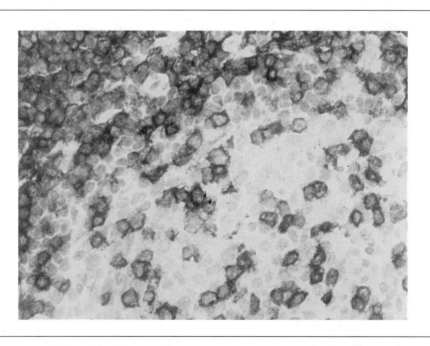

Figure 4. Monoclonal anti-CD3 (Novocastra) was used after AR treatment (citrate buffer for 20 min and trypsin 0.1% for 5 min) and TSA. CD3-Ab was used at 1/25th of the dilution used in the conventional ABC technique. Strong staining of CD3-positive T cells is seen in the mantle zone of a reactive germinal center; some scattered T cells are seen within the germinal center. **(See color plate A9).**

Materials and Reagents

Tissues

The tissue used for this work was surgically removed human tonsils ($n = 4$) showing follicular hyperplasia. Additionally, various lymph nodes ($n = 5$) were included from patients with hyperplasia of the T zones, mononucleosis, fatal EBV infection, sarcoidosis, and surgically removed organs ($n = 5$, colon: two cases of colitis ulcerosa, two cases of Crohn's disease and one case of adenocarcinoma; $n = 2$, spleen: one case of a systemic mycobacteria-negative granulomatous disease of unknown origin and one case with traumatic spleen rupture) from patients undergoing partial organ resection for cancer, progressive disease, or trauma. Part of each tissue specimen was routinely fixed in 4% buffered paraformaldehyde for 24 hours. Serial paraffin sections were made and placed on slides coated with 2% 3-(triethoxysilyl)propylamine (Merck, Darmstadt, Germany). The sections were dewaxed three times in xylene and rehydrated in a graded series of ethanols. Another part of the tissue was frozen in PBS in liquid nitrogen; 5-μm cryostat sections were cut and placed on coated slides.

Antibodies, Complexes, and Substrates

The indicated methods were tested in parallel runs on frozen sections, slides, and paraffin sections. As a general rule, the manufacturer's protocols were used. For digoxigenin (DIG)-labeled probes, F(ab)$_2$-anti-DIG-AP (Roche Molecular Biochemicals, Mannheim, Germany) was used, for FITC-labeled probes F(ab)$_2$-anti-FITC-AP

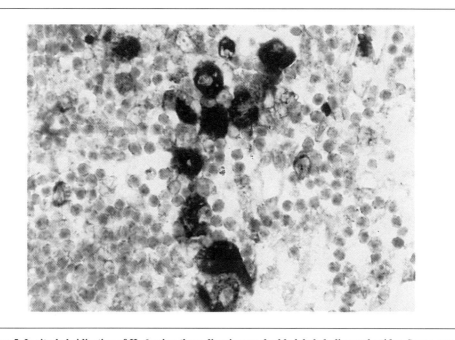

Figure 5. In situ hybridization of IL-6 using three digoxigenen double-labeled oligonucleotides. Strong cytoplasmic staining of Hodgkin cells and weaker staining of histiocytic cells in a case of Hodgkin's disease. The NBT-BCIP substrate was used. Morphology is not optimal; only proteolytic digestion with proteinase K was used. Although slides are slightly overdigested, there is a good signal-to-noise ratio. **(See color plate A10).**

(Roche Molecular Biochemicals) was used, and for biotin-labeled probes, the ABC-AP (DAKO) method was used according to the manufacturer's recommendations.

After hybridization, slides were pretreated with 10% normal rabbit/sheep serum depending on the detection system. The primary reagents were diluted in Tris-buffered saline with or without 0.05% casein. The monoclonal anti-DIG, anti-FITC-bridging biotin-bridging antibodies (Roche Molecular Biochemicals and DAKO) were diluted in 1% casein. The ABC-AP and ABC/HRP complexes were used as preadjusted solutions as prepared by the manufacturer (DAKO).

The substrate solutions for HRP was DAB (Sigma; 0.5 mg/mL + 0.003% H_2O_2) in 50 mmol/L Tris buffer, pH 8.0. For AP, the substrate was naphthol AS-BI phosphate (Sigma) and new fuchsin (Chroma). Sections were counterstained with hematoxylin and mounted with glycerin-gelatine.

Preparation of Tyramine Reporter Molecules

Biotinyl-tyramine was synthesized as mentioned above.

Oligonucleotides

The oligonucleotides used for hybridization were searched by computer analysis using the European Molecular Biology Laboratory (EMBL) genebank. Oligonucleotides should have a calculated melting point of 10° to 15°C higher than the hybridization temperature (here 37°C). Each oligonucleotide should specifically bind to the *ist* target without cross-hybridization to other possible targets. The oligonu-

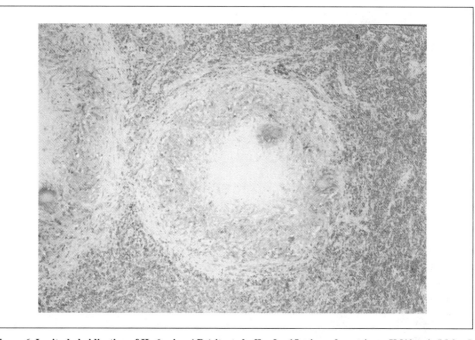

Figure 6. In situ hybridization of IL-6 using AR (citrate buffer for 15 min and proteinase K [10 µg/mL] for 5 min), three digoxigenen double-labeled oligonucleotides, and F(ab)$_2$-anti-Dig-POX and TSA. Here a case of tuberculosis was examined. The histiocytic and Langhan's giant cells are stained brown. DAB was used as substrate. **(See color plate A10).**

cleotides were synthesized commercially by MWG-Biotech (Ebersberg, Germany).
The important steps of the protocol are summarized below:

1. *AR technique*: Both enzyme digestion and microwave-based retrieval techniques, as well as the combination of both, were used for target (DNA/RNA) retrieval. The tissue sections were pretreated by microwave or pressure cooking and subsequent enzyme digestion before the probe was applied. We use proteinase-K in PBS (in various concentrations ranging from 1–25 µg/mL) at 37°C for 5 minutes. Protease digestion was stopped by rinsing slides in nuclease-free buffer. It is believed that enzyme digestion results in improved accessibility of the target to the probe on the one hand and in reduction of the activity of nucleases on the other hand, which will reduce false-negative results.

2. *In situ hybridization procedure*: For the demonstration of RNA (messenger RNA, EBV-encoded small nuclear RNAs) using complimentary oligonucleotide probes and viral DNA detection using oligonucleotide probes, we have successfully established an in situ hybridization and subsequent immunohistochemical detection protocol:

   a. *Probe labeling and testing*

      i. 5′ end labeling was performed after synthesis at the 5′ end of the oligonucleotide probe with an amino-linker phosphoramidite, creating a 5′ terminal amino function. FITC (Sigma) or digoxigenin-3-*O*-methylcarbonyl-ε-aminocaproic acid-*N*-hydroxy-succinimide ester (Roche Molecular Biochemicals), or d-biotinyl-ε-aminocaproic acid-*N*-hydroxy-succinimide ester (Roche Molecular Biochemicals) are introduced to the terminal amino function, forming stable amide bonds. Oligonucleotides were purified by high-performance liquid chromatography, quantified, and used for subsequent 3′ end labeling. Such modified oligonucleotides can be obtained commercially.

      ii. 3′ end labeling was performed with terminal transferase using DIG-11-dUTP or fluorescein-12-dUTP, fluorescein-15-dATP, and biotin-16-dUTP mixed with a threefold excess of unmodified nucleotides, e.g., dATP (all nucleotides and TdT were from Roche Molecular Biochemicals). The labeling was performed according to the manufacturer's protocol.

   b. *Quantification of oligonucleotide labeling efficiency*

      Equal amounts of serial dilutions of labeled oligonucleotides (10 ng, 1 ng, 100 pg, 10 pg, 1 pg, 100 fg, 10 fg, and water control) were mixed with salmon sperm carrier DNA and spotted onto nylon membranes (Hybond™-N+, Amersham Pharmacia Biotech, Piscataway, NJ, USA). Detection was performed with AP-labeled polyclonal anti-DIG antibodies (Roche Molecular Biochemicals) or with polyclonal anti-FITC-AP (Roche Molecular Biochemicals) or mouse anti-FITC (DAKO).

Only the labeled oligonucleotides that could be detected at 100 fg spots or less were used for further experiments. This low detection level suggests the incorporation of at least several modified nucleotides, allowing the detection of at least 1 pg mRNA on a dot-blot level after hybridization.

   c. *Prehybridization, hybridization, washing procedure, and hybrid detection*

      Cell, tissue pretreatment, hybridization, and posthybridization conditions are listed in the flow charts (Tables 3–5). All solutions were made with 0.1% diethyl pyrocarbonate (DEPC)-treated water. All procedures were performed at room temperature unless otherwise stated.

Table 3. InsituMax Technique: Tissue and Slide Pretreatment Steps

| Pre-treatment | Conventional Protocol | | Simplified Protocol | |
	Time (min)	Chemicals and Solutions	Time (min)	Chemicals and Solutions
2×	5	PBS, pH 7.5	1	PBS, pH 7.5
1×	5	0.1 mol/L glycine/PBS, pH 7.5	3 × 5	Microwaving in citrate or urea buffer
1×	5/10	Triton® X-100 0.3% in PBS (vol/vol), proteinase K 10 µg/mL, EDTA 5 mmol/L, pH 8.0, 37°C	5/10	Triton X-100 0.3% in PBS (vol/vol), proteinase K about 10 µg/mL[a], EDTA 5 mmol/L, pH 8.0, 37°C
1×	5	Paraformaldehyde 4% in PBS, pH 7.5	5	—
2×	1	PBS, pH 7.5	1	PBS, pH 7.5
1×	5	0.1 mol/L triethanolamine, pH 8.0, and 0.25% acetic anhydride (vol/vol)	—	0.1 mol/L triethanolamine, pH 8.0, and 0.25% acetic anhydride (vol/vol)
1×	30	Hybridization buffer, 37°C[b]	—	Hybridization buffer, 37°C[b]

[a]Proteinase K must be tested for activity and adjusted if necessary.
[b]25 µL hybridization buffer/slide; 4× SSC (1× SSC = 150 mmol/L NaCl, 15 mmol/L Na citrate, pH 7.5), 50% formamide, 10% dextran sulfate, 0.02% Ficoll®, 0.02% polyvinyl pyrolidone, 0.02% bovine serum albumin (BSA), 10 mmol/L dithiothreitol (DTT), 1 mg/mL yeast tRNA, 1 mg/mL denatured salmon sperm DNA (all reagents were from Sigma, Deisenhofen, or Roche Molecular Biochemicals).

3. *Immunological detection* of the hybrids was performed as shown in Table 6. Slides from posthybridization washings (Table 5) were used directly for the detection protocol beginning with step 1.

The DIG, FITC, and biotin molecules were detected in various protocols. An indirect approach was performed using only F(ab)$_2$-anti-DIG-POX/AP, F(ab)$_2$-anti-FITC-POX/AP, or ABC-POX/AP followed by color development. In addition, bridging steps may be included: the indirect step (which may use only unconjugated antibodies or ABC) is then followed by a bridging step as in conventional routine immunohistochemistry [for F(ab)$_2$-anti-DIG, F(ab)$_2$-anti-FITC a biotinylated monoclonal anti-sheep antibody was used and for ABC a biotinylated rabbit anti-avidin/streptavidin antibody was used]. These antibodies were followed by an ABC-POX/AP (or principally by APAAP or PAP) step and subsequent color development.

A high number of reporter molecules was deposited by the peroxidase activity. The reporter molecules were the targets for subsequent detection protocols; any detection protocol may be added at this step including additional bridging steps. To simplify and shorten the whole procedure, we used the ABC-POX/AP system directly after

Table 4. InsituMax Technique: Hybridization Steps

Hybridization	Time	Solution	Time	Solution
1×	5 min	20 µL hybridization buffer[a] and 5 ng oligonucleotide probe, 75°C	5 min	20 µL hybridization buffer[a,b] and 5 ng oligonucleotide probe, 75°C
1×	Overnight	Same as above, at 37°C	4 h	Same as above, at 37°C

[a]Hybridization solution as above including labeled (with either digoxygen, fluorescein isothiocyanate, or biotin) oligonucleotides. Slides were sealed with coverslips and incubated in a moist chamber.
[b]Without formamide.

amplification, but any system with increased sensitivity (e.g., anti-reporter-bridging antibody) may be used before the final enzyme and color development step.

Controls

To make sure that the enhancement achieved with the InsituMax technique is not an artifact, several controls were included in the experimental design.

1. Experiments were performed in which each of the reagents (antibodies or digoxygenated, FITC, or biotinylated tyramine solutions, and others) was individually omitted.

2. Sense and antisense oligonucleotides, as well as unlabeled oligonucleotides, were used for comparison.

3. Oligonucleotides were omitted from the hybridization solution as well.

4. Control cytospin preparations with a known cytokine expression pattern were enclosed as possible control slides.

5. The tissues used in our experiments were expected to have positive and negative cellular staining patterns for the defined probes (e.g., EBER staining was known to be expressed in only a few cells in cases of infectious mononucleosis). The staining pattern was compared with latent membrane protein positivity in immunohistochemical staining performed in parallel. The cytokine IL-6 is known to be expressed with the greatest likelihood by histiocytic cells. Il-9 was shown to be produced by Hodgkin and Sternberg-Reed cells in cases of Hodgkin's disease, while the nonneoplastic cellular components were almost completely negative. Interferon-γ was known to be produced by lymphocytes, especially T cells.

6. Finally, the tyramine reporter molecule enhancement step was tested in two ways: either H_2O_2 was omitted to ensure that peroxidase is necessary for the radicalization step, or excessive (nonlabeled = cold) tyramine was used to block biotinylated tyramine deposition.

General Discussion

Many different protocols have been established, each with its own advantages and disadvantages, frequently adjusted to the system and the question to be answered

Table 5. InsituMax Technique: Posthybridization Steps

Posthybrid-ization	Time (min)	Washing Solution	Time (min)	Washing Solution
1×	5	2× SSC to remove coverslips and excessive probe	5	2× SSC/Triton X-100 0.05% to remove coverslips and excessive probe
2×	30	2× SSC, 37°C	15	2× SSC/Triton X-100 0.05%, 37°C
1×	15	2× SSC, 42°C	5	2× SSC/Triton X-100 0.05%, 42°C[a]

[a]Has to be adjusted to the length of probe and its stickiness.

(32,33,51,64,65). Although commercially available probes and hybridization systems are readily at hand, the technique is still not as simple as some manufacturers suggest. Many hybridization experiments suffer from low reproducibility and a disappointing ratio of labor and results. Frequently, a panel of experimental adaptions have to be arranged for each probe.

The following considerations were important for the design of the experiments mentioned here.

According to our experience, the relative hybridization sensitivity may be ranked for different materials and labeling, hybridization, and detection strategies. This may be simplified in the following manner:

1. Cells > frozen tissue > paraffin tissue
2. (For RNA):antisense riboprobes > antisense single-stranded DNA probes > double-stranded DNA probes > synthetic oligonucleotides
   (For DNA): double-stranded DNA probes > synthetic oligonucleotides
3. Isotopes ($^{35}S > ^{33}P > ^{32}P > ^{3}H$) > nonisotopic (DIG > biotin > FITC)
4. Substrates (NBT/BCIP > DAB > naphthol-AS-bi-phosphate/neufuchsin)

Another important observation is the fact that the more the gene expression (e.g., RNA molecules/cell or DNA copy number) or the sequence length (DNA/RNA size) declines, the less frequently one can find published reports; although it is not frequently noted, severe difficulties have been inherently associated with the in situ hybridization technique.

Abundantly expressed genes, e.g., some housekeeping genes (β-actin) or EBV-encoded nuclear RNAs are easily detected by simple strategies such as oligonucleotide hybridization and subsequent indirect enzyme detection methods. Moderately abundantly expressed genes like those for hormones, immunoglobulins (in B cells), T-cell receptors, and some CD antigens (e.g., CD4, CD19) may still be detectable with a nonisotopic in situ hybridization histochemistry approach, while for genes expressed at a lower level such as inflammatory cytokine genes (IL-1, IL-6, tumor necrosis factor), the limit of this technique is reached. However, it seems to be almost impossible to demonstrate reproducibly certain genes (e.g., some cytokine genes like IL-2, IL-4, IL-7, and their receptors), which are expressed at a very low level. Figure 7 shows these considerations schematically.

The nonradioactive detection protocols using either indirect, APAAP, PAP, or ABC

Table 6. Immunologic Detection

Step	Conventional Immunologic Detection	InsituMax Amplification
	Method	
1	Blocking: H_2O_2, normal serum (rabbit, sheep, mouse)	
2	F(ab)₂-anti-DIG-POX, F(ab)₂-anti-FITC-POX, or ABC-POX	
3		Amplification: H_2O_2 + FITC-, DIG-, or biotinyl-tyramine
Optional:	Biotinylated-anti-sheep (for F(ab)₂-anti-DIG-AP, F(ab)₂-anti-FITC-AP, or a biotinylated bridging antibody for the ABC method	(Biotinylated) anti-DIG, anti-FITC, anti-biotin bridging antibody
Optional:	ABC system	ABC-AP/POX or F(ab)₂-anti-DIG-POX, F(ab)₂-anti-FITC-POX
4	Color development and counterstaining	

DIG, digoxygen; FITC, fluorescein isothiocyanate; ABC, avidin-biotin complex; AP, alkaline phosphatase.

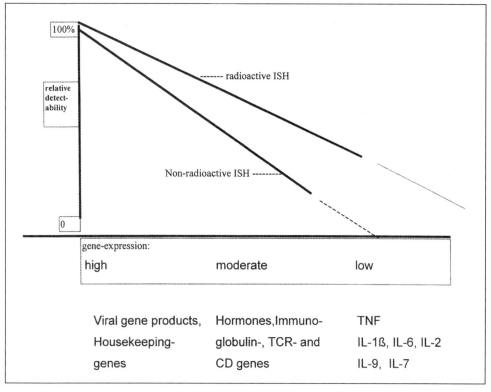

Figure 7. Gene expression and detectability.

methods, although optimized, still suffer from problems with background staining when used repeatedly or in higher concentrations. It was therefore desirable to find a way to increase the locally available number of enzyme or reporter molecules. In terms of chemically defined molecular interactions, it is clear that only a covalent linkage will result in a stable, background-free interaction. This was achieved by modifying the biotin-based amplification procedure at the target binding site, which resulted in a strong enhancement of the subsequent immunohistochemical staining method.

Effect of Labeling Oligonucleotides at both the 5' and 3' Ends and Use of Several Oligonucleotides for Hybridization

In preliminary experiments the efficiency of 5' end labeling of oligonucleotides compared with 5' plus 3' end labeling was established. In dot-blot dilution experiments, the sensitivity of 5' and 3' end-labeled oligonucleotides exceeded that of oligonucleotides labeled only at the 5' end; the detection limit was reduced from 3 pg to below 100 fg. This effect could also be demonstrated when the oligonucleotides were used in dot-blot hybridization experiments in which 1 pg of target DNA (a cloned and sequenced IL-6 probe) could be detected, while 10 to 30 pg of oligonucleotide labeled only at the 5' end were hardly detectable.

To enhance the sensitivity of the system further, we used three different oligonucleotides simultaneously, which allowed us to detect about 1 pg (5 amol of a 500-bp single-stranded DNA) of target DNA. The same holds true for some other probes tested (e.g., IL-9, EBER, etc.), suggesting that optimization of the labeling and a combination of a few oligonucleotides yield high and reproducible hybridization experiments (at least at the dot-blot level). Moreover, we could show in some instances that the use of oligonucleotide probes in the in situ hybridization procedure was more efficient than using antisense RNA probes because of an improved signal-to-noise ratio. These nonradioactively labeled antisense RNA probes frequently showed problems with a low signal-to-noise ratio due to severe background problems (also due to low stability, even after aliquoting and storing at -70°C). It is important that the expected melting point of the oligonucleotides can be calculated and therefore hybridization and washing can be much better controlled. This seems to be beneficial for hybridization on slides, which is more difficult to predict (as shown later).

The use of AP instead of peroxidase for the final color step allowed a moderate increase in sensitivity due to the possibility of using NBT/BCIP as a substrate; this could be exposed for a prolonged period without precipitating (but with the disadvantages of inferior morphology, dirty appearing slides, and making the use of hematoxylin for counterstaining impossible) (Figure 5). The use of an additional bridging step with monoclonal anti-biotin/FITC followed by AP-conjugated polyclonal rabbit anti-mouse antibody or by the more sensitive ABC system allowed the hybrids to be demonstrated with higher sensitivity.

With a single tyramine reporter enhancement step, nucleic acids may be detected by using only two or three labeled oligonucleotides. This was shown here for the cytokine IL-6 (but we were also able to detect other cytokines like IL-9 or interferon-γ; data not shown).

The presence of IL-6 in various cells of different tissues was demonstrated in cases of Hodgkin's disease and granulomatous lymphangitis caused by *Mycobacterium tuberculosis*. In Hodgkin's disease the signal could be localized on Hodgkin and Sternberg-Reed cells as well as on some mononuclear cells, e.g., histiocytes and lymphocytes; the same pattern of staining was demonstrated earlier with radioactive in situ hybridization. In tuberculosis, IL-6-positive cells could be visualized in the granulomatous tissue around the central necrosis. Langhans giant cells, epithelioid cells, and histiocytes could be stained.

When hybridizing the same tissue for interferon-γ, the distribution of staining was completely different: while the histiocytic cells were completely negative, the signal could be attributed to small and medium-sized lymphocytes between the granulomas. This staining pattern correlates with our expectations, because interferon-γ is only produced by T lymphocytes. Moreover, in cases of Hodgkin's disease and large cell anaplastic lymphoma the expression of IL-9 was mainly confined to the tumor cells; however, some surrounding small lymphocytes were also positive.

In summary, use of the in situ hybridization technique makes it possible to detect individual RNA or DNA molecules (Figure 8) with the aid of one to three double-labeled oligonucleotides. The results listed here demonstrate the power of the Insitu-Max technique, which attains a level of sensitivity that could previously only be achieved at the DNA/RNA level using PCR or ultrasensitive RNAse protection assays; these methods had the disadvantage of tissue disruption and lacked the possibility of morphologic correlation.

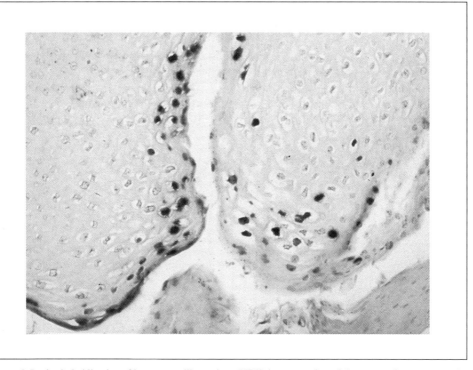

Figure 8. In situ hybridization of human papillomavirus (HPV) in a case of condyloma acuminatum. AR (citrate buffer for 30 min), three labeled oligonucleotides, and ABC/AP with neufuchsin/naphthol AS BI substrate were used. This is by far the most brilliant contrast; however, the counterstain is weak due to the boiling effect after microwave pretreatment of slides. **(See color plate A11).**

ULTRASENSITIVE FLUORESCENCE IN SITU HYBRIDIZATION EMPLOYING BIOTINYLATED TYRAMINE FOR PRECISE CHROMOSOMAL ASSIGNMENT OF SMALL DNA PROBES

In the past decade, fluorescence in situ hybridization (FISH) has been widely used to assign newly cloned genes and DNA markers to certain chromosomes and to determine the physical order of genes localized within the same chromosome band (22,37,38). Until recently, FISH was limited by the fact that only comparatively large DNA probes could be used. Small probes (less than 2 kb) rarely produced proper and reproducible hybridization signals on metaphase chromosomes and within interphase nuclei. Recently, highly sensitive immununostaining methods using tyramine-based enhancement methods for immunohistochemistry and FISH have been introduced. We and others have established an ultrasensitive tyramine-based FISH that allows detection of probes smaller than 2 kb (28,40,53). By combining this method with fluorescence R-banding, we were able to assign DNA probes as small as 0.8 kb to defined chromosome bands rapidly and precisely.

Materials and Reagents

The technique is summarized in the following steps:

1. *Metaphase preparations*: Metaphase spreads were prepared from cultured phytohemagglutin-stimulated peripheral blood lymphocytes from healthy donors according to routine protocols. Slides were air-dried and aged for 2 to 7 days at room temperature. Prior to hybridization, the slides were baked at 60°C overnight.

2. *Probes*: The characteristics of the probes used in this study are listed in Table 7. All probes were biotinylated by nick translation using a commercial kit (Life Technologies, Gaithersburg, MD, USA) according to the manufacturer's instructions. Unincorporated nucleotides were removed by ethanol precipitation.

3. *Hybridization*: The hybridization mixture contained 2 to 4 ng/µL DNA probe, 50% formamide, 10% dextrane sulfate, 10 µg/mL human Cot-1 DNA, and 2× standard saline citrate (SSC). One microliter of hybridization mixture was placed on cell-rich areas of the slides, covered with a 10-mm-round coverslip, and sealed with rubber cement. DNA probes and target DNA were simultaneously denatured at 72°C for 5 minutes and hybridized at 37°C for 1 to 2 days.

4. *Detection*: After hybridization, the slides were washed three times in 0.1× SSC at 60°C for 15 minutes, followed by washes in 1× SSC and 2× SSC at room temperature for 5 minutes each. To reduce the background staining caused by endogenous peroxidase, the slides were treated for 10 minutes with 3% H_2O_2 diluted in PBS buffer (pH 8.0). Thereafter, DNA probes were detected by incubation with mouse anti-biotin antibodies (DAKO) for 30 minutes, followed by incubation with biotinylated donkey anti-mouse antibodies (Jackson/Dianova, Hamburg, Germany) for 30 minutes. Both antibodies were diluted 1:1000 in PNM buffer (phosphate buffer, pH 8.0, with 5% nonfat dry milk). The slides were then incubated in ABC (Vector) for 30 minutes. The ABC complex was prepared 1 hour before use by adding 10 µL avidin solution and 10 µL peroxidase-conjugated biotin solution to 1 mL PBS buffer (pH 8.0). Then the slides were incubated for 10 minutes with biotinylated tyramine diluted approximately 1:200 in PBS containing 0.03% H_2O_2 followed by incubation with avidin-FITC (Jackson/Dianova) diluted 1:200 in PNM buffer for 30 minutes. Each incubation step was followed by three washes in phosphate buffer for 5 minutes each. After mounting

Table 7. Chromosomal Assignment Probes with Ultrasensitive Tyramine-Based FISH and Fluorescence

Name	Size (kb)	Locations	Metaphase Cells Hybridization Signals %			No. of Analyzed Cells	Interphase Cells Hybridization Signals			No. of Analyzed Cells
			0	1	2		0	1	2	
Partial cDNA of ALK gene	0.8	2p23	50	30	20	100	40	30	30	210
p210	1.2	11q13	40	33	27	120	35	26	39	230
Anonymous cDNA	2	1q42	5	19	76	120	5	8	87	200
759F6 YAC	1740	1q32	0	0	100	100	0	3	97	200

slides with antifade medium with 4'6-diamidine-2-phenylindole (DAPI) (20 ng/mL), hybridization signals were evaluated under the fluorescence microscope. The ISIS software (Metasystems, Althuissen, Germany) was applied for documentation.

5. *Fluorescence R-banding*: After ultrasensitive FISH, fluorescence R-banding employing chromomycin A3 and methyl green must be performed, as described previously (78). The results of chromosome banding may be documented with IKS3 software (Metasystems).

Results and Discussion

The optimum balance between intensive hybridization signals and the nonspecific background staining is achieved by adjusting the concentrations and incubation time of antibodies and/or biotinyl-tyramine. We found that a 1:1000 dilution of mouse anti-biotin antibodies and donkey anti-mouse serum shows the best results. Higher concentrations result in higher background activity and lower concentrations in less efficient hybridization. On the other hand, varying the concentration and incubation time of biotinyl-tyramine also leads to different results. Diluting biotinyl-tyramine to 1:200 and incubating it for 10 minutes at room temperature leads to satisfactory results in most experiments. However, one has to be aware of the fact that the concentration of the biotinyl-tyramine solution has to be adjusted each time a new lot of biotinyl-tyramine solution is used for the first time. It seems to be easier to obtain reproducible results by adjusting the concentration and incubation time of tyramine than by adjusting concentration and incubation time of the antibodies.

Small single-copy probes gave strong hybridization signals in many metaphase and interphase cells, while the background staining remained low. When using a 1.2-kb p210 probe, at least one hybridization signal could be obtained in 60% of metaphase cells and 65% of interphase cells. Two hybridization signals could be obtained in 27% of metaphase cells and 39% of interphase cells. FISH with a 0.8-kb partial cDNA of the ALK gene showed at least one hybridization signal in 50% of metaphase cells and 60% of interphase cells; 20% of metaphase cells and 30% of interphase cells displayed two hybridization signals.

After fluorescence R-banding, the 0.8-kb partial cDNA of the ALK gene and the

1.2-kb p210 probe, part of the bcl-1 locus [Dr. T.C. Meeker (San Francisco, CA, USA)], were localized to 2p23 and 11q13, respectively.

Similar techniques using biotinylated or fluorochrome-labeled tyramines that permit highly sensitive fiber FISH or multicolor FISH with single-copy probes as well as techniques for the sensitive detection of viral genomes have been described (2,23,66).

With our procedure, a remarkably high hybridization efficiency was achieved, while the background staining remained very low. Even with small single-copy probes, two strong hybridization signals were seen in a significant proportion of both metaphase and interphase cells. Moreover, the probe concentration was reduced to one-tenth of that applied in conventional FISH studies. Higher probe concentration caused cross-hybridization and high background staining. The same low probe concentration was used for small DNA probes as well as for cosmid, P1-derived artificial chromosomes (PAC), bacterial artificial chromosomes (BAC), and yeast artificial chromosomes (YAC) DNA probes.

FUTURE PERSPECTIVES

New or improved AR techniques are in development, the principles of AR are well accepted, and AR techniques are widely used in immunohistochemical studies and routine work. Standardization and general application are still problematic; unfortunately, there is not a single AR pretreatment applicable to all possible antigens, and many antigens cannot yet be properly detected.

The ImmunoMax technique is a combination of optimized AR with the amplification of immunohistochemical signals by catalyzed reporter deposition. It is of value for the detection of many antigens that cannot be detected routinely or that have been shown to cause problems and inconsistent staining. Finally, it may be applicable for those antigens for which only expensive primary reagents are available, resulting in a tremendous reduction of costs.

Hopefully, the ImmunoMax technique may allow further detection of previously formalin-resistant antigens and may also be transferred to the in situ hybridization techniques for detecting low quantities of RNA with nonradioactive techniques, which was shown here by the in situ hybrization experiments (InsituMax technique). The modified procedure may allow detection of rare transcripts that were previously undetectable by conventional in situ hybridization techniques. The method may be transferred to routine in situ hybridizations for reproducible diagnosis.

As shown here, the enhancement technique can be used for signal amplification of any immunohistochemical reaction including detection of hybridized probes to chromosomes. The simultaneous or sequential evaluation of hybridization signals and fluorescence R-banding makes it possible to assign the DNA probes directly to defined chromosomal bands, which has also been achieved by combining conventional FISH and high-resolution fluorescence R-banding (31).

ACKNOWLEDGMENTS

The catalyzed biotinyl-tyramine-based enhancement technique, which we originally termed the ImmunoMax-Method, is covered by US Patent 5 196 306 5 583 001 5731 158 and EPO 0465577. These patents are held by Dupont/NEN Co.

REFERENCES

1. **Adams, J.C.** 1992. Biotin amplification of biotin and horseradish peroxidase signals in histochemical stains. J. Histochem. Cytochem. *40*:1457-1463.
2. **Adler, K., T. Erickson, and M. Bobrow.** 1997. High sensitivity detection of HPV-16 in SiHa and CaSki cells utilizing FISH enhanced by TSA. Histochem. Cell. Biol. *108*:321-324.
3. **Atassi, M.Z.** 1975. Antigenic structure of myoglobin: the complete immunochemical anatomy of a protein and conclusions relating antigenic structures of proteins. Immunochemistry *12*:423-438.
4. **Baas, I.O., F.M. van den Berg, J.W. Mulder, M.J. Clement, R.J. Slebos, S.R. Hamilton, and G.J. Offerhaus.** 1996. Potential false-positive results with antigen enhancement for immunohistochemistry of the p53 gene product in colorectal neoplasms. J. Pathol. *178*:264-267.
5. **Balaton, A.J., F. Ochando, and M.H. Painchaud.** 1993. Use of microwaves for enhancing or restoring antigens before immunohistochemical staining. Ann. Pathol. *13*:188-189.
6. **Barlow, D.J., M.S. Edwards, and J.M. Thornton.** 1986. Continuous and discon-tinuous protein antigenic determinants. Nature *322*:747-748.
7. **Battifora, H. and M. Kopinski.** 1986. The influence of protease digestion and duration of fixation on the immunostaining of keratins. A comparison of formalin and ethanol fixation. J. Histochem. Cytochem. *34*:1095-1100.
8. **Bigbee, J.W., J.C. Kosek, and L.F. Eng.** 1977. Effects of primary antiserum dilution on staining of antigen rich tissues with peroxidase-antiperoxidase techniques. Histochem. Cytochem. *25*:443-447.
9. **Bobrow, M.N., T.D. Harris, K.J. Shaughnessy, and G.J. Litt.** 1989. Catalyzed reporter deposition, a novel method of signal amplification. Application to immunoassays. J. Immunol. Methods *125*:279-285.
10. **Bobrow, M.N., K.J. Shaughnessy, and G.J. Litt.** 1991. Catalyzed reporter deposition, a novel method of signal amplification. II. Application to membrane immunoassays. J. Immunol. Methods *137*:103-112.
11. **Bobrow, M.N., G.J. Litt, K.J. Shaughnessy, P.C. Mayer, and J. Conlon.** 1992. The use of catalyzed reporter deposition as a means of signal amplification in a variety of formats. J. Immunol. Methods *150*:45-49.
12. **Bromley, L., S.P. McCarthy, J.E. Stickland, C.E. Lewis, and J.O. McGee.** 1994. Non-isotopic in situ detection of mRNA for interleukin-4 in archival human tissue. J. Immunol. Methods *167*:47-54.
13. **Coons, A.H., H.J. Creech, and R.N. Jones.** 1941. Immunological properties of an antibody containing a fluorescent group. Proc. Soc. Experim. Biol. Med. *47*:200-202.
14. **Cordell, J.L., B. Falini, W.N. Erber, A.K. Ghosh, Z. Abdulaziz, S. MacDonald, K.A. Pulford, H. Stein, and D.Y. Mason.** 1984. Immunoenzymatic labeling of monoclonal antibodies using immune complexes of alkaline phosphatase and monoclonal anti-alkaline phosphatase (APAAP complexes). J. Histochem. Cytochem. *32*:219-229.
15. **Farr, A.G. and P.K. Nakane.** 1981. Immunohistochemistry with enzyme labeled antibodies: a brief review. J. Immunol. Methods *47*:129-144.
16. **Flenghi, L., B. Bigerna, M. Fizzotti, S. Venturi, L. Pasqualucci, S. Pileri, B.H. Ye, M. Gambacorta, R. Pacini, C.D. Baroni, et al.** 1996. Monoclonal antibodies PG-B6a and PG-B6p recognize, respectively, a highly conserved and a formol-resistant epitope on the human BCL-6 protein amino-terminal region. Am. J. Pathol. *148*:1543-1555.
17. **Fox, C.H., F.B. Johnson, J. Whiting, and P.P. Roller.** 1985. Formaldehyde fixation. J. Histochem. Cytochem. *33*:845-853.
18. **Fraenkel-Conrat, H., B.A. Brandon, and H.S. Olcott.** 1947. The reaction of formaldehyde with proteins. IV. Participation of indole groups. Gramicidin. J. Biol. Chem. *168*:99-118.
19. **Fraenkel-Conrat, H. and H.S. Olcott.** 1948. Reaction of formaldehyde with proteins. VI. Cross-linking of amino groups with phenol, imidazole, or indole groups. J. Biol. Chem. *174*:827-843.
20. **Fraenkel-Conrat, H. and H.S. Olcott.** 1948. The reaction of formaldehyde with proteins. V. Cross-linking between amino and priary amide or guanidyl groups. J. Am. Chem. Soc. *70*:2673-2684.
21. **Grody, W.W., R.A. Gatti, and F. Naeim.** 1989. Diagnostic molecular pathology. Mod. Pathol. *2*:553-568.
22. **Heppell-Parton, A.C., D.G. Albertson, R. Fishpool, and P.H. Rabbitts.** 1994. Multicolor fluorescence in-situ-hybridization to order small, single-copy probes on metaphase chromosomes. Cytogenet. Cell Genet. *66*:42-47.
23. **Hopman, A.H., F.C. Ramaekers, and E.J. Speel.** 1998. Rapid synthesis of biotin-, digoxigenin-, trinitrophenyl, and fluorochrome-labeled tyramides and their application for In-situ-hybridization using CARD amplification. J. Histochem. Cytochem. *46*:771-777.
24. **Horobin, R.W.** 1998. Problems and artifacts of microwave accelerated procedures in neurohistotechnology and resolutions. Methods *15*:101-106.
25. **Hsu, S.M.** 1988. The use of monoclonal antibodies and immunohistochemical techniques in lymphomas: review and outlook. Hematol. Pathol. *2*:183-197.
26. **Hsu, S.M., L. Raine, and H. Fanger.** 1981. Use of avidin-biotin-peroxidase complex (ABC) in immunoperoxidase techniques: a comparison between ABC and unlabeled antibody (PAP) procedures. J. Histochem. Cytochem. *29*:577-580.
27. **Imam, S.A., L. Young, B. Chaiwun, and C.R. Taylor.** 1995. Comparison of two microwave based antigen-retrieval solutions in unmasking epitopes in formalin-fixed tissue for immunostaining. Anticancer Res. *15*:1153-

1158.

28. **Kerstens, H.M., P.J. Poddighe, and A.G. Hanselaar.** 1995. A novel in-situ-hybridzation signal amplification method based on the deposition of biotinylated tyramine. J. Histochem. Cytochem. *43*:347-352.

29. **Khan, G., R.K. Gupta, P.J. Coates, and G. Slavin.** 1993. Epstein-Barr virus infection and bcl-2 proto-oncogene expression. Separate events in the pathogenesis of Hodgkin's disease? Am. J. Pathol. *143*:1270-1274.

30. **Komminoth, P. and M. Werner.** 1997. Target and signal amplification: approaches to increase the sensitivity of in-situ-hybridization. Histochem. Cell Biol. *108*:325-333.

31. **Korenberg, J.R. and X.N. Chen.** 1995. Human cDNA mapping using a high-resolution R-banding technique and fluorescence in-situ-hybridzation. Cytogenet. Cell Genet. *69*:196-200.

32. **Lan, H.Y., W. Mu, Y.Y. Ng, D.J. Nikolic-Paterson, and R.C. Atkins.** 1996. A simple, reliable, and sensitive method for nonradioactive in-situ-hybridzation: use of microwave heating to improve hybridization efficiency and preserve tissue morphology. J. Histochem. Cytochem. *44*:281-287.

33. **Landry, M. and T. Hokfelt.** 1998. Subcellular localization of preprogalanin messenger RNA in perikarya and axons of hypothalamo-posthypophyseal magnocellular neurons: an in-situ-hybridization study. Neuroscience *84*:897-912.

34. **Leong, A.S. and J. Wright.** 1987. The contribution of immunohistochemical staining in tumour diagnosis. Histopathology *11*:1295-1305.

35. **Leong, A.S. and J. Milios.** 1990. Accelerated immunohistochemical staining by microwaves. J. Pathol. *161*:327-334.

36. **Leong, A.J. and J. Milios.** 1993. An assessment of the efficacy of the microwave antigen retrieval procedure on a range of tissue antigens. Appl. Immunohistochem. *1*:267-274.

37. **Lichter, P., C.J. Tang, K. Call, G. Hermanson, G.A. Evans, D. Housman, and D.C. Ward.** 1990. High-resolution mapping of human chromosome 11 by in-situ-hybridzation with cosmid clones. Science *247*:64-69.

38. **Lichter, P. and D.C. Ward.** 1990. Is non-isotopic in-situ-hybridization finally coming of age? Nature *345*:93-94.

39. **Lu, Q.L., P. Lawson, and J.A. Thomas.** 1995. Criteria for consistent and high sensitivity of DNA in-situ-hybridzation on paraffin sections: optimal proteolytic enzyme digestion. J. Clin. Lab. Anal. 9:285-292.

40. **Macechko, P.T., L. Krueger, B. Hirsch, and S.L. Erlandsen.** 1997. Comparison of immunologic amplification vs enzymatic deposition of fluorochrome-conjugated tyramide as detection systems for FISH. J. Histochem. Cytochem. *45*:359-363.

41. **Malisius, R., H. Merz, B. Heinz, E. Gafumbegete, B.U. Koch, and A.C. Feller.** 1997. Constant detection of CD2, CD3, CD4, and CD5 in fixed and paraffin embedded tissue using the peroxidase mediated deposition of biotin-tyramide. J. Histochem. Cytochem. *45*:1665-1672.

42. **Marani, E.** 1995. Spotting hot microwave problems (editorial). Eur. J. Morphol. *33*:149-153.

43. **McCormick, D., H. Chong, C. Hobbs, C. Datta, and P.A. Hall.** 1993. Detection of the Ki-67 antigen in fixed and wax-embedded sections with the monoclonal antibody MIB1. Histopathology *22*:355-360.

44. **McDougall, J.K., A.R. Dunn, and K.W. Jones.** 1972. In-situ-hybridization of adenovirus RNA and DNA. Nature *236*:346-348.

45. **Merz, H., O. Rickers, S. Schrimel, K. Orscheschek, and A.C. Feller.** 1993. Constant detection of surface and cytoplasmic immunoglobulin heavy and light chain expression in formalin-fixed and paraffin-embedded material. J. Pathol. *170*:257-264.

46. **Merz, H., R. Malisius, S. Mannweiler, R. Zhou, W. Hartmann, K. Orscheschek, P. Moubayed, and A.C. Feller.** 1995. IMMUNOMAX—A Maximized Immunohistochemical Method for the Retrieval and Enhancement of Hidden Antigens. Lab. Invest. *73*:149.

47. **Mighell, A.J., P.A. Robinson, and W.J. Hume.** 1995. Patterns of immunoreactivity to an anti-fibronectin polyclonal antibody in formalin-fixed, paraffin-embedded oral tissues are dependent on methods of antigen retrieval. J. Histochem. Cytochem. *43*:1107-1114.

48. **Mullis, K.B. and F.A. Faloona.** 1987. Specific synthesis of DNA in vitro via a polymerase-catalyzed chain reaction. Methods Enzymol. *155*:335-350.

49. **Munakata, S. and J.B. Hendricks.** 1993. Effect of fixation time and microwave oven heating time on retrieval of the Ki-67 antigen from paraffin-embedded tissue. J. Histochem. Cytochem. *41*:1241-1246.

50. **Norton, A.J., S. Jordan, and P. Yeomans.** 1994. Brief, high-temperature heat denaturation (pressure cooking): a simple and effective method of antigen retrieval for routinely processed tissues. J. Pathol. *173*:371-379.

51. **Pardue, M.L., J.J. Bonner, J. Lengyel, and A. Spradling.** 1977. In-situ-hybridization for the study of chromosome structure and function, p. 217-232. *In* R.S. Sparkes, D.E. Comings, and C.F. Fox (Eds.), Molecular Human Cytogenetics. Academic Press, New York.

52. **Pileri, S.A., G. Roncador, C. Ceccarelli, M. Piccioli, A. Briskomatis, E. Sabattini, S. Ascani, D. Santini, P.P. Piccaluga, O. Leone, et al.** 1997. Antigen retrieval techniques in immuno-histochemistry: comparison of different methods. J. Pathol. *183*:116-123.

53. **Raap, A.K., M.P. van de Corput, R.A. Vervenne, R.P. van Gijlswijk, H.J. Tanke, and J. Wiegant.** 1995. Ultrasensitive FISH using peroxidase-mediated deposition of biotin- or fluorochrome tyramides. Hum. Mol. Genet. *4*:529-534.

54. **Sano, T., T. Hikino, Y. Niwa, K. Kashiwabara, T. Oyama, T. Fukuda, and T. Nakajima.** 1998. In-situ-hybridzation with biotinylated tyramide amplification: detection of human papillomavirus DNA in cervical neo-

plastic lesions (see comments). Mod. Pathol. *11*:19-23.

55. **Satoh, S., H. Tatsumi, K. Suzuki, and N. Taniguchi.** 1992. Distribution of manganese superoxide dismutase in rat stomach: application of Triton X-100 and suppression of endogenous streptavidin binding activity. J. Histochem. Cytochem. *40*:1157-1163.

56. **Schaer, J.C., B. Waser, G. Mengod, and R.C. Reubi.** 1997. Somatostatin receptor subtypes sst1, sst2, sst3 and sst5 expression in human pituitary, gastroenteropan-creatic and mammary tumors: comparison of mRNA analysis with receptor autoradio-graphy. Int. J. Cancer *70*:530-537.

57. **Shi, S.R., M.E. Key, and K.L. Kalra.** 1991. Antigen retrieval in formalin-fixed, paraffin-embedded tissues: an enhancement method for immunohistochemical staining based on microwave oven heating of tissue sections. J. Histochem. Cytochem. *39*:741-748.

58. **Shi, S.R., C. Cote, K.L. Kalra, C.R. Taylor, and A.K. Tandon.** 1992. A technique for retrieving antigens in formalin-fixed, routinely acid-decalcified, celloidin-embedded human temporal bone sections for immunohistochemistry. J. Histochem. Cytochem. *40*:787-792.

59. **Shi, S.R., B. Chaiwun, L. Young, R.J. Cote, and C.R. Taylor.** 1993. Antigen retrieval technique utilizing citrate buffer or urea solution for immunohistochemical demonstration of androgen receptor in formalin-fixed paraffin sections. J. Histochem. Cytochem. *41*:1599-1604.

60. **Shi, S.R., S.A. Imam, L. Young, R.J. Cote, and C.R. Taylor.** 1995. Antigen retrieval immunohistochemistry under the influence of pH using monoclonal antibodies. J. Histochem. Cytochem. *43*:193-201.

61. **Shi, S.R., R.J. Cote, C. Yang, C. Chen, H.J. Xu, W.F. Benedict, and C.R. Taylor.** 1996. Development of an optimal protocol for antigen retrieval: a 'test battery' approach exemplified with reference to the staining of retinoblastoma protein (pRB) in formalin-fixed paraffin sections. J. Pathol. *179*:347-352.

62. **Shi, S.R., R.J. Cote, L. Young, S.A. Imam, and C.R. Taylor.** 1996. Use of pH 9.5 Tris-HCl buffer containing 5% urea for antigen retrieval immunohistochemistry. Biotech. Histochem. *71*:190-196.

63. **Shi, S.R., R.J. Cote, and C.R. Taylor.** 1997. Antigen retrieval immunohistochemistry: past, present, and future. J. Histochem. Cytochem. *45*:327-343.

64. **Sibony, M., F. Commo, P. Callard, and J.M. Gasc.** 1995. Enhancement of mRNA in-situ-hybridization signal by microwave heating. Lab. Invest. *73*:586-591.

65. **Speel, E.J., B. Schutte, F.C. Ramaekers, and A.H. Hopman.** 1992. The effect of avidin-biotin interactions in detection systems for in-situ-hybridzation. J. Histochem. Cytochem. *40*:135-141.

66. **Speel, E.J., F.C. Ramaekers, and A.H. Hopman.** 1997. Sensitive multicolor fluorescence in-situ-hybridzation using catalyzed reporter deposition (CARD) amplification. J. Histochem. Cytochem. *45*:1439-1446.

67. **Sperry, A., L. Jin, and R.V. Lloyd.** 1996. Microwave treatment enhances detection of RNA and DNA by in-situ-hybridzation (see comments). Diagn. Mol. Pathol. *5*:291-296.

68. **Sternberger, L.A.** 1974. Immunocytochemistry. Prentice-Hall, Englewood Cliffs, NJ.

69. **Suurmeijer, A.J. and M.E. Boon.** 1993. Notes on the application of microwaves for antigen retrieval in paraffin and plastic tissue sections. Eur. J. Morphol. *31*:144-150.

70. **Taylor, C.R., S.R. Shi, B. Chaiwun, L. Young, S.A. Imam, and R.J. Cote.** 1994. Strategies for improving the immunohistochemical staining of various intranuclear prognostic markers in formalin-paraffin sections: androgen receptor, estrogen receptor, progesterone receptor, p53 protein, proliferating cell nuclear antigen, and Ki-67 antigen revealed by antigen retrieval techniques (see comments). Hum. Pathol. *25*:263-270.

71. **Taylor, C.R., S.R. Shi, C. Chen, L. Young, C. Yang, and R.J. Cote.** 1996. Comparative study of antigen retrieval heating methods: microwave, microwave and pressure cooker, autoclave, and steamer. Biotech. Histochem. *71*:263-270.

72. **Teo, C.G., S.Y. Wong, and P.V. Best.** 1989. JC virus genomes in progressive multifocal leukoencephalopathy: detection using a sensitive non-radioisotopic in-situ-hybridization method. J. Pathol. *157*:135-140.

73. **van de Corput, M.P., R.W. Dirks, R.P. van Gijlswijk, E. van Binnendijk, C.M. Hattinger, R.A. de Paus, J.E. Landegent, and A.K. Raap.** 1998. Sensitive mRNA detection by fluorescence in-situ-hybridzation using horse-radish peroxidase-labeled oligodeoxy-nucleotides and tyramide signal amplification. J. Histochem. Cytochem. *46*:1249-1259.

74. **von Wasielewski, R., M. Werner, M. Nolte, L. Wilkens, and A. Georgii.** 1994. Effects of antigen retrieval by microwave heating in formalin-fixed tissue sections on a broad panel of antibodies. Histochemistry *102*:165-172.

75. **Wilkens, L., R. von Wasielewski, M. Werner, M. Nolte, and A. Georgii.** 1996. Microwave pretreatment improves RNA-ISH in various formalin-fixed tissues using a uniform protocol. Pathol. Res. Pract. *192*:588-594.

76. **Wong, S.S.** 1991. Chemistry of protein conjugation and cross-linking, p. 1-48. CRC Press, Boca Raton.

77. **Yu, C.C., A.L. Woods, and D.A. Levison.** 1992. The assessment of cellular proliferation by immunohistochemistry: a review of currently available methods and their applications. Histochem. J. *24*:121-131.

78. **Zhang, Y., P. Matthiesen, R. Siebert, S. Harder, M. Theile, S. Scherneck, and B. Schlegelberger.** 1998. Detection of 6q deletions in breast carcinoma cell lines by fluorescence in-situ-hybridzation. Hum. Genet. *103*:727-729.

Antigen Retrieval Versus Amplification Techniques in Diagnostic Immunohistochemistry

15

Kenji Kawai and Robert Y. Osamura

Department of Pathology, Tokai University School of Medicine, Japan

INTRODUCTION

One of the recent technologic developments in immunohistochemistry (IHC) has focused on the retrieval of antigenicity, particularly using paraffin-embedded sections. To retrieve antigenicity, the following methods were used: *(i)* heat-induced antigen retrieval (AR), *(ii)* retrieval by enzyme digestion, or *(iii)* amplification methods, such as dextran polymer histochemistry, or tyramide signal amplification (TSA). In the practice of diagnostic pathology, when antibodies for IHC cannot detect antigens without retrieval techniques, such antibodies may be classified into the following groups: (group 1) those for which only heat-induced AR can retrieve stainability; (group 2) those for which amplification techniques perform as well as the heat-induced method; and (group 3) the few antigens that can be unmasked better by enzyme digestion than by high-temperature heating AR.

The antibodies belonging to group 1 include MIB-1, and those in group 2 include p53, vimentin, and bcl-2. From our experience, antibodies against CD30 (Ki-1) and keratin (AE1 and AE3) can detect the antigens better after enzyme (trypsin) digestion and belong to group 3. The antibodies against leu2 and leu3 could not retrieve antigenicity by these methods and can stain only on fresh frozen sections. For group 2, it could be speculated that a trivial amount of antigenicity may remain, although most of it could be masked by fixation and embedding procedures. For groups 1 and 3, the available antigenicity may be completely masked by tissue processing. The effectiveness of heat or enzyme digestion suggests different mechanisms of retrieval. Antigens such as leu2 and leu3 may be damaged structurally or extracted during tissue processing.

For diagnostic use of AR-IHC on paraffin sections, as has been well documented,

Antigen Retrieval Techniques
Edited by Shan-Rong Shi, Jiang Gu, and Clive R. Taylor
©2000 Eaton Publishing, Natick, MA

249

heat-induced AR may be the technique of choice. In other instances, however, it is important to know whether stainability can be restored by amplification techniques (such as TSA) and that enzyme digestion must be used in certain situations. This review emphasizes the advantages and applications of heat-induced AR in conjunction with TSA amplification for routine IHC.

BACKGROUND

The heat-induced AR technique is a nonenzymatic antigen unmasking method that is used prior to IHC staining on formalin-fixed, paraffin-embedded tissue sections or ethanol-fixed cytologic specimens. Because of its ease and excellent results, it is widely used in diagnostic IHC (1–4,6,8–10). TSA is a new approach toward detecting masked antigenicity and enhancing the sensitivity of IHC staining with or without AR. Here, we compare heat-induced AR and TSA, emphasizing the potentials of TSA using several monoclonal antibodies.

AMPLIFICATION AND HEAT-INDUCED ANTIGEN RETRIEVAL

Tyramide Signal Amplification

TSA is an extremely sensitive IHC staining procedure that is based on biotin-labeled tyramide and peroxidase methodologies. In comparison with the standard streptavidin-biotin method, TSA is about 50 to 100 times more sensitive (7). This procedure results in greater amplification of IHC signals and allows us to detect extremely small quantities of the masked target antigens. In the present study, the Catalyzed Signal Amplification (CSA) system (DAKO, Carpinteria, CA, USA) was used without heating to detect masked target antigenicity.

Antigen Retrieval

High-temperature heating of tissue is a critical factor in AR (8,9). The pH of the AR solution also influences the degree of unmasking of epitopes (9,10), as has been pointed out previously (5,6,9,10). In addition, different AR solutions are optimal for enhancement of different antigens with different antibodies (6,9,10).

In the present study of heat-induced AR using an autoclave, we investigated various pH values for their IHC sensitivity using different AR solutions (Table 1).

After pretreatment with AR solutions and then autoclave heating, IHC staining was performed by the indirect peroxidase-labeled antibody method.

DETECTION OF ANTIGENS

We used monoclonal antibodies to detect the following nuclear and membrane antigens: nuclear antigens—p53, estrogen receptor (ER), progesterone receptor, and MIB-1 (Ki-67); membrane antigens—CD8, CD79a, CD56, and epithelium-specific antigen (MOC-31). Tissue sections were obtained from routinely processed formalin-fixed, paraffin-embedded tissues of colon cancer, breast cancer, tonsils, nephroblastoma of the kidney, and gastric cancer.

Table 1. Antigen Retrieval Solutions Tested

Solution	pH value
Glycine-HCl	2.2
Acetate buffer	4.0
Citrate buffer	6.0
Phosphate-buffered saline	7.2
Tris buffer	8.0
Carbonate-bicarbonate buffer	10.0

p53

In the detection of p53 antigen, both heat-induced AR and TSA showed good detection sensitivity for IHC staining. The enhancement of staining intensity by heating was influenced by the pH value of the AR solution.

Estrogen Receptor

In the detection of the ER antigen, both heat-induced AR and TSA improved IHC staining results (Figure 1, a and b). Heating techniques are influenced by the pH value of the AR solution, and IHC staining using pH 6.0 showed excellent sensitivity for ER. Heat-induced AR also reduced background staining.

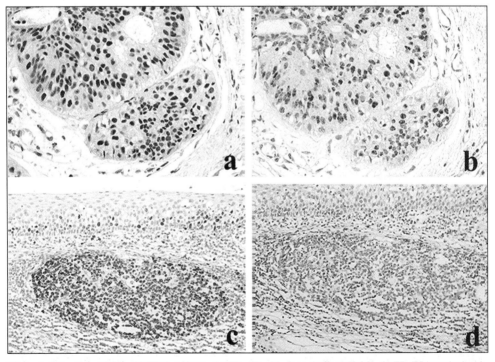

Figure 1. Detection of ER and MIB-1 antigens. (a) ER, AR with citrate buffer (pH 6.0), (b) ER, TSA method without AR, (c) MIB-1, AR with citrate buffer (pH 6.0), and (d) MIB-1, TSA method without AR. It should be noted that ER can be comparably detected by TSA method, but AR is mandatory for MIB-1 (no staining by TSA method). **(See color plate A11).**

TSA is also sensitive for detection of the ER antigen, but IHC showed a granular pattern and background staining, which occasionally obscured the target localization of the antigen. This was an important problem in TSA.

MIB-1

It should be emphasized that TSA did not detect MIB-1 antigenicity, for which only heat-induced AR was effective (2–4,9) (Figure 1, c and d). Among our limited AR solutions tested (Table 1), citrate buffer, pH 6.0, was effective for detection of MIB-1, and other solutions tested were insufficient. However, we did not test AR solutions at pH 1.0, EDTA-NaOH (pH 8.0), or any of the other solutions that have been documented as satisfactory in the literature (6,9).

CD79a

In the detection of membrane antigen CD79a, both heat-induced AR and TSA showed good sensitivity and enhanced IHC staining results. However, positive immunostaining products of heat-induced AR technique were finer than those obtained by TSA, as mentioned earlier.

CD56

In the detection of CD56 antigens, both heat-induced AR and TSA improved IHC staining results; results from heat-induced AR were significantly influenced by the pH value of the AR solution. TSA was sensitive for the detection of CD56. The staining pattern of heat-induced AR was finer and clearer than that of TSA.

CONCLUSION

Heat-induced AR gave reliable and excellent IHC staining results with various monoclonal antibodies. Heat-induced AR for routine IHC may not only enhance the intensity of staining but may also decrease background staining. Staining results for some antigens were dependent on the pH value of the AR solution. TSA may improve detection limits compared with the standard IHC detection system. TSA showed good sensitivity for various antigens and also enhanced the signal intensity of IHC staining, except for MIB-1; however, this technique frequently causes increased background staining with dense granular brown deposits that sometimes obscure the target localization of antigens. This phenomenon was especially prominent in the detection of nuclear antigens.

In conclusion, whereas TSA has the potential ability to detect masked membrane antigens in the daily practice of diagnostic IHC, heat-induced AR under optional conditions is a more reliable procedure for demonstrating masked antigenicity and for the evaluation of target localization.

REFFERENCES

1. **Battifora, H., R. Alsabeh, K. Jenkins, and A. Gown.** 1995. Epitope retrieval (unmasking) in immunohistochemistry. Adv. Pathol. Lab. Med. 8:101-118.

2. **Cattoretti, G. and A. Suurnmeijer.** 1994. Antigen unmasking on formalin-fixed paraffin-embedded tissues using microwaves: a review. Adv. Anat. Pathol. *2*:2-9.

3. **Gown, A.M., N. DeWever, and H. Battifora.** 1993. Microwave-based antigenic unmasking: a revolutionary new technique for routine immunohistochemistry. Appl. Immunohistochem. *1*:256-266.

4. **Leong, A.S.Y. and J. Milios.** 1993. An assessment of the efficacy of the microwave antigen-retrieval procedure on a range of tissue antigens. Appl. Immunohistochem. *1*:267-274.

5. **Morgan, J.M., H. Navabi, and B. Jasani.** 1997. Role of calcium chelation in high-temperature antigen retrieval at different pH valves. J. Pathol. *182*:233-237.

6. **Pileri, S.A., G. Roncador, C. Ceccarelli, M. Piccioli, A. Briskonatis, E. Sabattini, S. Ascani, D. Santini, P.P. Piccaluga, O. Leone, et al.** 1997. Antigen retrieval techniques in immunohistochemistry: comparison of different methods. J. Pathol. *183*:116-123.

7. **Sanno, N., A. Teramoto, M. Sugiyama, Y. Itoh, and R.Y. Osamura.** 1996. Application of catalyzed signal amplification in immunodetection of gonadotropin subunits in clinically nonfunctioning pituitary adenomas. Am. J. Clin. Pathol. *106*:16-21.

8. **Shi, S.-R., M.E. Key, and K.L. Kalra.** 1991. Antigen retrieval in formalin-fixed paraffin-embedded tissues: an enhancement method for immunohistochemical staining based on microwave oven heating of tissue sections. J. Histochem. Cytochem. *39*:741-748.

9. **Shi, S.-R., J. Gu, K.L. Kalra, T. Chen, R.J. Cote, and C.R. Taylor.** 1995. Antigen retrieval technique: a novel approach to immunohistochemistry on routinely processed tissue sections. Cell Vision *2*:6-22.

10. **Taylor, C.R., S.-R. Shi, and R.J. Cote.** 1996. Antigen retrieval for immunohistochemistry. Status and need for greater standardization. Appl. Immunohistochem. *4*:144-166.

Standardization of Routine Immunohistochemistry: Where to Begin?

16

Shan-Rong Shi[1], Jiang Gu[2], Richard J. Cote[1], and Clive R. Taylor[1]

[1]Department of Pathology, University of Southern California Keck School of Medicine, Los Angeles, CA, and [2]Department of Biomedical Sciences, University of South Alabama, Mobile, AL, USA

INTRODUCTION

The widespread application of immunohistochemistry (IHC) has transformed diagnostic surgical pathology "from something resembling an art into something more closely resembling a science" (48). However, all is not entirely well.

The standardization of immunohistochemistry has become a critical issue, as emphasized by the First National Cancer Institute Workshop on the standardization of immunoreagents in 1977 (13). Efforts to improve standardization have focused on three principal areas: antibodies and reagents, technical procedures, and the interpretation of immunohistochemical findings for use in diagnostic pathology (48). Several proposals have emanated from the work of the Biological Stain Commission since early 1991 (47) and have contributed both to an increased understanding of the problem and to real practical improvements.

In the early days of IHC, the major application of the method in pathology was in the detection of cellular (lineage) markers, to diagnose poorly differentiated malignant tumors, exemplified by the use of antibodies to intermediate filaments for the classification of undifferentiated or anaplastic tumors. In these circumstances, IHC was used as a qualitative procedure, not strictly quantitative, and rigorous standardization of IHC was less critical. Interpretation was a matter of present or not present, positive or negative, which was in itself a sufficient technical challenge, but much less so than an attempt to compare degrees of staining (differences in intensity).

Antigen Retrieval Techniques
Edited by Shan-Rong Shi, Jiang Gu, and Clive R. Taylor
©2000 Eaton Publishing, Natick, MA

Today, the demand for quantitative IHC, or at least a more reliable semiquantitative form of IHC, is ever more pressing, due to the emergence of a new field of pathology that requires demonstration of the differential expression of various prognostic markers for cancer. The recognition of these prognostic markers follows translational research, which has in a remarkably short time adapted knowledge derived from basic science studies of oncogenes, tumor suppressor genes, and cell cycle regulation into a series of stains of potential diagnostic or prognostic value.

For these reasons, standardization of IHC in terms of semiquantitative or quantitative methods has received increasing attention in both basic and clinical research. This type of translational research relied heavily on retrospective studies, allowing use of specimens and clinical data from previously published series in which clinical outcome was known and long-term follow-up available. In particular, application of the method to archival tissues stored in pathology files worldwide played a critical role in facilitating IHC studies of prognostic markers, leading to exponential increase in publications in recent years (49). One much heralded example was the development of a tumor-targeted therapeutic agent, a monoclonal antibody named Herceptin, as a treatment for certain categories of breast cancer. Approval for clinical trials by the Food and Drug Administration (FDA) was contingent on the development of a quantitative test to evaluate HER-2/neu expression in breast tumors. Standardized test kits such as the HerceptTest (DAKO, Carpinteria, CA, USA), and the INFORM DNA probe test (Ventana Medical Systems, Tucson, AZ, USA) have been approved by the FDA to meet this need, although the accuracy and comparability of these methods remain controversial (60). Similar controversial issues abound in other studies of diverse prognostic markers including p53, estrogen receptor (ER), progesterone receptor (PR), MIB-1, etc., as is described elsewhere (Chapters 9, 11, 12, and 13).

Standardization is a great challenge, easier said than done, because many factors play a part, from fixation and processing of the tissue through antigen retrieval (AR), the selection of the IHC staining reagents and protocol to the final step of scoring and evaluating the significance of the findings (Figure 1). One approach to the standardization of IHC is to adopt a Total Test strategy, as advocated by our group at The University of Southern California (49). In essence, this approach requires that the pathologist pay attention to each and every step of the whole procedure from the moment that the biopsy is taken, including type and duration of fixation, AR method employed, selection of reagents, performance of IHC staining, incorporation of proper controls, and interpretation and validation of the staining result. These issues, which have been discussed elsewhere, are summarized in Table 1 and form part of the forthcoming National Committee for Clinical Laboratory Standards guidelines for proper IHC testing. As we have pointed out previously (48,49,51), much of the variability in staining that may be attributed to differences in fixatives or fixation times (or staining methods) may be reduced, if not eliminated, by use of an optimized AR protocol. Exactly how to develop an optimized protocol is a major topic in the remainder of this chapter.

Having addressed the Total Test approach and done whatever is possible to ensure consistent fixation, the starting point for improving IHC results may be optimization of the AR technique based on test battery approach. Once this step has been achieved, the investigator may turn his or her attention to further enhancement of sensitivity, if necessary, by simplification of the immunostaining method, with a more highly sensitive one-step detection or signal amplification method.

Three major interrelated issues, namely, standardization of the AR technique,

Table 1. Components of the Total Test in Immunohistochemistry

Element of Testing Process	Quality Assurance Issues	Responsibility
Clinical question/test selection	Indications for immunohistochemistry; selection of stain(s)	Surgical pathologist; sometimes clinician
Specimen acquisition and management	Specimen collection, fixation processing, sectioning	Pathologist/technologist
Analytic issues	Qualifications of staff; intra- and interlaboratory proficiency testing of procedures	Pathologist/technologist
Results of validation and reporting	Criteria for positivity/negativity in relation to controls; content and organization of report; turnaround time	Pathologist/technologist
Interpretation, significance	Experience/qualifications of pathologist; proficiency testing of interpretational aspects; diagnostic, prognostic significance; appropriateness/correlation	Surgical pathologist and/or clinician
Reprinted with permission from Reference 47a.		

simplification of IHC staining method, and quantitative IHC, are discussed in the remainder of this chapter.

STANDARDIZATION OF THE ANTIGEN RETRIEVAL TECHNIQUE: A POTENTIAL WAY TO STANDARDIZE ROUTINE IMMUNOHISTOCHEMISTRY

From a practical point of view, one of the most difficult issues in the standardization of IHC for use on archival tissues may be the adverse influence of formalin, the most commonly used fixative worldwide, and the effects of processing the tissue for embedding in paraffin (14,24). It has been recognized that formalin fixation is a time-dependent or clock reaction (4,15). In routine hospital practice, tissues are placed in formalin as they are removed from patients and then submitted to the laboratory in formalin, leading to fixation for variable periods ranging from 12 hours to days or even weeks (autopsy). Not surprisingly, the preservation of antigenicity in archival paraffin tissues may vary greatly and may result in variable intensity of immunostaining for formalin-sensitive antigens. Battifora and Kopinski (4) reported a careful study on the duration of formalin fixation and the influence of enzymatic digestion on immunostaining; they pointed out a critical issue: the digestion period should be adjusted according to the length of exposure to the fixative. Because accurate information regarding the duration of fixation for most, if not all, paraffin blocks is not available even in a single hospital, it is extremely difficult to set the exact time of enzymatic digestion for each individual sample tested. In addition, the period of enzymatic digestion must not be overly long in order to retain acceptable morphology. Furthermore, overdigestion may significantly reduce immunostaining intensity for some antigens. The authors recommended a pilot test of enzymatic digestion for periods ranging from 1 to 3 hours in order to find the optimal time of digestion for each specimen, a procedure that is not practical for hospital laboratories handling hundreds of tissue samples during the day-to-day workload.

Extensive use of the AR technique for IHC in both clinical and research histopathology has demonstrated that AR is superior to enzymatic digestion, not only for increasing the intensity of IHC for a greater variety of antigens, but also for maintaining better morphology (8,36,37,50). Based on numerous reports that AR-IHC

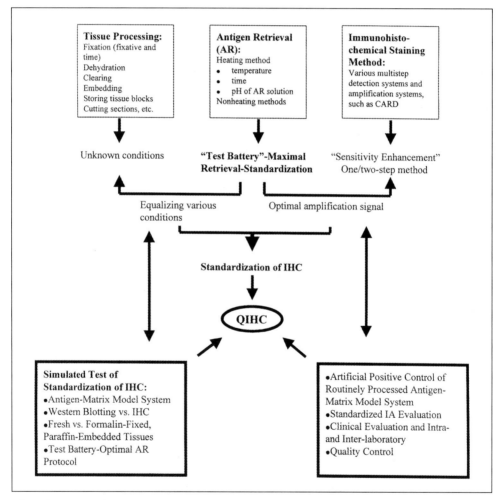

Figure 1. Diagram of our suggested plan of standardization of routine IHC described in text. The upper three boxes indicate the potential approach to standardization of IHC staining results based on the AR technique using the test battery method to equalize various conditions of tissue fixation and processing in terms of unknown conditions, in addition to simplification of the IHC staining method to reach optimal amplification signal, which may result in standardization of IHC. Based on this condition, quantitative IHC may be performed using our proposed establishment of an artificial antigen-matrix model system (AMMS), and a simulated test for standardization may be carried out to reach the goal as indicated in the lower two boxes. CARD, catalyzed reporter deposition; IA, image analysis; QIHC, quantitative IHC.

gives excellent results for many of the markers used in diagnostic pathology (37,40,51), the possibility of improving the standardization of IHC through the use of AR has been suggested by Taylor, "...but if we cannot have uniform fixation, let us at least strive toward a more uniform approach to retrieval by using standardized and well-described antigen retrieval procedures" (48). As discussed elsewhere (in the Appendix), the use of a test battery approach has been advocated in order to find an optimal protocol for AR-IHC (37,39). This approach is based on monitoring the two major factors [the heating condition (temperature and duration of heating) and the pH value of the AR solution] that influence the effectiveness of AR-IHC. In our experience, a maximal retrieval level, showing the strongest intensity of AR-IHC, can be obtained by using this test battery approach (37,39,51), which may therefore have value in the standardization of IHC.

One important question was whether or not an optimal AR protocol, established by a test battery, could produce comparable AR-IHC results for a variety of archival tissues that had been fixed in formalin for widely different time periods.

We recently conducted an experiment to examine this question. We explored the possibility of standardizing the results of IHC staining based on establishment of an optimal protocol of AR, to obtain maximal retrieval for a particular antigen/antibody combination, under which conditions a similar intensity of immunostaining might be achieved for archival paraffin-embedded tissues subjected to varying periods of formalin fixation (Figure 2). Once established, this optimized protocol may then be applied to other antibodies, often with good results. If initial results are not satisfactory for any particular antibody, then the performance of further test batteries, varying heating time, pH, etc., allows rapid modification to optimize results for the antibody in question (41).

In our experiment, tests were conducted using monoclonal antibodies to AE1, MIB-1, and p53 (Pab-1801, DO7, and BP53-12-1) for AR-IHC on formalin-fixed, paraffin-embedded tissues of renal and breast carcinoma that had been fixed in formalin for different periods: 4, 12, and 24 hours and 3, 7, 14, and 30 days. Using the test battery approach, varying the buffer solution, pH, and heating time, an optimal AR protocol was established. Results of this test are summarized in Tables 2 to 4, in which the intensity of positive immunostaining is graded as ++++, +++, ++, +, and – for extremely strong, strong, moderate, weak, and negative, respectively, and a grade of ± is used to represent focal or questionable weakly positive cells in tissue sections. As previously shown, the effectiveness of AR-IHC for certain antigens is pH dependent. The greatest intensity of immunostaining (maximal retrieval) for MIB-1 and p53-1801

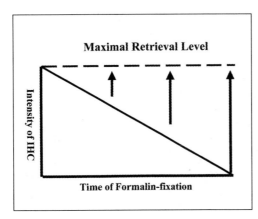

Figure 2. Diagram explaining standardization of IHC based on AR using a test battery to achieve maximal retrieval level by an optimal AR protocol. The intensity of IHC (y axis) is reversely correlated with the time of formalin-fixation (x axis), as indicated by a reduced slope. The three arrows indicate a potential maximal retrieval level that may equalize the intensity of IHC to a comparable result for routinely processed paraffin-embedded tissues with various times of fixation. Reprinted with permission from Reference 41a.

Table 2. Comparison of Antigen Retrieval Immunohistochemistry Protocols for MIB-1 under Microwave Heating at 100°C for 10 Minutes

AR protocol	Periods of formalin-fixation (h)						
	4	12	24	3×24	7×24	14×24	30×24
None	-	-	-	-	-	-	-
CB6	+	+	+	-	±	±	-
T-H1	++++	+++	+++	++	+++	+++	+++
T-H10	++	++	+	+	+	+	±

Tissue was renal carcinoma routinely paraffin-embedded.
None, without AR; CB6, citrate buffer, pH 6.0; T-H1, Tris-HCl buffer, pH 1.0; T-H10, Tris-HCl buffer, pH 10.0.
Reprinted with permission from Reference 41.

was obtained while using buffer solution at pH 1.0. A similar high intensity of immunostaining for p53-1801 could also be achieved by using Tris-HCl buffer at pH 10.0. High staining intensity of AE1 was also obtained when using pH 10.0 and pH 1.0 Tris-HCl buffer solutions, particularly for tissues overfixed in formalin (Tables 2–4).

In general, either a higher pH value (Tris-HCl buffer, pH 10.0–11.0), or a lower pH value (Tris-HCl, pH 1–2) yielded a stronger intensity of AR-IHC than the more usual pH 6.0 value buffer reported in the literature (antibodies p53-1801 and keratin AE1; Tables 3 and 4). This effect was particularly apparent for tissues overfixed in formalin (7 days and more). Weak false nuclear background staining was occasionally observed with low pH buffer as the AR solution. In sections not subjected to AR, MIB-1 was negative for all tissues. The immunostaining intensity of all antibodies was fixation time dependent: the longer the fixation time, the weaker the intensity of the final stain (Tables 2–4, first rows labeled None) (38,41).

Recently, Pileri et al. (28) performed a comparative study of different AR-IHC methods of using 16 antibodies for both formalin- and B5-fixed, paraffin-embedded tissue sections; they demonstrated that EDTA-NaOH (pH 8.0) and Tris-HCl buffer (pH 8.0) were superior to citrate buffer (pH 6.0). Our study also indicated that citrate buffer at pH 6.0 was less satisfactory. Thus, another potential approach toward obtaining the maximal retrieval level for MIB-1 may be the selection of different AR solutions, such as EDTA-NaOH, for inclusion in any new test battery. Although the possibility of standardization of routine IHC through adaption of the AR technique is supported by this study and others (25), practical standardization of IHC, particularly for routine clinical use requires further evaluation.

One interesting conclusion is that there is a clear need for reevaluation of the clinical interpretation of AR-IHC results by the pathologist, based on the pre-AR literature or on personal experience with preretrieval IHC staining. For example, the use of monoclonal antibody to estrogen receptor ER-1D5 using AR on routine paraffin sections gives consistently good staining, in both intensity and number of positive cells, equaling or surpassing the previously used monoclonal antibody ER-ICA on paraffin sections, and also bettering the results obtained with frozen sections (3). Indeed in the early days,

Table 3. Comparison of Antigen Retrieval Immunohistochemistry for p53-1801 under Microwave Heating at 100°C for 10 Minutes

AR protocol	Periods of formalin-fixation (h)						
	4	12	24	3×24	7×24	14×24	30×24
None	+++	++	++	+	+	+(BG+)	+(BG+)
CB6	+++	+++	+++	+++	++	++	++
T-H1	++++	++++	++++	++++	++++	++++	++++
T-H10	++++	++++	++++	++++	++++	++++	++++

Tissue was breast carcinoma routinely paraffin-embedded.
None, without AR; CB6, citrate buffer, pH 6.0; T-H1, Tris-HCl buffer, pH 1.0; T-H10, Tris-HCl buffer, pH 10.0.
Reprinted with permission from Reference 41.

Table 4. Comparison of Antigen Retrieval Immunohistochemistry for Monoclonal Antibody to Keratin AE1 under Microwave Heating at 100°C for 10 Minutes

AR protocol	Periods of formalin-fixation (h)						
	4	12	24	3×24	7×24	14×24	30×24
None	++	+	±	±	-	-	-
CB6	+++	+++	+++	+++	+++	+++	++
T-H1	++++	++++	++++	++++	++++	++++	++++
T-H10	++++	++++	++++	++++	++++	++++	++++

Tissue was renal carcinoma routinely paraffin-embedded.
None, without AR; CB6, citrate buffer, pH 6.0; T-H1, Tris-HCl buffer, pH 1.0; T-H10, Tris-HCl buffer, pH 10.0.
Reprinted with permission from Reference 41.

ER staining could not be accomplished in formalin paraffin sections; now it is routine with AR. Goulding et al. (17) reevaluated the clinical significance of ER-1D5 based on a comparison among the three different IHC staining methods mentioned above; they concluded that it was necessary to reevaluate the clinical data with respect to ER status as determined by the new paraffin section AR-IHC methodology. A recent study by Pertschuk et al. (27) revealed a similar conclusion, that paraffin section AR-IHC (with ER-1D5) is the method of choice for evaluation of ER status in predicting prognosis.

This approach to improved standardization of routine IHC, as demonstrated by our study, has been supported by the recent literature. For example, Lambkin et al. (22) conducted an interlaboratory comparative study of 16 Irish histopathology laboratories using monoclonal antibody to ER-1D5, with high-temperature heating AR pretreatment for all archival paraffin sections. Although there were some variable results among the16 participants in terms of intensity, the percentage of ER-positive tumor cells, the background, and the overall results were quite similar: (*i*) most participants achieved a low score in the case exhibitng low ER expression; (*ii*) all showed negative ER staining results for the negative control case; and (*iii*) most participants achieved comparable ER-positive staining for six cases that had high expression of ER. This study demonstrated the potential approach to routine IHC standardization through AR standardization. Pertschuk and Axiotis (see Chapter 9) also advocated AR as a potential way to standardize of AR-IHC for ER staining. They found little difference in staining result if the specimens are fixed for 4 to 48 hours, since the AR technique permits consistent identification of ER under these variable conditions of fixation.

To summarize:

- The test battery is a practical approach to standardize the AR technique in order to establish an optimal AR protocol for certain antigens.
- Standardization of routine IHC may be based on use of optimized AR protocols to reach the maximal retrieval level.
- Effective AR provides a potential approach to the challenge of variable fixation and processing of archival paraffin tissues (Figure 2).
- For many laboratories, optimized AR with standardized (especially automated) protocols may be sufficient to achieve consistent high-quality staining. For those requiring greater sensitivity, it may be necessary to resort to additional strategies as described below.

ENHANCED SENSITIVITY OF IMMUNOHISTOCHEMISTRY: SIMPLIFICATION OF DETECTION AND SIGNAL AMPLIFICATION SYSTEM

One of the critical issues in the early days of IHC development related to the need to achieve greater sensitivity, leading from the simplest one-step direct conjugate method to multiple-step detection techniques such as peroxidase-anti-peroxidase (PAP), avidin-biotin conjugate (ABC), and biotin-streptavidin detection (BSA) systems. The major advantage of these multi-step detection systems is an amplification of signal, resulting primarily from the fact that more molecules of enzyme are localized to the antigen/antibody binding site (50). The availability of these more sensitive detection systems contributed to the initial success of rendering immunoperoxidase methods more widely applicable to routine formalin-fixed, paraffin-embedded tissues. Further improvements in sensitivity followed the use of various antigen retrieval procedures (40).

In general, signal amplification is critical in the development of more effective detection systems for immunohistochemical staining. Numerous different approaches have been proposed for the development of more efficient staining techniques, variously promoted as sensitive or super-sensitive detection systems (50). For simplicity, we have grouped these into three categories (Table 5), namely, the predetection phase (before primary incubation), the detection phase (from primary incubation to label incubation), and the postdetection phase (after label incubation) amplification. This simple classification facilitates an understanding of the possible mechanisms of amplification and provides a convenient approach to the comparison of different

Table 5. Classification of Three Basic Signal Amplification Approaches for Immunohistochemistry

Classification	Basic principles and mode of action	Advantages and problems
1. Predetection amplification: AR	Restoration of formalin-induced modification of protein structure, resulting in dramatic amplification of signal, while reducing the background simultaneously	Simplest and cheapest procedure (heating) among all methods of amplification; not effective for some antibodies/antigens.
2. Detection amplification: A. Multistep detection systems: PAP, ABC, APAAP, BSA B. Stepwise amplification C. Polymeric and polylabeling amplification	Increase in accumulation of labeling signal (enzyme or others) A. PAP: 2–50-fold, ABC: 2–100-fold of increase B. Repeating cycles of detection C. Currently available kits: EnVision, PowerVision, and EPOS. Average further dilution of primary antibody: 2–5; our test: 1:160 further dilution of PCNA (42)	The polylabeling technique and polymer-based amplification systems are simpler, cheaper, and faster than other multistep detection systems. As a biotin-free detection system, this avoids the problem of the endogenous biotin reaction.
3. Postdetection amplification: A. Enhanced DAB by metal, imidazol, etc. B. CARD C. Anti-end product (EP) D. Gold-silver enhancement method	A. Enhance the color reaction B. HRP catalyzes deposition of biotinylated tyramine at the site of HRP C. Anti-EP + biotinylated link + HRP label, 16-fold increase of signal D. Silver enhancement	Procedures are complicated, involving repeating cycles of reactions. Labor and costs may be a drawback to widespread application. Background staining increases with amplification of signal.

EPOS, enhanced polymer one-step staining; CARD, catalyzed reporter deposition; HRP, horseradish peroxidase; AR, antigen retrieval; PAP, peroxidase-anti-peroxidase; ABC, avidin-biotin complex; APAAP, alkaline phosphatase-antialkaline phosphatase; BSA, biotin-streptavidin; PCNA, proliferating cell nuclear antigen.

Reprinted, with permission from Reference 42.

methods, which in turn may promote the development of more efficient and practical methods for standardization of IHC.

Postdetection Amplification

Methods of postdetection phase amplification seek to intensify the chromogen reaction. The two principal drawbacks are an increase in the complexity of the immunostaining procedure (with additional steps that are difficult to control) and a general increase in nonspecific background staining. This latter effect often means that while the intensity of the stain is increased, the signal-to-noise ratio is not improved, and interpretation may even be more difficult.

Detection Phase Amplification

Development and innovation of staining methods have continued apace, reflective of drawbacks intrinsic to the currently available three-step detection systems, including complex time-consuming protocols, difficulties in standardization, inefficient demonstration of certain hard to detect antigens, and endogenous biotin or endogenous enzyme activity. Several computer-assisted automated stainers have been manufactured to address the issues of consistency, high labor intensity, and cost and have led to remarkable improvements in reproducibility. However, multistep techniques continue to pose problems for standardization and control, a problem that is to some extent compounded by the proliferation of automated stainers, because now any laboratory can perform immunostaining with little underlying basic knowledge, forcing total reliance on the automated staining protocols and quality control methods.

The demand for more sensitive, more reliable, and simpler methodologies for IHC thus continues to escalate. Simplification of conventional multistep detection systems, producing shorter protocols without compromising detection sensitivity, has long been desirable but is technically challenging. In practice, any reduction of the number of steps has always been accompanied by reduced sensitivity. New approaches, such as catalyzed reporter deposition or tyramine signal amplification (1,5), immunopolymerase chain reaction (PCR) (35), and end-product amplification (9), which give improved detection sensitivity, are accompanied by even more complicated protocols, and by high or unacceptable nonspecific staining. Other methods that use natural or synthetic polymer carriers to increase the numbers of enzymes or ligands that are coupled to linker antibodies have also been reported. These polymer carriers include dextran (6,21,23), polypeptides (45), dendrimers (2,32,43), and DNA branches (7). The applicability of these technologies for IHC remain untested.

In 1995, a polymer-enhanced two-step IHC detection system (EnVision™; DAKO) was reported and subsequently evaluated (20,34,55), providing a potential solution to the long awaited need for simplification. However, the high molecular weight of the dextran carrier employed for the conjugation of enzymes to linker antibodies appears to create spatial hindrance, thus compromising the penetrative ability of the detection reagent. Consequently, sensitivities of the polymer- enhanced system vary greatly for different antibodies and antigens. For example, significantly lower sensitivity has been reported for the staining of nuclear antigens (55).

Utilizing polymer carriers dramatically increases the number of enzymes that can be conjugated to linker antibodies. However, because such conjugates also increase dramatically in size, the enzyme density per unit surface may not be increased to the degree that would be expected. A desirable goal would be to prepare a more compact enzyme-antibody conjugate, with a high number of enzyme molecules attached to each linker antibody, but minimal increase in molecular size. To achieve such goal, it was postulated that small molecules of linear or minimally branched multifunctional reagents, which are able to polymerize with linker antibodies and enzymes in a tight, compact configuration, should be employed. In this context, polymerization of many small organic monomeric molecules such as acrylic acid, bisacrylic acid, and their derivatives can be initiated reproducibly under mild or physiological conditions. It was reasoned that an admixture of the enzyme horseradish peroxidase (HRP), together with linker antibodies and polymerizable small molecules may allow for the preparation of enzyme-antibody conjugates, characterized by a tight compact shape, with a high enzyme-to-antibody ratio. Unlike the polymerization process for a pure preparation of small molecules, which inevitably leads to high degree of polymerization, and consequently a low penetrability of the end product, the degree of polymerization with admixed proteins may be much lower, given the fact that HRP has only one amino group that is readily accessible.

We have recently evaluated a new detection system based on a controlled polylabeling technology using the approach described above. This reagent is effective in a two-step detection system for IHC (PowerVision™; ImmunoVision Technologies, Daly City, CA, USA) (42). The results of IHC staining studies indicate that these conjugates combine compact molecular shape and small size, yielding superior detection efficiency, for both cell surface and nuclear antigens, compared with other conjugates prepared with more orthodox polymerized linkers. The PowerVision two-step detection system was compared with three currently available multistep detection systems, ChemMate (Ventana), LSAB2 (DAKO), and Super Sensitive (BioGenex, San Ramon, CA, USA) kits. All immunohistochemical staining was performed on routinely formalin-fixed, paraffin-embedded tissue sections, under identical conditions, including use of the microwave AR technique.

The experimental design incorporated three sets of experimental conditions in order to facilitate comparison of the different methods. Experimental set 1, comparing the immunostaining results obtained using a panel of 15 antibodies, revealed that the sensitivity of the PowerVision detection system was significantly greater than that of the other three methods, as evidenced by the greater intensity of immunostaining achieved for all 15 antibodies. Experimental set 2, an efficiency test, employed further serial dilutions of a commercial prediluted, ready-to-use monoclonal antibody to proliferating cell nuclear antigen (PCNA). Dilutions ranged from 1:10 to 1:640. The detection efficiency of the PowerVision reagent was superior to that of the other detection systems, as exemplified by the observation that at a dilution of 1:320, a moderate staining intensity could be achieved by using the PowerVision system, while the other methods showed faintly positive or negative results. Experimental set 3 demonstrated that the immunoreactivity of long-term-stored archival paraffin sections for monoclonal antibody to p27^{Kip1} could be restored to a level similar to that obtained using fresh-cut paraffin sections, when combining an optimized AR protocol (using an EDTA-NaOH solution of pH 8.0) with the PowerVision system, whereas other reagents gave unsatisfactory results. Other two-step and one-step detection systems are currently under development, such as EPOS, a one-step method manufactured by DAKO (52). This reflects an encouraging trend toward simplification, which should facilitate standardization of IHC, and is consistent with the overall philosophy that, all other things being equal, simple techniques are better than complicated ones.

Predetection Amplification

AR is an effective and simple technique for predetection phase amplification, which has found general acceptance as a means of increasing the efficiency of IHC staining of routinely formalin-fixed, paraffin-embedded tissue sections (40). It is generally accepted, although not well understood, that AR-induced amplification of signal is the result of increased antigenicity contingent on restoration of certain epitopes in the formalin-modified protein structure (40). To the extent that the AR technique serves to restore the natural antigen-antibody reaction, it favors specific binding and does not aggravate nonspecific background staining, providing the potential for an enhanced signal-to-noise ratio. This situation provides the ideal milieu for the use of highly sensitive detection methods, as illustrated in the present study.

In theory, the successful application of an ultrasensitive two-step detection system raises the possibility that it may be possible to develop sensitive one-step immunohistochemical staining methods based on use of the controlled polylabeling technique with primary antibodies. This approach may permit the creation of bifunctional adaptors as bridges to connect the primary antibody with large numbers of enzymatic molecules, yielding a single-step reagent that may achieve a satisfactory IHC results in routinely processed formalin paraffin sections.

QUANTITATIVE IMMUNOHISTOCHEMISTRY

Although quantitative immunohistochemistry (QIHC), including both manual and computer-assisted image analysis quantitative studies, has been explored for more than three decades (16,26), it has not been adopted routinely. Until recently, manual estimation of intensity and percentage of IHC staining was the most commonly used method of evaluation. Development of various image analysis systems has provided an objective measurement of IHC staining results, and has yielded interesting information on the clinical evaluation of ER staining, as described in Chapter 9.

However, clinical application of automated image analysis is still controversial, for a variety of reasons, including (*i*) variable results of immunostaining consequent on lack of standardization of IHC; (*ii*) variable results obtained by various image analysis systems, even with consistent staining; (*iii*) manual estimation (often termed semi-quantitative), which has provided a practical and satisfactory approach in some areas of research and in some clinical applications; (*iv*) the high cost of image analysis systems; and (*v*) the relative slowness of image analysis coupled with the ungoing need for active intervention by the pathologist, all of which hampers efficiency. Hendricks (19), in summarizing this issue, raised questions focusing on comparison of the information obtained by both manual evaluation and automated image analysis. It seems that no significant difference may exist between the two kinds of evaluation from the point of clinical relevance, as exemplified by recent numerous translational studies of cancer research that are predominantly based on manual semi-QIHC (11,12,46).

Methodology

Manual method. This is the most commonly used method for a semi-QIHC and is based on visual estimation of the intensity and percentage of positive staining of IHC. A frequently used grading system provides a visual aggregate of intensity/percentage as follows: ++++, +++, ++, +, and -, representing extremely strong, strong, moderate, weak, and negative staining, respectively. Scoring of the percentage of positive cells (staining intensity above a control threshold), more frequently used for nuclear staining, purports to assign the positive populations to four groups, based on an estimate of positive cells among total cells observed, as follows: -, less than 1% or less than 5%; +, less than one-quarter or one-third; ++, less than one-half; +++, more than one-half. The chosen cutoff percentages are arbitrary, but may be adjusted with reference to clinical data or outcome analysis. The H-SCORE is based on a product of intensity of

ER staining that is graded as negative (score 0), weakly positive (score 1), positive (score 2), strongly positive (score 3), and very strongly positive (score 4), as well as the estimated percentage of positive cells (50). In numerous studies of ER, this H-SCORE has been shown to be proportional to biochemical assay [dextran-coated charcoal (DCC)] and correlates well with response to hormonal therapy.

Stereology based-systemic random sampling method. This is a mathematic principle used for both manual methods and automated image analysis for QIHC or semi-QIHC. Because counting all cells manually is hardly feasible, an efficient sampling method based on stereologic principles has been recommended for QIHC to obtain the maximal amount of quantitative morphologic information with minimal but feasible counting requirements (18). This stereologic principle has been usefully employed in recent neurobiologic studies (10) and has the advantages of simplicity combined with more accurate quantitative counting results, compared with other methods such as profile counts or assumption-based methods. According to the original description of the interactive stereologic immunoscoring method, based on systematic random sampling (54), the essential principle is similar to that of the traditional method of counting blood cells by using a specified grid; counting randomly selected areas using a point grid, 200 cells sampled from 50 to 100 fields of vision may allow a coefficient of variation of less than 5% (29). This method is useful to assess the percentage of positive cells (above a defined visual threshold of intensity) but is not useful for evaluation of variations in intensity of IHC in a population.

Image analysis systems. The main steps in image analysis are image capture, image storage (compression), correction of imaging defects (e.g., nonuniform illumination, electronic noise, glare effect), image enhancement, segmentation of objects in the image, and image measurement. The main tools of image processing include image digitization and shading correction. For review of the basic image analysis systems (IA) technique, readers are refered to a recent review article (26). Several commercial IA systems are available, among which the CAS 200 system (Cell Analysis Systems, Lombard, IL, USA) is perhaps the most popular one in current use. The CAS 200 system employs two video cameras, one coupled with a 500-nm bandpass filter and, the other coupled with a 650-nm filter. Images of the nuclei of all cells in the field are captured by one camera using the 650-nm filter, while the other camera captures images of the reaction product [brown for diaminobenzidine (DAB)] at 500 nm. The optical density of the reaction product can be determined by converting the light transmission (gray level) to optical density using a calibrated look-up table, and the relative area of the staining reaction can be calculated. Simple thresholding methods are used to establish the gray levels for capturing the cell nuclei and for setting the lower limit for detection of DAB, based on a slide stained with control antibody. Combinations other than methyl green (nuclear staining) and DAB may be used, restricted only by the spectral overlap of the reagents and the availability of suitable filter combinations.

Quantitation of percentage of stained cells (positive area or population statistics) is a more common measurement approach for QIHC, for many of the markers of interest, such as p53, Ki-67, MIB-1, etc., which makes a great deal of sense biologically. It appears obvious that the percentage values obtained by using an IA system should be more accurate (certainly more reproducible) than those obtained by manual estimation. Using the CAS system, the positive area is measured by a nuclear masking method with the use of two filters (650 and 500 nm), as mentioned above. The threshold for positive staining is established using a slide stained with control antibody. However, for accurate measurement of percentage of positive area as a percentage, some critical issues must be considered. Field selection or sampling strategies are as important as the counting method itself. An equal opportunity rule must be followed such that all fields have an equal opportunity of being sampled. Therefore, it may not be reasonable to count the positive percentage based only on the areas of strongest positivity, as pointed out by Weinberg (58). A recent study by Polkowski et al. (29) demonstrated satisfactory reproducibility of QIHC for p53 and Ki-67 using stereology-based systematic random sampling (QPRODIT 5.2) with the CAS 200/486 system.

It is obvious that heterogeneity of antigen expression, and staining in tissue sections is a major cause of lack of reproducibility of QIHC; how to deal with this issue, short of counting every event, is the problem. Complicated approaches have been devised (with limited success) to circumvent heterogeneity, such as receptogram analysis (44). Currently, it is often the practice to select the field by manual observation, based on perceived requirements of different markers tested, all of which vary subjectively, which rather defeats the overall goal of obtaining objective reproducible data by automated methods.

Measurement of amount of antigen (protein) by QIHC. This approach is of value when seeking a cutoff point for clinical decision, based on the level of expression of a certain prognostic marker. It may also be useful in comparative studies of IHC, in which accurate comparison of intensity of staining is necessary to evaluate a new protocol or method, with reference to the existing standard. Efforts have been made to circumvent this persisting major weak point of IHC, namely, the subjective nature of estimating amounts of antigen present based on evaluation of intensity.

To measure the exact amount of protein tested in tissue section, parallel controls are required to monitor the numerous factors that influence the perceived intensity of immunostaining, including something as simple as variation in thickness of a section (e.g., from 4–6 μm—producing an intensity change of 50%, all other factors being equal). Several approaches have been described. For example, Press et al. (30) published an article concerning QIHC of Her-2/neu in formalin-fixed, paraffin-embedded tissue sections. Their quantitation of Her-2/neu in tissue was referenced to Western blotting of cell lines and various quantities of purified Her-2/neu protein. In their method, the assumption was made that the reduction in immunostaining intensity of archival paraffin sections might be close to that observed in paraffin-embedded cell lines, because they were fixed and processed in a similar way. A similar principle is embodied in the Quicgel method developed by Battifora's group (31). They created an internal artificial tissue control block using the breast cancer cell line that is then added to the tissue cassette containing the clinical biopsy specimen. Based on a study of 55 cases, they could measure the ER content of test specimens using a CAS 200 IA system, through a conversion factor, based on comparison of ER-positive staining results between a cell line and the specimen tested. They concluded that the Quicgel method may serve as a control in IHC analysis for ER, to minimize intralaboratory and interlaboratory variation in this field.

Other research groups have also reported methods of QIHC based on the IA system. Watanabe et al. (57) documented a method based on Western blotting to calculate the molar antigen content in tissue sections, offering the following formula: AgC = (SIPab-SIPns)/[Σ(AISab - AISns)/Nab] × AgBC, where AgC = molar antigen content in each portion in mol/L; Σ(AISab - AISns) = a sum of specific staining intensity measured in the widely defined area, corresponding to the antigen content in the tissue; Nab = number of sections used for the measurement of AISab or AISns; AgBC = antigen content in tissues measured by biochemical methods; AISab = the average gray

268

level-based absorbance in widely defined areas of the sections (0.95×0.95 mm); SIPab = absorbance in the same portions measured by the IA method (3.9×3.9 mm); AISns = the average gray level-based absorbance in a widely defined area of the adjacent section incubated with normal serum; and SIPns = absorbance in corresponding portions. In addition, several articles have documented detailed methods to calculate the amount of antigen (protein) in tissue sections based on Western blotting (30,56,59).

Midwestern assay. Roth et al. (33) developed an enzyme-based assay for simultaneous antigen localization and quantitation in tissue sections by employing two enzyme-chromogen reaction systems sequentially, to obtain both soluble and insoluble reaction products at the same location of tissue section. The soluble reaction products were then spectrophotometrically quantifiable, while the deposited insoluble products were visualized and evaluated by microscopy. This simple technique has considerable promise and allows for some interesting conclusion and approaches to QIHC.

CONCLUSION

- Accurate measurement of the amount of antigen (protein) in the tissue section may be possible in comparing with intensities of stain achieved on Western blots of the same kind of antigen in known amounts, in order to calculate a conversion factor for intensity and amount of protein.
- To control all factors that may influence the intensity of immunostaining, it is necessary that any artificial cell or tissue control system (or Western blot) be subjected to the influence of all possible factors that induce variation during the fixation, processing, and staining procedure, following the basic principles incorporated in the Quicgel method.
- IA systems may be standardized by optimal field selection using stereology-based systematic random sampling and an equal opportunity principle.
- The idea of applying two simultaneous protocols, with soluble and insoluble reaction products, warrants further exploration; quantitative spectroscopic analysis of the eluate could be provided for comparison with QIHC of the insoluble reaction product in situ.

Development of Reference Standards and Standard Curves for Calculation of Antigen Content in Tissue Section

It may be easier and cheaper to develop preparations of purified protein (antigen tested), which can be diluted to produce a series of known reference standards for both Western blotting and IHC (when suitably prepared). The technique of matrix models (53) may be applied to create what is in effect an artificial control tissue for the protein (antigen) in question (see below). In this way, a conversion formula may be developed from a standard curve of exact amount of the antigen under investigation for formalin-fixed, paraffin-embedded tissue sections, under various conditions of immunostaining, including AR pretreatment. Such antigen preparations may be employed as a pretest to establish a standardized IHC protocol for the antigen and as a practical reference standard for quality control and solubilization of IHC staining of test specimens.

Antigen Matrix Model: Artificial Positive Tissue Control

To control the quality of immunostaining performed at different times and in different laboratories by different technicians, it is essential to have available a universal positive control or reference standard. A simulated tissue that could serve in this capacity may be prepared using the purified protein-matrix model system to produce a faux-tissue that may be formalin-fixed, paraffin-embedded, and processed in a manner identical to unknown test specimens for each batch of IHC staining. The intensity of IHC of this positive control tissue section (containing known amounts of antigen) may then be used for calculation of the amount of antigen in test sections.

This proposal has several advantages over the Quicgel method: (*i*) Quicgel can not be used for retrospective studies, because it requires embedding an artificial control cell line with each specimen as the paraffin block is prepared; (*ii*) Quicgel requires the availability of suitable cell lines, expressing the antigen in question, which must show consistent behavior under cell culture and storing; and (*iii*) the purified protein-matrix model has the potential for achieving great consistency in terms of amount of antigen present, based on exact determinations of quantity at various dilutions. In addition, this artificial model can be processed and stored in the same way as routine paraffin-embedded specimens in the pathology laboratory. This concept is described briefly in Figure 1.

REFERENCES

1. **Adams, J.C.** 1992. Biotin amplification of biotin and horseradish peroxidase signals in histochemical stains. J. Histochem. Cytochem. *40*:1457-1463.
2. **Barth, R.F., D.M. Adams, A.H. Soloway, F. Alam, and M.V. Darby.** 1994. Boronated starburst dendrimer-monoclonal antibody immunoconjugates: evaluation as a potential delivery system for neutron capture therapy. Bioconjugate Chem. *5*:58-66.
3. **Battifora, H.** 1994. Immunocytochemistry of hormone receptors in routinely processed tissues (editorial). Appl. Immunohistochem. *2*:143-145.
4. **Battifora, H. and M. Kopinski.** 1986. The influence of protease digestion and duration of fixation on the immunostaining of keratins. A comparison of formalin and ethanol fixation. J. Histochem. Cytochem. 34:1095-1100.
5. **Bobrow, M.N., T.D. Harris, K.J. Shaughnessy, and G.J. Litt.** 1989. Catalyzed reporter depositin, a novel method of signal amplification. Application to immunoassays. J. Immunol. Methods *125*:279-285.
6. **Bocher, M., T. Giersch, and R.D. Schmid.** 1992. Dextran, a hapten carrier in immunoassays for s-trazines. A comparison with ELISAs based on hapten-protein conjugates. J. Immunol. Methods *151*:1-8.
7. **Boeckh, M. and G. Boivin.** 1998. Quantitation of cytomegalovirus: methodologic aspects and clinical applicaitons. Clin. Microbiol. Rev. *11*:533-554.
8. **Boon, M.E. and L.P. Kok.** 1995. Breakthrough in pathology due to antigen retrieval. Mal. J. Med. Lab. Sci. *12*:1-9.
9. **Chen, B.-X., M.J. Szabolcs, A.Y. Matsushima, and B.F. Erlanger.** 1996. A strategy for immunohistochemical signal enhancement by end-product amplification. J. Histochem. Cytochem. *44*:819-824.
10. **Coggeshall, R.E. and H.A. Lekan.** 1996. Methods for determining numbers of cells and synapses: a case for more uniform standards of review. J. Comp. Neurol. *364*:6-15.
11. **Cote, R.J., M.D. Dunn, S.J. Chatterjee, J.P. Stein, S.-R. Shi, Q.-C. Tran, S.X. Hu, H.J. Xu, S. Groshen, C.R. Taylor et al.** 1998. Elevated and absent pRB expression is associated with bladder cancer progression and has cooperative effects with p53. Cancer Res. *58*:1090-1094.
12. **Cote, R.J., Y. Shi, S. Groshen, A.-C. Feng, C. Cordon-Cardo, D. Skinner, and G. Lieskovosky.** 1998. Association of p27Kip1 levels with recurrence and survival in patients with stage C prostate carcinoma. J. Natl. Cancer Inst. *90*:916-920.
13. **DeLellis, R.A., L.A. Sternberger, R.B. Mann, P.M. Banks, and P.K. Nakane.** 1979. Immunoperoxidase technics in diagnostic pathology. Report of a workshop sponsored by the National Cancer Institute. Am. J. Clin. Pathol. *71*:483-488.
14. **Esteban, J.M., C. Ahn, H. Battifora, and B. Felder.** 1994. Quantitative immunohistochemical assay for hormonal receptors: technical aspects and biological significance. J. Cell Biochem. *19*(Suppl):138-145.
15. **Fox, C.H., F.B. Johnson, J. Whiting, and P.P. Roller.** 1985. Formaldehyde fixation. J. Histochem. Cytochem. *33*:845-853.
16. **Fritz, P., H. Multhaupt, J. Hoenes, D. Lutz, R. Doerrer, P. Schwarzmann, and H.V. Tuczek.** 1992. Quantitative immunohistochemistry. Theoretical background and its application in biology and surgical pathology. Prog. Histochem. Cytochem. *24*:1-53.

17. Goulding, H., S. Pinder, P. Cannon, D. Pearson, R. Nicholson, D. Snead, J. Bell, C.W.E. Elston, J.F. Robertson, R.W. Blamey, and I.O. Ellis. 1995. A new immunohistochemical antibody for the assessment of estrogen receptor status on routine formalin-fixed tissue samples. Hum. Pathol. *26*:291-294.

18. Gundersen, H.J.G. and R. Osterby. 1981. Optimizing sampling efficiency of stereological studies in biology: or 'Do more less well!'. J. Microsc. *121*:65-73.

19. Hendricks, J.B. 1996. Quantitative immunohistochemistry: a look in the crystal ball. J. Histotechnol. *19*:293-294.

20. Heras, A., C.M. Roach, and M.E. Key. 1995. Enhanced polymer detection system for immunohistochemistry (abstr). Mod. Pathol. *8*:165A.

21. Hurwitz, E., R. Kashi, R. Arnon, M. Wilchek, and M. Sela. 1985. The covalent linking of two nucleotide analogues to antibodies. J. Med. Chem. *28*:137-140.

22. Lambkin, H.A., P. Dunne, and P.M. McCarthy. 1998. Standardization of estrogen-receptor analysis by immunohistochemistry – an assessment of interlaboratory performance in Ireland. Appl. Immunohistochem. *6*:103-107.

23. Manabe, Y., T. Trubota, Y. Haruta, M. Odazaki, S. Haisa, K. Nakamura, and I. Kimura. 1983. Production of a monoclonal antibody-bleomycin conjugate utilizing dextran T-40 and the antigen-targeting cytotoxicity of the conjugate. Biochem. Biophys. Res. Commun. *115*:1009-1014.

24. Mighell, A.J., W.J. Hume, and P.A. Robinson. 1998. An overview of the complexities and subtleties of immunohistochemistry. Oral Dis. *4*:217-223.

25. Munakata, S. and J.B. Hendricks. 1993. Effect of fixation time and microwave oven heating time on retrieval of the Ki-67 antigen from paraffin-embedded tissue. J. Histochem. Cytochem. *41*:1241-1246.

26. Oberholzer, M., M. Ostreicher, H. Christen, and M. Bruhlmann. 1996. Methods in quantitative image analysis. Histochem. Cell Biol. *105*:333-355.

27. Pertschuk, L.P., J.G. Feldman, Y.-D. Kim, L. Braithwaite, F. Schneider, A.S. Braverman, and C. Axiotis. 1996. Estrogen receptor immunocytochemistry in paraffin embedded tissues with ER1D5 predicts breast cancer endocrine response more accurately than H222Spr in frozen sections or cytosol-based ligand-binding assays. Cancer *77*:2514-2519.

28. Pileri, S.A., G. Roncador, C. Ceccarelli, M. Piccioli, A. Briskonatis, E. Sabattini, S. Ascani, D. Santini, P.P. Piccaluga, O. Leone, et al. 1997. Antigen retrieval techniques in immunohistochemistry: comparison of different methods. J. Pathol. *183*:116-123.

29. Polkowski, W., G.A. Meijer, J.P.A. Baak, F.J.W. ten Kate, H. Obertop, G.J.A. Offerhaus, and J.J.B. van Lanschot. 1997. Reproducibility of p53 and Ki-67 immunoquantitation in Barrett's esophagus. Anal. Quant. Cytol. Histol. *19*:246-254.

30. Press, M.F., M.C. Pike, V.R. Chazin, G. Hung, J.A. Udove, M. Markowicz, J. Danyluk, W. Godolphin, M. Sliwkowski, R. Akita, et al. 1993. Her-2/neu expression in node-negative breast cancer: direct tissue quantitation by computerized image analysis and association of overexpression with increased risk of recurrent disease. Cancer Res. *53*:4960-4970.

31. Riera, J., J.F. Simpson, R. Tamayo, and H. Battifora. 1999. Use of cultured cells as a control for quantitative immunocytochemical analysis of estrogen receptor in breast cancer. The Quicgel method. Am. J. Clin. Pathol. *111*:329-335.

32. Roberts, J.C., Y.E. Adams, D. Tomalia, J.A. Mercer-Smith, and D.K. Lavallee. 1990. Using starburst dendrimers as linker molecules to radiolabel antibodies. Bioconjug. Chem. *1*:305-308.

33. Roth, K.A., J.W. Brenner, L.A. Selznick, M. Gokden, and R.G. Lorenz. 1997. Enzyme-based antigen localization and quantitation in cell and tissue samples (Midwestern assay). J. Histochem. Cytochem. *45*:1629-1641.

34. Sabattini, E., K. Bisgaard, S. Ascani, S. Poggi, M. Piccioli, C. Ceccarelli, F. Pieri, G. Fraternali-Orcioni, and S.A. Pileri. 1998. The EnVision™ system: a new immunohistochemical method for diagnostics and research. Critical comparison with the APAAP, ChemMate™, CSA, LABC, and SABC techniques. J. Clin. Pathol. *51*:506-511.

35. Sano, T., C.L. Smith, and C.R. Cantor. 1992. Immuno-PCR: very sensitve antigen detection by means of specific antibody-DNA conjugates. Science *258*:120-122.

36. Shi, S.-R., M.E. Key, and K.L. Kalra. 1991. Antigen retrieval in formalin-fixed, paraffin-embedded tissues: an enhancement method for immunohistochemical staining based on microwave oven heating of tissue sections. J. Histochem. Cytochem. *39*:741-748.

37. Shi, S.-R., J. Gu, K.L. Kalra, T. Chen, R.J. Cote, and C.R. Taylor. 1995. Antigen retrieval technique: a novel approach to immunohistochemistry on routinely processed tissue sections (review). Cell Vision *2*:6-22.

38. Shi, S.-R., A. Imam, L. Young, R.J. Cote, and C.R. Taylor. 1995. Antigen retrieval immunohistochemistry under the influence of pH using monoclonal antibodies. J. Histochem. Cytochem. *43*:193-201.

39. Shi, S.-R., R.J. Cote, C. Yang, C. Chen, H.-J. Xu, W.F. Benedict, and C.R. Taylor. 1996. Development of an optimal protocol for antigen retrieval: a 'test battery' approach exemplified with reference to the staining of retinoblastoma protein (pRB) in formalin-fixed paraffin sections. J. Pathol. *179*:347-352.

40. Shi, S.-R., R.J. Cote, and C.R. Taylor. 1997. Antigen retrieval immunohistochemistry: past, present, and future. J. Histochem. Cytochem. *45*:327-343.

41. Shi, S.-R., R.J. Cote, B. Chaiwun, L.L. Young, Y. Shi, D. Hawes, T. Chen, and C.R. Taylor. 1998. Standardization of immunohistochemistry based on antigen retrieval technique for routine formalin-fixed tissue sections. Appl. Immunohistochem. *6*:89-96.

41a. Shi, S.-R., R.J. Cote, and C.R. Taylor. 1999. Standardization and further development of antigen retrieval

271

immunohistochemistry: strategies and future goals. J. Histotechnol. *22*:177-192.

42. **Shi, S.-R., J. Guo, R.J. Cote, L.L. Young, D. Hawes, Y. Shi, S. Thu, and C.R. Taylor.** 1999. Sensitivity and detection efficiency of a novel two-step detection system (PowerVision) for immunohistochemistry. AIMM *7*:201-208.

43. **Singh, P., F. Moll, S.H. Lin, C. Ferzli, K.S. Yu, R.K. Koski, R.G. Saul, and P. Cronin.** 1994. Starburst™ dendrimers: enhanced performance and flexibility for immunoassays. Clin. Chem. *40*:1845-1849.

44. **Sklarew, R.J., S.C. Bodmer, and L.P. Pertschuk.** 1990. Quantitative imaging of immunocytochemical (PAP) estrogen receptor staining patterns in breast cancer sections. Cytometry *11*:359-378.

45. **Slinkin, M.A., C. Curtet, C. Sai-Maurel, J.F. Gestin, V.P. Torchilin, and J.F. Chatal.** 1992. Site-specific conjugation of chain-terminal chelating polymers to Fab' fragments of anti-CEA mAb: effect of linkage type and polymer size on conjugate biodistribution in nude mice bearing human colorectal carcinoma. Bioconjug. Chem. *3*:477-483.

46. **Stein, J.P., D.A. Ginsberg, G.D. Grossfeld, S.J. Chatterjee, D. Esrig, M.G. Dickinson, S. Groshen, C.R. Taylor, P.A. Jones, D.G. Skinner, and R.J. Cote.** 1998. Effect of p21WAF1/CIP1 expression on tumor progression in bladder cancer. J. Natl. Cancer Inst. *90*:1072-1079.

47. **Taylor, C.R.** 1992. Report of the Immunohistochemistry Steering Committee of the Biological Stain Commission. "Proposed Format: Package Insert for Immunohistochemistry Products". Biotech. Histochem. *67*:323-338.

47a. **Taylor, C.R.** 1992. Quality assurance and standardization in immunohistochemistry. A proposal for the annual meeting of the Biological Stain Commission, June, 1991. Biotech. Histochem. *67*:110-117.

48. **Taylor, C.R.** 1994. An exaltation of experts: concerted efforts in the standardization of immunohistochemistry. Hum. Pathol. *25*:2-11.

49. **Taylor, C.R.** 1994. The current role of immunohistochemistry in diagnostic pathology. Adv. Pathol. Lab. Med. *7*:59-105.

50. **Taylor, C.R. and R.J. Cote. (Eds.).** 1994. Immunomicroscopy: A Diagnostic Tool for the Surgical Pathologist. 2nd ed., p. 1-70. W.B. Saunders, Philadelphia.

51. **Taylor, C.R., S.R. Shi, and R.J. Cote.** 1996. Antigen retrieval for immunohistochemistry. Status and need for greater standardization. Appl. Immunohistochem. *4*:144-166.

52. **Trutrumi, Y., A. Serwaza, and K. Kawai.** 1995. Enhanced polymer one-step staining (EPOS) for proliferating cell nuclear antigen (PCNA) and Ki-67 antigen: application to intra-operative frozen diagnosis. Pathol. Int. *45*:108-115.

53. **van der Ploeg, M., and W.A.L. Duijndam.** 1986. Matrix models. Essential tools for microscopic cytochemical research. Histochemistry *84*:283-300.

54. **van Diest, P.J., P. van Dam, S.C. Henzen-Lognans, E. Berns, M.E.L. van der Burg, J. Green, and I. Vergote.** 1997. A scoring system for immunohistochemical staining: consensus report of the task force for basic research of the EORTC-GCCG. J. Clin. Pathol. *50*:801-804.

55. **Vyberg, M. and S. Nielsen.** 1998. Dextran polymer conjugate two-step visualization system for immunohistochemistry. Appl. Immunohistochem. *6*:3-10.

56. **Watanabe, J., K. Kanai, and S. Kanamura.** 1991. Measurement of NADPH-ferrihemoprotein reductase content in sections of liver. J. Histochem. Cytochem. *39*:1635-1643.

57. **Watanabe, J., Y. Asaka, and S. Kanamura.** 1996. Relationship between immunostaining intensity and antigen content in sections. J. Histochem. Cytochem. *44*:1451-1458.

58. **Weinberg, D.S.** 1994. Quantitative immunocytochemistry in pathology, p. 235-260. *In* A.M. Marchevsky and P.H. Bartels (Eds.), Image Analysis: A Primer for Pathologists. Raven Press, New York.

59. **Wicht, H., E. Maronde, J. Olcese, and H.-W. Korf.** 1999. A semiquantitative image-analytical method for the recording of dose-response curves in immunocytochemical preparations. J. Histochem. Cytochem. *47*:411-419.

60. **Wisecarver, J.L.** 1999. HER-2/neu testing comes of age. Am. J. Clin. Pathol. *111*:299-301.

Section V

Nonheating Antigen Retrieval Technique

Nonheating Antigen Retrieval Techniques for Light and Electron Microscopic Immunolabeling

17

Jürgen Roth, Martin Ziak, and Bruno Guhl

Division of Cell and Molecular Pathology, Department of Pathology, University of Zürich, Zürich, Switzerland

INTRODUCTION

Immunohistochemical localization of protein and carbohydrate epitopes by monoclonal and polyclonal antibodies in cells and tissues has become an indispensable routine technique in research and diagnostics. For the preservation of the cellular and histologic details, chemical fixation by aldehydes represents the most commonly used procedure. Furthermore, combined aldehyde-osmium tetroxide fixation is generally applied in diagnostic electron microscopy. The adverse effects on protein conformation of chemical fixation, as well as of tissue dehydration by nonpolar and polar organic solvents at ambient temperature and embedding in wax or resins at elevated temperatures, are well known. As a consequence, the reactivity of antibodies with their respective protein antigens can be influenced at varying degrees and may be abolished in extreme cases (6,13,27). Hence, much effort has been directed to work out conditions that would at least partially overcome the deleterious effects of fixation, dehydration, and embedding. Thus, polyclonal antibodies were raised against the formaldehyde-treated antigen to improve their reactivity toward formaldehyde-exposed cellular components (16). Furthermore, low-denaturing dehydration and embedding protocols have been developed using various Lowicryl (9,10,43,45) and LR resins (36,37) for aldehyde-fixed materials. The adverse effects of dehydration and embedding can be circumvented by the preparation of frozen tissue sections, but usually at the expense of recognition of tissue structure details. Although they provide the least of denaturing conditions, the techniques of physical fixation by ultra-rapid freezing, followed by freeze substitution and resin embedding at low temperature, are not suitable for routine immunolabeling (18,21,31,33). Last but not least, to overcome the various negative effects of tissue processing for immunohistochemistry, various approaches to signal amplification have been published and applied sucess-

Antigen Retrieval Techniques
Edited by Shan-Rong Shi, Jiang Gu, and Clive R. Taylor
©2000 Eaton Publishing, Natick, MA

fully (1,2,19,32,47,53).

A completely different strategy was introduced in 1991 by Shi and colleagues (49) for reversing the effects of formaldehyde fixation and paraffin embedding. They subjected tissue sections to microwave oven heating prior to immunohistochemical staining. Currently, it is the most widely employed technique for antigen retrieval in paraffin sections and as such has permitted a breakthrough in the application of immunohistochemistry to diagnostic pathology (50,53).

This chapter presents various nonheating antigen retrieval techniques and their application to light and electron microscopic immunolabeling. These procedures can be classified as antigen demasking techniques and may provide tools complementary to those of antigen retrieval by heating.

PROTOCOLS

Protocol for Protease Digestion of Paraffin Sections

As a consequence of formaldehyde-induced cross-linking of proteins, a highly dense protein scaffold results, which can sterically hinder the accessibility of antigens for antibodies. Treatment of deparaffinized and rehydrated sections with proteases has been applied to render the protein-masked antigens accessible (11,20,41).

Materials and Reagents

Prepare the pepsin solution by dissolving 40 mg of pepsin in 100 mL 0.01 N HCl. Likewise, dissolve 10 mg of trypsin in 100 mL of 0.1 mol/L Tris-buffered saline (pH 7.8).

Procedure

1. Deparaffinize sections.
2. Place sections in water.
3. Incubate sections with protease solution for 20 to 30 minutes at 37°C.
4. Wash sections in three changes of Tris-buffered isotonic saline (pH 7.4).

Comments

No special precautions need to be taken. Tests with varying periods of digestion times are recommended.

Protocol for Etching Techniques for Resin Sections

Many embedding resins, such as epoxide- or conventional methacrylate-based ones, are chemically highly reactive and will also form covalent links with the biologic matter to be embedded. In semithin and ultrathin sections, due to the high degree of cross-linking between the resin and the tissue, exposure of antigenic sites on the section surface may therefore be highly limited. To reverse this effect, different etching techniques for partial or complete removal of the resin are available, using hydrogen peroxide or alcoholic sodium hydroxide and alcoholic potassium hydroxide (4,12,26,28,30,35). The procedures can be applied to both semithin and ultrathin sections.

Materials and Reagents

The hydrogen peroxide solution should be freshly prepared from 30% hydrogen peroxide stored in plastic bottles in a refrigerator. Alkaline alcohol solutions are prepared as follows. Two grams of KOH pellets are dissolved in 10 mL of absolute methanol and 5 mL of propylenoxide in a glass beaker using a magnetic stirrer. Likewise, 2 g of NaOH pellets are dissolved in 10 mL of ethanol and 5 mL of propylenoxide. The mixture is then filtered through ordinary filter paper and used.

Procedure

1. Semithin sections are mounted on glass slides and dried at 40°C in an oven overnight. Adherence of the semithin sections may be improved by using Superfrost Plus glass slides (Merck, Darmstadt, Germany). Ultrathin sections are placed on parlodion/carbon-coated nickel or copper grids.

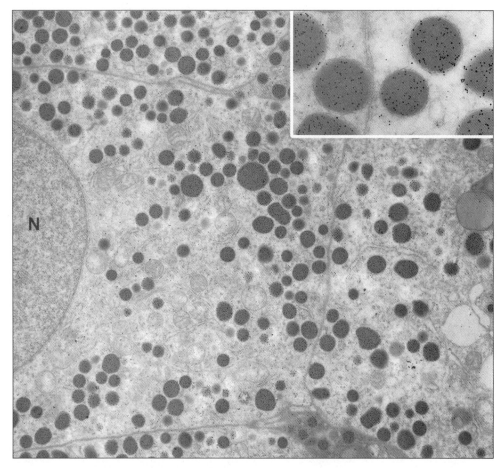

Figure 1. Human pituitary adenoma fixed with 2% glutaraldehyde and 1% osmium tetroxide and embedded in Epon. Ultrathin sections were pretreated with 1% periodic acid for 4 minutes and then incubated with an antibody to reveal growth hormone with the protein A-gold technique (44). Gold particle labeling is concentrated over electron-dense core secretory granules. The inset shows double protein A-gold labeling to reveal growth hormone (large gold particles) and prolactin (small gold particles).

2. Semithin sections on glass slides are covered with a large volume of 10% hydrogen peroxide for 5 to 10 minutes at ambient temperature, or one of the above-described alkaline alcohol solutions for 2 to 5 minutes. Grids with the attached ultrathin sections are floated on a large droplet of etching solution for 5 to 10 minutes (hydrogen peroxide) or only a few seconds (alkaline alcohol solutions).
3. After hydrogen peroxide etching, semithin and ultrathin sections are rapidly washed with isotonic phosphate-buffered saline (PBS; 10 mmol/L phosphate buffer, pH 7.2 to 7.4, 0.15 mol/L NaCl). Following etching with either of the alkaline alcohol solutions, grids with the attached ultrathin sections are rapidly washed by transferring them to a series of droplets of PBS. However, semithin sections are first rinsed with 50% alcohol and then with PBS, to prevent detachment of the semithin sections.

Comments

Appropriate precautions should be taken when working with hydrogen peroxide. Due care should be exercised in the preparation and use of the alkaline alcohol solutions, since the reaction is exothermic and the mixture highly volatile. Only freshly prepared mixtures should be used. Prevent any contact with the highly agressive alkaline solution. Furthermore, the etching (removal) of the resin must be carefully controlled, since prolonged treatment will result in damage of the tissue structure, decreased immunolabeling, and increased background staining. This may be especially critical for the treatment of ultrathin sections. Establishment of the optimal conditions is recommended, depending on the embedding resin and the antigen to be demonstrated.

The etching procedures are not applicable for sections of Lowicryl K4M-embedded tissues, because the UV irradiation-initiated polymerization results in a saturated vinyl type of carbon-to-carbon backbone (9) that is resistant to any of the above-mentioned etching solutions. However, an important aspect of the free radical polymerization is the very weak bonding of the resin with the biologic material. This results in a section surface relief with exposed biologic matter (24), which permits highly favorable conditions for immunolabeling on semithin and ultrathin sections (25,43,45,51).

Protocol for Oxidation Techniques

Double fixation with glutaraldehyde and osmium tetroxide, followed by Epon embedding, usually precludes any possibility of immunolabeling. However, pretreatment of sections with strongly oxidizing reagents offers a possibility of overcoming this problem in many instances and provides a means to perform retrospective studies (4,5,12,46). The mechanism by which the oxidizing agents reverse the effect of osmium tetroxide fixation is unclear.

Materials and Reagents

Prepare a saturated solution of sodium metaperiodate in distilled water, and store it at room temperature. Wrap the glassware containing the solution with aluminum foil to protect it from light. The sodium metaperiodate solution should be freshly prepared every 2 weeks. A 1% periodic acid solution in distilled water should be freshly prepared before use.

Procedure

1. Place grids with attached thin sections on a droplet of a saturated aqueous solution of sodium metaperiodate for 30 to 60 minutes at ambient temperature, or on a droplet of 1% periodic acid for 4 minutes at ambient temperature.
2. Wash sections thoroughly with distilled water (5–10 changes for 5 min each).

Comments

Due care should be exercised when working with strong oxidants. Crystalline sodium metaperiodate ages with time of storage.

The procedure has been shown to be most effective in the demonstration of enzymes and hormones (Figure 1) stored at high concentrations in secretory granules (5,17,46) but has also provided excellent results in the demonstration of low-molecular-weight neurotransmitters (39).

Protocol for Sodium Dodecyl Sulfate Treatment

Based on the observation that antibodies may react with sodium dodecyl sulfate (SDS)-denatured proteins on immunoblots but only weakly or not at all when applied to immunohistochemistry, Brown and colleagues (8) have explored the effect of SDS treatment of sections and cell cultures for immunohistochemistry. They found that SDS treatment of cryostate sections from paraformaldehyde-lysine periodate-fixed tissues, and of cell cultures, resulted in a dramatic increase in staining intensity. Meanwhile, the technique has been applied to ultrathin cryosections of formaldehyde-fixed tissue for immunogold labeling (29).

Materials and Reagents

Prepare a 1% solution of SDS in PBS (pH 7.2).

Procedure

1. Encircle tissue sections with a peroxidase-anti-peroxidase (PAP) pen to prevent spreading of the incubation solutions.
2. Cover cryostate sections with 1% SDS in PBS for 5 minutes at ambient temperature. Cell cultures grown on coverslips are SDS-treated face down on Parafilm® for 5 minutes after optional permeabilization with 0.1% Triton® X-100. Ultrathin cryosections attached to grids are placed on droplets of 1% SDS in PBS containing 1% bovine serum albumin for 1 minute.
3. Wash the sections three times for 5 minutes each in PBS in a Coplin jar and proceed as for immunolabeling. Coverslips with the cultured cells are washed either in petri dishes filled with PBS or on droplets of PBS on Parafilm. Ultrathin cryosections are washed three times with PBS containing 1% bovine serum albumin.

Comments

Brown and colleagues (8) emphasize that due care should be exercised to prevent drying of the sections or cell cultures, since SDS treatment makes them hydrophobic.

For this reason, the slides are placed horizontally during the entire procedure. They also point out that thorough washing of the sections is required to remove any SDS remaining free in solution, which otherwise may denature the antibodies. Control slides not exposed to SDS have to be washed in separate containers. Adverse effects of SDS treatment were occasionally observed, such as loss of Golgi staining for the AE1 anion exchanger in kidney epithelia and prevention of rhodamine-phalloidin binding to actin.

Protocol for Low-pH Treatment

Formaldehyde at concentrations above 2%, as commonly used for tissue fixation, exists in two forms: partially as the hydrated monomer and partially in the form of divalent reactive polyacetals of different lengths (13,40,52). While the monomer reacts with neighboring amino groups of amino acids to form methylene bridges, the polyacetals react preferentially with the ε-amino groups of lysine to form polymethylether cross-links. Although these links are stable against heat at pH 7.0, polymethylether cross-links depolymerize in an acidic mileu (3,42,52). Recently, acidic milieu treatment of ultrathin cryosections, prepared from formaldehyde-glutaraldehyde-fixed tissue, has been shown to improve the intensity of immunogold labeling (14) (Figure 2).

Materials and Reagents

Prepare a 50 mmol/L phosphate buffer, pH 5.5.

Procedure

1. Place grids with attached ultrathin cryosections on droplets of 50 mmol/L phosphate buffer (pH 5.5) for 2 hours at 37°C in a moist chamber.
2. Wash the sections by floating the grids on three consecutive droplets of PBS (pH 7.4).

Comments

Although phosphate buffer adjusted to pH 5.5 has only limited buffering capacity, its use over citrate and acetate buffers was advantageous, since the use of these buffers frequently resulted in the formation of disturbing electron-dense precipitates. Thus far, the low-pH pretreatment has been applied to the study of membrane proteins by immunogold electron microscopy, and its general usefulness remains to be demonstrated. Likewise, its effect on only formaldehyde-fixed tissue remains to be further explored and extended to sections of paraffin-embedded tissues. By applying silver-intensified immunogold labeling to paraffin sections, no improvement of immunolabeling intensity for megalin could be observed. It is not clear, however, whether the retrieval effect of the low-pH treatment was obscured by the enhancement of the immunogold labeling by silver intensification.

Protocol for N-glycosidase F Treatment

Aberrant glycosylation, due to simplified synthesis of O-linked oligosaccharides of glycoproteins, has been observed in a variety of cancers (15,34,38). Some of these glycotopes have become of importance since they are used in the diagnosis of carcinoma and may have a value as prognosticators (7,22,23). In general, such *O*-linked oligosaccharides are not as elaborate in structure as *N*-linked oligosaccharides and might be hidden, so that antibody binding may be sterically hindered. That such an effect exists could be demonstrated, since enzymatic removal of *N*-linked oligosaccharides brought about a dramatic increase in specificity and intensity of immunolabeling of a sugar moiety present in *O*-linked oligosaccharides (14).

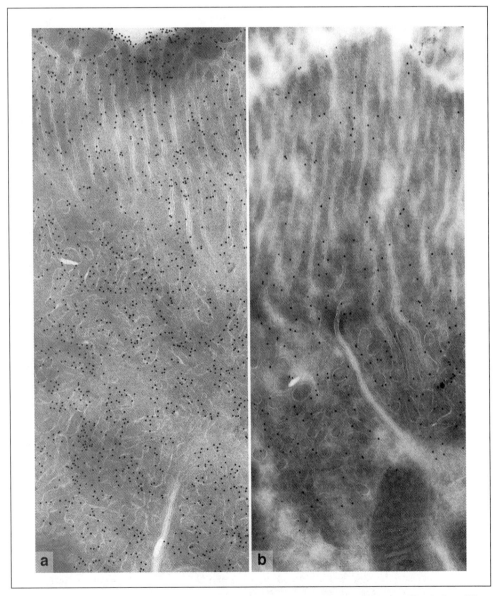

Figure 2. Demonstration of megalin in rat proximal tubular epithelia with the protein A-gold technique. Ultrathin frozen sections were prepared from 3% formaldehyde/0.01% glutaraldehyde perfusion-fixed kidney. (a) This section was subjected to low-pH pretreatment at pH 5.5 and exhibits a much stronger labeling for megalin in the brush border and tubulovesicular endosomal system than the section shown in panel b. (b) This section was not subjected to low-pH treatment.

Materials and Reagents

Prepare a solution of 0.25 or 0.5 U of *N*-glycosidase F of *Flavobacterium meningosepticum* from recombinant *Escherichia coli* (Roche Molecular Biochemicals, Mannheim, Germany) in phosphate buffer (50 mmol/L, pH 7.4), as recommended by the manufacturer.

Procedure

1. Incubate tissue sections with *N*-glycosidase F in a moist chamber at 37°C. Deparaffinized and rehydrated tissue sections are incubated with 0.25 U enzyme/mL overnight and ultrathin cryosections with 0.5 U enzyme/mL for 4 hours.
2. Wash sections first briefly with enzyme incubation buffer and condition with PBS containing 1% bovine serum albumin, 0.05% Triton X-100, and 0.05% Tween® 20 for 20 minutes. (Use 0.01% of both Triton X-100 and Tween 20 for ultrathin cryosections.)

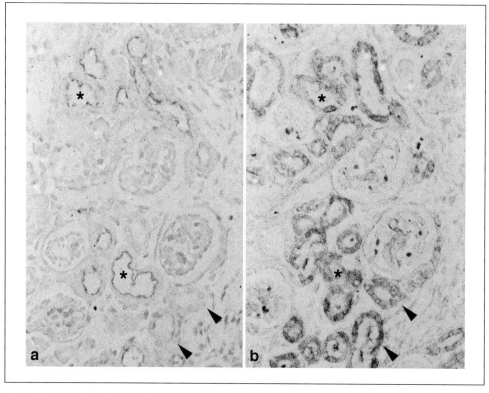

Figure 3. Immunohistochemical demonstration of oligo/poly α2,8 KDN in consecutive serial paraffin sections of 5-day-old rat kidney with the use of an IgM type monoclonal antibody. (a) Pretreatment of a paraffin section with *N*-glycosidase F results in a distinct labeling of the brush border region and apical cytoplasm of convoluted proximal tubules, some of which are labeled by an asterisk. (b) A section not pretreated with *N*-glycosidase F, but otherwise incubated like the section shown in panel a, exhibits diffuse cytoplasmic labeling in the convoluted proximal tubules (asterisks) and additional nonspecific labeling over other tubular profiles, some of which are labeled with arrowheads. Note that these tubules are unlabeled in the section pretreated with *N*-glycosidase F (arrowheads in panel a).

Comments

Treatment of sections with *N*-glycosidase F results in complete removal of *N*-linked oligosaccharide side chains, since the enzyme acts at the asparagine–*N*-acetyl-glucosamine core linkage, leaving the *O*-linked oligosaccharide side chains intact and exposed. Consequently, the binding of monoclonal anti-carbohydrate antibodies reacting with moities present in *O*-linked oligosaccharide side chains seems to be facilitated, especially if they are of IgM type. In addition to an increase in labeling intensity for oligo/poly α2,8 KDN present on *O*-linked oligosaccharide side chains of megalin (54), a remarkable improvement in localization specificity was observed (Figure 3). The efficiency of the *N*-glycosidase F treatment can be controlled by incubation of an enzyme-treated section with concanavalin A (48).

CONCLUDING REMARKS

The spectrum of nonheating antigen retrieval techniques described in this chapter represent procedures that result in the unmasking of hidden antigens. They have been successfully applied in many laboratories for immunohistochemical studies applying indirect immunofluorescence, indirect immunoperoxidase, and indirect immunogold labeling. The latter approach, in conjunction with oxidation techniques, has the advantage of being useful not only for light but also for electron microscopic studies and allows retrospective studies on aldehyde-osmium-fixed and Epon-embedded surgical specimens. Altogether, the techniques covered in this chapter provide useful methods that are complementary to heating retrieval techniques.

REFERENCES

1. **Adams, J.** 1981. Heavy metal intensification of DAB-based HRP reaction product. J. Histochem. Cytochem. *29*:775.
2. **Adams, J.** 1992. Biotin amplification of biotin and horseradish peroxidase signals in histochemical stains. J. Histochem. Cytochem. *40*:1457-1463.
3. **Baschong, W., C. Baschong-Prescianotto, and E. Kellenberger.** 1983. Reversible fixation for the study of morphology and macromolecular composition of fragile biological structures. Eur. J. Cell Biol. *32*:1-6.
4. **Baskin, D., S. Erlandsen, and J. Parsons.** 1979. Influence of hydrogen peroxide or alcoholic sodium hydroxide on the immunohistochemical detection of growth hormone and prolaction after osmium fixation. J. Histochem. Cytochem. *27*:1290-1292.
5. **Bendayan, M. and M. Zollinger.** 1983. Ultrastructural localization of antigenic sites on osmium-fixed tissues applying the protein A-gold technique. J. Histochem. Cytochem. *31*:101-109.
6. **Brandtzaeg, P.** 1982. Tissue preparation methods for immunohistochemistry, p. 275. *In* G.R. Bullock and P. Petrusz (Eds.), Techniques in Immunocytochemistry, Vol. 1. Academic Press, London.
7. **Brockhausen, I.** 1993. Clinical aspects of glycoprotein biosynthesis. Crit. Rev. Clin. Lab Sci. *30*:65-151.
8. **Brown, D., J. Lydon, M. McLaughlin, S.A. Tilley, R. Tyszkowski, and S. Alper.** 1996. Antigen retrieval in cryostat tissue sections and cultured cells by treatment with sodium dodecyl sulfate (SDS). Histochem. Cell Biol. *105*:261-267.
9. **Carlemalm, E., R.M. Garavito, and W. Villiger.** 1982. Resin development for electron microscopy and an analysis of embedding at low temperature. J. Microsc. *126*:123-143.
10. **Carlemalm, E. and W. Villiger.** 1989. Low temperature embedding, p. 29-45. *In* G.R. Bullock and P. Petrusz (Eds.), Techniques in Immunocytochemistry, Vol. 4. Academic Press, London.
11. **Curran, R. and J. Gregory.** 1977. Demonstration of immunoglobulin in cryostat and paraffin sections of human tonsil by immunofluorescence and immunoperoxidase rtechniques. Effects of processing on immunohistochemical performance of tissues and the use of proteolytic enzymes to unmask antigens in sections. J. Clin. Pathol. *31*:974-983.
12. **Erlandsen, S., J. Parsons, and C. Rodning.** 1979. Technical parameters of immunostaining of osmicated tissue in epoxy sections. J. Histochem. Cytochem. *27*:1286-1289.

13. **Griffiths, G.** 1993. Fine Structure Immunocytochemistry. Springer-Verlag, Berlin.

14. **Guhl, B., M. Ziak, and J. Roth.** 1998. Unconventional antigen retrieval for carbohydrate and protein antigens. Histochem. Cell Biol. *110*:603-611.

15. **Hakomori, S.-I.** 1996. Tumor-associated carbohydrate antigens and modified blood group antigens, p. 243-276. *In* J. Montreuil, J. Vliegenthart, and H. Schachter (Eds.), Glycoproteins and Disease. Elsevier, Amsterdam.

16. **Harrach, B. and K. Robeneck.** 1990. Polyclonal antibodies against formaldehyde-modified apolipoprotein A-1. An approach to circumvent fixation-induced loss of antigenicity in immunohistochemistry. Arteriosclerosis *10*:564-576.

17. **Heitz, P., A. Landolt, H. Zenklusen, M. Kasper, J. Reubi, M. Oberholzer, and J. Roth.** 1987. Immunocytochemistry of pituitary tumors. J. Histochem. Cytochem. *35*:1005-1011.

18. **Heuser, J., T. Reese, M. Dennis, Y. Jan, C. Jan, and L. Evans.** 1979. Synaptic vesicle exocytosis captured by quick freezing and correlated with quantal transmitter release. J. Cell Biol. *81*:275-300.

19. **Holgate, C.S., P. Jackson, P.N. Cowen, and C.C. Bird.** 1983. Immunogold-silver staining: new method of immunostaining with enhanced sensitivity. J. Histochem. Cytochem. *31*:938-944.

20. **Huang, S., H. Minassian, and J. More.** 1976. Application of immunofluorescent staining on paraffin sections improved by trypsin digestion. Lab. Invest. *35*:383.

21. **Humbel, B. and H. Schwarz.** 1989. Freeze-substitution for immunochemistry, p. 115-134. *In* A. Verkleij and J. Leunissen (Eds.), Immuno-Gold Labeling in Cell Biology. CRC Press, Boca Raton.

22. **Itzkowitz, S.H., E.J. Bloom, W.A. Kokal, G. Modin, S. Hakomori, and Y.S. Kim.** 1990. Sialosyl-Tn. A novel mucin antigen associated with prognosis of colorectal cancer patients. Cancer *66*:1960-1966.

23. **Karlen, P., E. Young, O. Brostrom, R. Lofberg, B. Tribukait, A. Ost, C. Bodian, and S. Itzkowitz.** 1998. Sialyl-Tn antigen as a marker of colon cancer risk in ulcerative colitis: relation to dysplasia and DNA aneuploidy. Gastroenterology *115*:1395-1404.

24. **Kellenberger, E., W. Villiger, and E. Carlemalm.** 1986. The influence of the surface relief of thin sections of embedded, unstained biological material on image quality. Micron Microsc. Acta *4*:331-348.

25. **Kellenberger, E., M. Dürrenberger, W. Villiger, E. Carlemalm, and M. Wurtz.** 1987. The efficiency of immunolabel on Lowicryl sections compared to theoretical predictions. J. Histochem. Cytochem. *35*:959-969.

26. **Kuffler, D., J. Nicholls, and P. Drapeau.** 1987. Transmitter localization and vesicle turnover at a serotinergic synapse between identified leech neurons in culture. J. Comp. Neurol. *256*:516-526.

27. **Larsson, L.** 1988. Immunocytochemistry: Theory and Practice. CRC Press, Boca Raton.

28. **Mar, H. and T. White.** 1988. Colloidal gold immunostaining on deplasticized ultra-thin sections. J. Histochem. Cytochem. *36*:1387-1395.

29. **Maunsbach, A. and B. Afzelius.** 1999. Biomedical Electron Microscopy. Illustrated Methods and Interpretations. Academic Press, San Diego.

30. **Maxwell, M.** 1978. Two rapid and simple methods used for the removal of resins from 1.0 μm thick epoxy sections. J. Microsc. *112*:253-255.

31. **McCann, J., D. Maddox, S.L. Mount, R. Hong, and D. Taatjes.** 1996. Cryofixation, cryosubstitution, and immunoelectron microscopy: potential role in diagnostic pathology. Ultrastruct. Pathol. *20*:223-230.

32. **Merz, H., R. Malisius, S. Mannweiler, R. Zhou, W. Hartmann, K. Orscheschek, P. Moubayed, and A. Feller.** 1995. Immunomax: a maximized immunohistochemical method for the retrtieval and enhancement of hidden antigens. Lab. Invest. *73*:149-156.

33. **Müller, M. and H. Moor.** 1984. Cryofixation of thick specimens by high pressure freezing, p. 131-181. *In* J. Revel, T. Barnard, and G. Haggis (Eds.), The Science of Biological Specimen Preparation. SEM Inc., AMF O'Hare, Chicago.

34. **Muramatsu, T.** 1993. Carbohydrate signals in metastasis and prognosis of human carcinomas. Glycobiology *3*:294-296.

35. **Nakane, P.** 1971. Application of peroxidase-labeled antibodies to the intracellular localization of hormones. Acta Endocrinol. *153* (Suppl):190-204.

36. **Newman, G.R., B. Jasani, and E.D. Williams.** 1983. A simple post-embedding system for the rapid demonstration of tissue antigens under the electron microscope. Histochem. J. *15*:543-555.

37. **Newman, G. and J. Hobot.** 1987. Modern acrylics for post-embedding immunostaining techniques. J. Histochem. Cytochem. *35*:971-981.

38. **Orntoft, T.F. and E.M. Vestergaard.** 1999. Clinical aspects of altered glycosylation of glycoproteins in cancer. Electrophoresis *20*:362-371.

39. **Ottersen, O.** 1987. Postembedding light- and electron microscopic immunocytochemistry of amino acids: description of a new model system allowing identical conditions for specificity testing and tissue processing. Exp. Brain Res. *69*:167-174.

40. **Puchtler, H. and S. Meloan.** 1985. On the chemistry of formaldehyde fixation and its effects on immunohistochemical reactions. Histochemistry *82*:201-204.

41. **Reading, M.** 1977. A digestion technique for the reduction of background staining in the immunoperoxidase method. J. Clin. Pathol. *30*:88-90.

42. **Ris, H.** 1978. Preparation of chromatin and chromosomes for electron microscopy, p. 229-246. *In* G. Stein, J. Stein, and I.I. Kleinsmiths (Eds.), Meth. Cell Biol., Vol. XVIII. Academic Press, New York.

43. **Roth, J.** 1989. Postembedding labeling on Lowicryl K4M tissue sections: detection and modification of cellular components, p. 513-551. *In* A.M. Tartakoff (Ed.), Meth. Cell Biol., Vol. 31. Academic Press, San Diego.

44. **Roth, J., M. Gendayan, and L. Orci.** 1978. Ultrastructural localization of intracellular antigens by the use of protein A-gold complex. J. Histochem. Cytochem. *26*:1074-1081.

45. **Roth, J., M. Bendayan, E. Carlemalm, W. Villiger, and M. Garavito.** 1981. Enhancement of ultrastructural preservation and immunocytochemical staining in low temperature-embedded pancreatic tissue. J. Histochem. Cytochem. *29*:633-671.

46. **Roth, J., M. Kasper, P.U. Heitz, and F. Labat.** 1985. What's new in light and electron microscopic immunocytochemistry? Application of the protein A-gold technique to routinely processed tissue. Pathol. Res. Pract. *180*:711-717.

47. **Roth, J. and M.J. Warhol.** 1992. Immunogold silver staining techniques for high resolution immunohistochemistry in clinical materials, p. 2-23. *In* G. Bullock, D. Van Velzen, and M.J. Warhol (Eds.), Techniques in Diagnostic Pathology, Vol. 3. Academic Press, London.

48. **Roth, J., C. Zuber, T. Sata, and W.-P. Li.** 1998. Lectin-gold histochemistry on paraffin and lowicryl K4M sections using biotin and digoxigenin-conjugated lectins, p. 41-53. *In* J.M. Rhodes and J.D. Milton (Eds.), Methods Molecular Biology Series. Humana Press, Totowa, NJ.

49. **Shi, S.-R., M. Key, and K. Kalra.** 1991. Antigen retrieval in formalin-fixed, paraffin-embedded tissues: an enhancement method for immunohistochemical staining based on microwave oven heating of tissue sections. J. Histochem. Cytochem. *39*:741-748.

50. **Shi, S.-R., R. Cote, and C. Taylor.** 1997. Antigen retrieval immunohistochemistry: past, present, and future. J. Histochem. Cytochem. *45*:327-343.

51. **Taatjes, D.J., U. Schaub, and J. Roth.** 1987. Light microscopical detection of antigens and lectin binding sites with gold-labelled reagents on semi-thin Lowicryl K4M sections: usefulness of the photochemical silver reaction for signal amplification. Histochem. J. *19*:235-245.

52. **Tomé, D., N. Naulet, and G.J. Martin.** 1982. Application de la RMN à l'étude des réactions du formaldehyde avec les fonctions aminées de l'alanine et de la lysine en fonction du pH du milieu. J. Chim. Phys. *79*:361-368.

53. **Werner, M., R. Von Wasielewski, and P. Komminoth.** 1996. Antigen retrieval, signal amplification and intensification in immunohistochemistry. Histochem. Cell Biol. *105*:253-260.

54. **Ziak, M., D. Kerjaschki, M.G. Farquhar, and J. Roth.** 1999. Identification of megalin as the sole rat kidney sialoglycoprotein containing poly alpha 2,8 deaminomeuraminic acid. J. Am. Soc. Nephrol. *10*:203-209.

Antigen Retrieval Immuno-histochemistry Used for Routinely Processed Celloidin-Embedded Human Temporal Bone Sections

18

Shan-Rong Shi, Richard J. Cote, and Clive R. Taylor

Department of Pathology, University of Southern California Keck School of Medicine, Los Angeles, CA, USA

INTRODUCTION

Human temporal bone collection has contributed invaluable knowledge of otopathology in terms of etiology, diagnosis, and therapy of ear diseases since early in this century (58,60). Following the work of early pioneers, Schuknecht (57–61) established a productive temporal bone laboratory and made significant morphologic observations linked to clinicopathologic interpretations extending over more than 30 years. His achievements have been summarized in the second edition of *Pathology of the Ear* (60), an excellent book illustrating his philosophical contribution to the development of modern otopathology based on translation of research information from the basic sciences to the clinical study of ear disease. The importance of immunohistochemistry (IHC) as applied in human temporal bone study was emphasized at the Human Temporal Bone Research Workshop in 1988 (12).

IHC was first applied to otopathology in 1976 (38). Subsequent studies of cytoskeletal elements were carried out in animal or human materials by using fresh tissue and modified fixation and processing methods (4,5,11,18,35,54,62,64,65,75). The range of immunohistochemical stains was expanded to the study of neurotransmitters of auditory and vestibular nerve systems (3,6,17,28,88,89), immunoglobulins and immunocompetent cells in the endolymphatic sac (2,13,22,31,36,79,98,), viruses and other proteins in otosclerosis, etc. (7,8,10,16,26,39,43,56,90,92,94).

Antigen Retrieval Techniques
Edited by Shan-Rong Shi, Jiang Gu, and Clive R. Taylor
©2000 Eaton Publishing, Natick, MA

In the search for successful immunohistochemical staining of human temporal bone, investigation was related to modified methods of fixation and tissue processing, including microdissection and frozen sections (10,28,92). Wackym et al. (94) used immunoelectron microscopy with a protein A-colloidal gold method and a single antibody (to type I collagen) based on a technique of re-embedding celloidin sections of human temporal bone (53,59). However, this method was not adaptable to the performance of IHC studies on routine formalin-fixed, acid-decalcified, celloidin-embedded human temporal bone tissue by light microscopy. Thus, an urgent need existed to develop an immunohistochemical staining technique that could be used for routinely processed, celloidin-embedded human temporal bone sections.

In the early 1990s, the antigen retrieval (AR) technique, both high-temperature heating and a nonheating AR method of immersing celloidin sections in a sodium hydroxide-methanol solution, was successfully developed, as described in Chapter 1.

Application of AR-IHC to routinely processed celloidin-embedded human temporal bone sections began at the House Ear Institute in Los Angeles promptly after the AR technique was published in the early 1990s (66,67). Several serially designed studies were carried out to standardize AR methods, including the development of a combined heating and nonheating AR method. In addition, several interesting projects were carried out by using the AR-IHC on celloidin human temporal bone sections based on principles of both surgical pathology and translational research between clinical and basic sciences under the guidance of Dr. Linthicum. The nonheating AR technique has also been employed successfully in celloidin-embedded human brain tissue sections by Dr. Jean K. Moore at the House Ear Institute (48,49).

ANTIGEN RETRIEVAL TECHNIQUE

Materials and Reagents

- Commercial charged slides (Fisher Scientific, Pittsburgh, PA, USA), Fisherbrand Superfrost/Plus microscope slides (Fisher)

- 0.1% poly-L-lysine (Sigma, St. Louis, MO, USA)

- Microwave oven: domestic cooking used with maximal energy around 1000 W

- Slide holder and container: Coplin jar or larger plastic or glass containers

- Buffer solutions: citrate, Tris-HCl buffer, or EDTA-NaOH solutions (refer to the Appendix)

Basic Principles of Tissue Section Preparation

Adhesion of celloidin section on slide. Commercial charged slides are recommended for better adhesion of the tissue. Slides coated with either poly-L-lysine or 3-aminopropyltriethoxysilane (APES) are also available. For paraffin-embedded tissue sections, mount the thin section on charged or coated slides and dry the slides at 60°C for 1 hour to ensure adherence of the tissue section. Since the celloidin-embedded tissue section is too thick to stick on the slide, we recommend the following protocol:

1. Wash celloidin-embedded tissue sections in distilled water for 10 minutes and

mount on either 0.1% poly-L-lysine or APES-coated slides by pressing the section down with filter paper and trimming the tissue along the edges of the slides.

2. Place a few drops of 0.1% poly-L-lysine on the slide to cover the whole section,
and dry briefly in an oven. Pay attention to control the optimal time of drying the
sections in the oven. Do not dry excessively.

3. If a heating AR method is desired, mount celloidin sections on charged or coated slides, and set slides in a jar horizontally by overlapping each other. One plain
glass slide is set on the top of the overlapped sections, and a Coplin jar or a glass
bottle filled with distilled water is set on the top of all overlapped slides to prevent tissue sections from detaching by boiling. Then add AR solutions (buffer
solutions at designed pH values or other solutions including distilled water) to a
sufficient volume. After heating, repeat step 2 to stick the heated tissue section
on a slide for the subsequent nonheating AR treatment.

Optimal AR protocol. Although a single AR protocol using either heating or nonheating may yield improved immunostaining results for many antibodies, optimal
protocols may be developed for the strongest immunostaining intensity. For certain
antibodies AR conditions are critical, particularly for quantitative IHC or standardization of routine IHC. This important issue has been addressed elsewhere in this
book (see Chapter 16 and the Appendix).

Control groups. Although most studies report satisfactory results without false
positivity, use caution when performing AR-IHC, to rule out any false positivity or
artificial alteration of the immunostaining pattern (9,72,73,78,85). For example, we
found that weakly positive nuclear staining may be seen with a low-pH AR solution
for monoclonal antibody to MIB-1 (Ki-67) (71–73,82,83,85). Other articles have
reported nonspecific staining or unwanted immunoreactivity with AR-IHC (24,47,
63). Thus, for any antibody tested, knowledge of immunolocalization of the antigen in
frozen fresh tissue is valuable as a gold standard. Otherwise, a frozen tissue section
should be stained simultaneously to validate the immunolocalization obtained in
paraffin section by using AR-IHC. In addition, using celloidin-embedded tissues as
positive and negative controls is important to demonstrate the accuracy of AR-IHC.

Because celloidin-embedded human temporal bone is a limited resource, we recommend establishing a bank of other human tissues processed in the same way as
human temporal bone and embedded in celloidin, to provide a basis for methodologic studies. The advantages of such a control tissue bank include the following: *(i)* a
variety of tissue components can be tested with different antibodies of interest to find
an optimal AR-IHC protocol; and *(ii)* human temporal bone collections can be
reserved for more valuable distinctive usage in IHC or molecular biology studies.

Penido, Tseng, and Kao (unpublished data) reported an interesting study concerning standardization and development of AR methods, based on comparison between
celloidin-embedded human temporal bone and other human tissues, and routinely
processed paraffin-embedded tissues. They demonstrated that the bank of control tissues embedded in celloidin was a valuable AR-IHC resource for comparative studies.
Keithley and Tian (32) studied fibronectin-like immunoreactivity of the basilar membrane of the cochlea of celloidin-embedded human temporal bone sections using a
control tissue of rat cochlea embedded in celloidin or routinely processed and embedded in paraffin. By using this control rat tissue, they developed an optimal AR protocol to study fibronectin immunolocalization for archival celloidin sections of human
temporal bone and to preserve human temporal bone collections for further study.

Nonheating Antigen Retrieval Method

Based on studies by Fraenkel-Conrat and coworkers (19–21), we developed a non-heating AR technique by using sodium hydroxide (NaOH)-methanol as the AR solution for IHC staining on routinely formalin-fixed, acid-decalcified, celloidin-embedded human temporal bone sections. The method is simple and effective for retrieval of a variety of antigens in celloidin-embedded tissue sections. The NaOH-methanol AR solution is prepared by adding 50 to 100 g of NaOH to 500 mL methanol in a brown-colored bottle and mixing vigorously. The solution can be stored at room temperature for longer periods. The clear, saturated solution is diluted 1:3 or 1:5 by the addition of methanol prior to use. Celloidin-embedded tissue sections, prepared as described above, are immersed in the freshly diluted NaOH-methanol solution for 30 minutes. The slides are then rinsed in 100% methanol for 15 minutes twice, 70% methanol for 15 minutes twice, phosphate-buffered saline (PBS) for 15 minutes twice, 0.3% Triton® X-100 for 10 minutes and PBS for 15 minutes. The slides are then ready for the immunostaining procedure (73).

Heating Antigen Retrieval Method

The heating AR technique is a simple method, as described in other chapters and the Appendix. Briefly, immerse the formalin-fixed tissue sections in solution (various buffer solutions used as the AR solution as described in the Appendix and other chapters) and boil slides by microwave, conventional heating, autoclave, pressure cooker, or steamer (84). Critical points for using this heating AR method are as follows: *(i)* never dry the slides during the heating process, *(ii)* maintain the same condition every time in order to have consistent results, and *(iii)* a cooling time is required for better results and for retention of tissue morphology.

Preparation of celloidin sections for heating were performed as mentioned above. Microwave heating time was counted from the boiling point (100°C) for 10 minutes, or for adjusted periods of time according to the optimal protocol.

Combined Antigen Retrieval Method

Combined heating and NaOH-methanol treatment used for celloidin-embedded human temporal bone sections was first documented in 1993 (70). For a sequential AR protocol, first heat the slides by microwave as mentioned above, followed by the adhesion procedure of the celloidin section on a slide, and the nonheating NaOH-methanol treatment described above. Penido, Tseng, and Kao (unpublished data) compared the intensity of AR-IHC between single nonheating AR and combined AR methods and found that 10 of 17 antibodies tested showed stronger AR-IHC intensity by using the combined method (Table 1). Ganbo et al. (23), from Dr. Sando's laboratory, tested the combined method in archival celloidin temporal bone sections using cluster differentiation (CD) markers and demonstrated the following principles: *(i)* in using a reversed sequence of the combined method for the nonheating followed by the heating method, most tissue sections were damaged even at a lower temperature (60°C); and *(ii)* the nonheating AR method of NaOH-methanol solution followed by 0.1% trypsin containing 0.1% $CaCl_2$ (pH 7.8) incubation at 37°C for 5 minutes could improve IHC staining of CD68 and CD3. (Better results of CD3 were obtained with additional AR heating for 5 min prior to trypsin digestion, but this approach was inferior for CD68).

FACTORS THAT INFLUENCE THE EFFECT OF ANTIGEN RETRIEVAL-IMMUNOHISTOCHEMISTRY

Heating Antigen Retrieval Method

Please refer to Chapter 2 for details.

Nonheating Antigen Retrieval Method

Penido, Tseng, and Kao (unpublished data) conducted a study of standardization and development of AR-IHC using routinely celloidin-embedded tissues of human temporal bone, kidney, liver, spleen, adenoids, lung, skin, and intestine, as well as baboon temporal bone. A total of 603 celloidin sections were used. Factors that influenced the results of the nonheating AR method may be summarized as follows:

1. *Concentration of AR solution (NaOH-methanol) and immersion time:* A series of concentrations of NaOH-methanol solutions ranging from 1:3 to 1:160 diluted by 100% methanol was carefully analyzed. The results are summarized in Figure 1. In general, the immunostaining reactivity was correlated with both the concentration and the immersion time in NaOH-methanol solution. The correlation between concentration *(C)* and immersion time *(t)* may be similar to that between heating temperature *(T)* and heating time *(t)*, i.e., $C \times t$ versus $T \times t$. Since the stronger concentration of NaOH-methanol may damage the fine structure of inner ear tissue, more diluted AR solutions with elongated immersion times may be useful for better results. Based on our experiments, we recommend using an NaOH-methanol solution at a ratio of 1:5 for 30 minutes. Although a stronger NaOH-methanol solution such as 1:2 or 1:3 may yield satisfactory intensity of AR-IHC for some antibodies (keratin AE1 and NCL-5D3), comparable results were obtained by the combined method. For some antibodies such as IgG, the combined method showed better immunostaining reactivity than the single nonheating method, even if a stronger NaOH-methanol solution was used. In addition, the stronger NaOH-methanol solution showed damage to the tissue section, or resulted in detachment of the sections from the slides.

2. *Methanol is a better solvent for AR solution of NaOH-methanol:* A comparative study of AR-IHC on celloidin tissue sections used three solutions: NaOH-methanol, NaOH-ethanol, and NaOH-water at the same ratio of 1:5. After immersing the slides in each AR solution for 30 minutes, the slides were rinsed for 20 minutes in two changes of methanol, ethanol, or distilled water, respectively. The immunostaining reactivity obtained by using the NaOH-methanol solution showed the strongest intensity, and the reactivity obtained by ethanol showed a moderate intensity. Immunostaining reactivity was not detected for the celloidin tissue sections treated by the NaOH-water solution. However, a similar strong intensity was achieved by rinsing the slides in methanol with the three different AR solutions (Table 2).

Methanol plays an important role in the de-celloidin from the celloidin-embedded tissue to improve antigen-antibody recognition.

3. *Optimal incubation time of immunostaining on celloidin tissue section after AR:* A comparison of AR-IHC for celloidin tissue sections using different incubation times is summarized in Figure 2. The study demonstrated that an elongated incubation time was necessary to achieve satisfactory results, a finding similar to that incorporated in our protocol documented previously (67–69), i.e., overnight incubation for primary antibody, and 60 minutes for linking and labeling reagents. The reason why

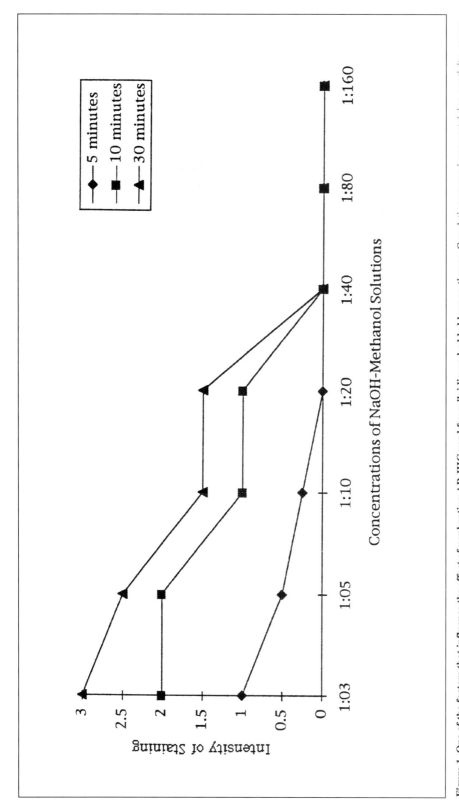

Figure 1. One of the factors that influence the effect of nonheating AR-IHC used for celloidin-embedded human tissues. Correlation among immunostaining reactivity, concentration of the NaOH-methanol solution, and immersion time of celloidin sections (C × t). The stronger the concentration, the shorter the immersion time. Reprinted with permission from Reference 74a.

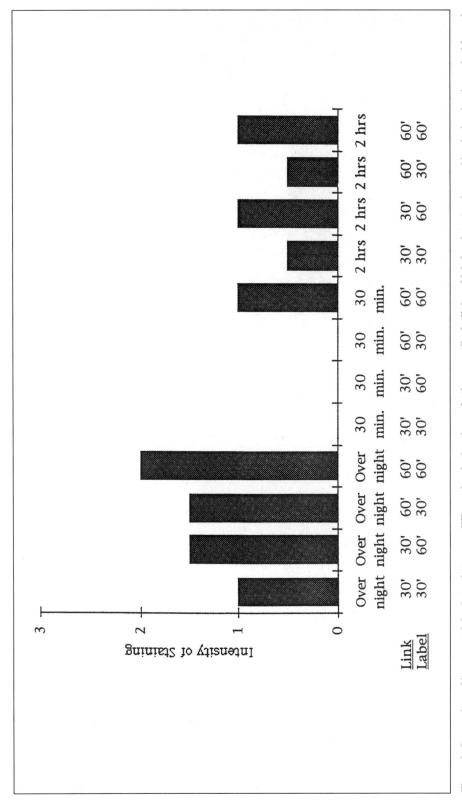

Figure 2. Comparison of immunostaining intensity among different incubation times of primary antibody, link and label moiety. An elongated incubation time is required for each step of incubation to achieve the best result. Reprinted with permission from Reference 74a.

Table 1. Comparison of Immunostaining Intensity between the Nonheating NaOH-Methanol and Combined Methods of Antigen Retrieval

Antibody[a]	Clone	Nonheating Method	Combined Method
Keratin 10, 14/15, 16/17, 19	AE1	+	++
Keratin 8, 18, 19	NCL-5D3	++	+++
Keratin 7	OV-TL 12/30	+	+++
Vimentin	V9	++	+++
Pan-cytokerain	F12-19	++	+++
Keratin (P)		++	+++
SMA	1A4	++	++
α-Tubulin	DM1A	++	+++
β-Tubulin	DM1B	++	++
β-Tubulin II	JDR3B8	+	+++
Lysozyme (P)		++	+++
IgG (P)		+	+++
IgA (P)		+	+
IgM (P)		++	++
CD20	L26	+	+
T cell	MT1	+	+
LCA	2B11&PD7/26	-	-

[a](P), polyclonal antibody (others are monoclonal antibodies); SMA, smooth muscle-specific actin; LCA, leukocyte common antigen. All antibodies were purchased from BioGenex Laboratories (San Ramon, CA, USA), except for IgG from Sigma (St. Louis, MO, USA) and keratin (P) from DAKO (Carpenteria, CA, USA).

a longer incubation time is necessary may relate to the thickness of the celloidin section (20 μm). Remodeling routinely processed celloidin sections into thin sections may permit the incubation time to be shortened, leading to better results of AR-IHC.

APPLICATIONS

Surgical Pathology: Antigen Retrieval Permits Immunohistochemical Staining of Fixed and Archival Tissues

IHC has become an important tool in surgical pathology, as evidenced by the accumulation of literature concerning the application of IHC in diagnosis and research. More than 10 000 articles regarding IHC staining of paraffin sections were written in 1992. A further explosion of publications on IHC has resulted from recent advances of molecular biology (15,80,81). However, the application of IHC in otopathology, in terms of surgical pathology or analytical morphology, is less well developed and largely anecdotal. For example, using AR-IHC of antibodies to keratin in celloidin-embedded human temporal bone sections in a case of otosclerosis from the collection

Table 2. Comparison of Immunostaining Results of Nonheating Antigen Retrieval Method Using Three Solvents

Protocol[a]	NaOH-methanol	NaOH-ethanol	NaOH-water
A	+++	++	-
B	+++	+++	+++

[a]Protocol A, Nonheating AR treatment of each solution, followed by rinsing of the slides in methanol, ethanol, and distilled water, respectively, for each group; Protocol B, Nonheating AR treatment of each solution, followed by rinsing of the slides in methanol for all groups. This test was performed using the monoclonal antibody to keratin of NCL-5D3 as the primary antibody.

at the House Ear Institute (74), an unusual epithelial cell-lined cyst was revealed in the scala tympani of the basal turn of the cochlea. The lesion, together with other pathologic findings, such as clearly defined extended Reissner's membrane and ruptures of the membranous labyrinth, could not be demonstrated precisely by the routine hematoxylin and eosin staining method (Figures 3–6). This single case demonstrates the feasibility and clinicopathologic analysis of otopathologic tissues, somewhat analogous to the much more extensive use of IHC in surgical pathology (15,80,81). The advantages occurring from the ability to utilize AR-IHC for archival human temporal bone collections housed in temporal bone banks have already been demonstrated.

To our knowledge, there have been no prior reports on an epithelial cell-lined cyst in the scala tympani in otosclerosis. Although some pathologic changes, predominantly atrophy of the spiral ligament, have been well documented (1,34,57,97), existence of cysts in the scala tympani may have been overlooked in the absence of IHC staining. Based on previous studies on the pathology of spiral ligament, which were found in otosclerosis and our human temporal bone data, we have proposed a mechanism for development of this epithelial cell-lined cyst in the scala tympani, as illustrated in Figure 7. Three major factors may be involved in the pathogenesis of epithelial cyst formation in the scala tympani.

The first proposed factor is space formation or cavitization in the spiral ligament caused by atrophy; atrophy is the most common pathologic change in the cochlea during otosclerosis, as emphasized by Schuknecht et al. (57). Kelemen and Linthicum (34) pointed out the possibility of larger cyst formation in the spiral ligament caused by deformation of the bony labyrinth as a result of compression from the advancing new bone. They also mentioned that differentiation of the cyst from artifacts caused by fixation in the spiral ligament is not readily achieved. The case described here clearly reveals a cyst lined by epithelial cells in the scala tympani (Figure 6), a true pathologic lesion (epithelial cell-lined cyst), and not an artifact. Although a small fragment of calcification could be seen in the lower wall of the cyst in the scala tympani (Figure 6B, arrow), there was no otosclerotic bone protruding into the scala tympani. No significant deformity of the bony cochlear duct could be found except the round window niche, which was partially obliterated by new bone formation.

The second hypothesis is that the cyst-like space protruding into the scala tympani is related to a disturbance of the inner ear fluid that results from obstruction of both the endolymphatic duct and the cochlear aqueduct. Theoretically, it is reasonable to

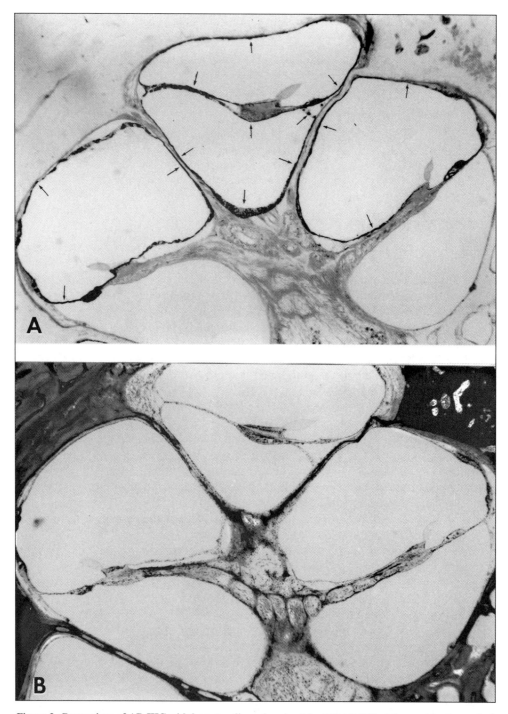

Figure 3. Comparison of AR-IHC with hematoxylin and eosin stain. (A) AR-IHC of the combination method using cocktail keratin monoclonal antibodies of AE1 and NCL-5D3 as the primary antibodies with the AR-IHC technique described in the text for archival celloidin-embedded human temporal bone sections of a patient with otosclerosis from the House Ear Institute (same data and method used in Figures 3–6). Extremely extended Reissner's membrane caused by severe endolymphatic hydrops of the left temporal bone was clearly demonstrated by keratin immunohistochemistry (arrows), in contrast to the adjacent serial section stained by hematoxylin and eosin (B), which does not indicate the same findings. Original magnification 20×. Reprinted with permission from Reference 74.

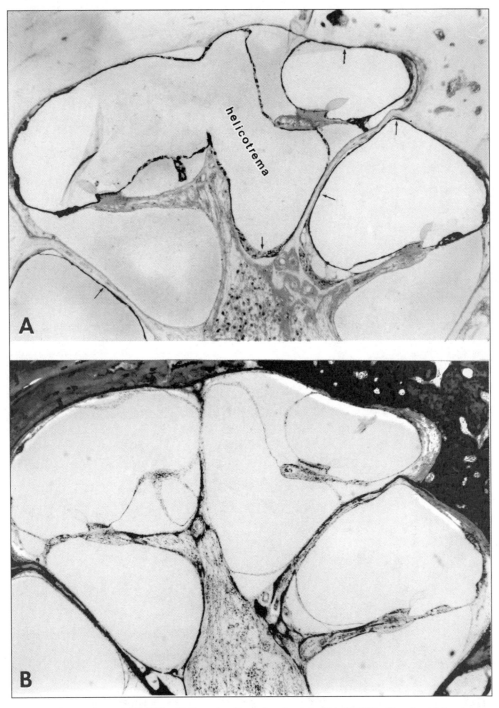

Figure 4. Comparison of AR-IHC with hematoxylin and eosin stain. (A) AR-IHC of keratin staining demonstrates herniation of Reissner's membrane in the apical turn of the left cochlea and extremely extended Reissner's membrane (arrows). (B) Hematoxylin and eosin-stained adjacent slide of the same case did not show these significant findings. Original magnification 20×. Reprinted with permission from Reference 74.

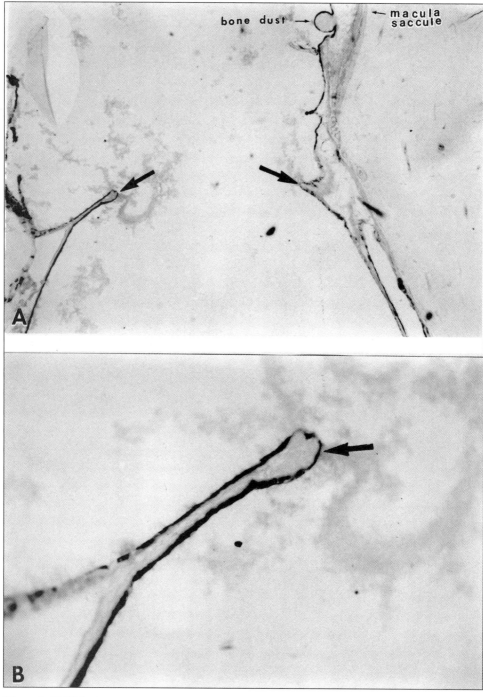

Figure 5. AR-IHC of keratin staining. (A) Rupture of the saccule resulted in endolymphatic hydrops. A strong keratin-labeled epithelium surrounding the edge of the rupture (arrows) allows one to exclude artifact. Bone dust produced by an operation is lined with keratin-labled epithelium as indicated. (B) Higher magnification of the rupture shows the keratin-positive cells (arrow). Original magnification for panel A, 63×; in panel B, 160×. Reprinted with permission from Reference 74.

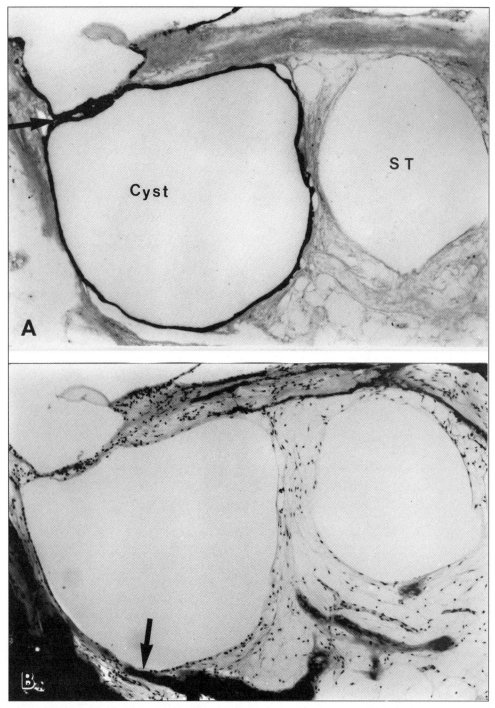

Figure 6. AR-IHC staining of keratin compared with hematoxylin and eosin stain. (A) Cyst lined by epithelial cells in the scala tympani (Cyst), in contrast to another space (ST) in the scala tympani that represents lack of keratin-labeling. Note the possible epithelial migration from the supporting cells of the organ of Corti (arrow) through a rupture of the basilar membrane. (B) Hematoxylin and eosin staining of the adjacent slide from the same case cannot provide the same information. Hyalination and ossification are seen near the lower part of the cyst (arrow). Original magnification 63×. Reprinted with permission from Reference 74.

propose that this factor may be the major cause of protruding cysts in the scala tympani, as there may be an additive effect based on increased endolymphatic pressure (caused by obliteration of the endolymphatic duct) and decreased perilymphatic pressure (caused by obliteration of the cochlear aqueduct) (55). The present case showed severe endolymphatic hydrops in the left membranous labyrinth, characterized by several ruptures of the membrane, a finding not frequently seen in otosclerosis.

The third proposed factor contributing to cyst formation is epithelial cell migration from the keratin-positive supporting cells of the organ of Corti, through the holes in the ruptured basilar membrane. Rupture of the cochlear basilar membrane has been demonstrated by both serial human temporal bone section and the method of microdissection and surface preparations (30,61). This case showed a close relationship between the basilar membrane and cyst formation (Figure 6A, arrow), revealing a possible adhesive lesion existing in the area of basilar membrane deformity. In addition, the epithelial lining cells showed negative immunostaining for keratin 7, which is the same keratin pattern as the supporting cells of the organ of Corti (11,69). Another observation that may support the notion of epithelial cell migration through the basilar membrane is that only the cyst closely adjacent to the basilar membrane was lined by epithelial cells; another cyst-like space, separated from the basilar membrane, was devoid of keratin immunostaining (Figure 6A). The cyst may have contained perilymph fluid, as the intercellular spaces of the spiral ligament communicate with the perilymphatic space, a condition that has been demonstrated by electron microscopy (1).

In general, the utility of AR-IHC for archival routinely processed celloidin-embedded human temporal bone sections is likely to open a new field in otopathology, not only for studying elemental components of the tissues at a molecular level, but also for differential diagnosis based on clinicopathologic analysis. Temporal bone studies concerning congenital deformities as well as some anatomic measurements such as the cochlear aqueduct may be more exactly demonstrated and measured by using keratin-IHC, as the epithelial cell-lined abnormal and normal structures should be recognized more readily. Currently, there are hundreds of monoclonal antibodies available commercially, providing almost limitless opportunities for research using human temporal bone collections.

Irreplaceable Resource of Information for Study of Otopathology

Abundant data from IHC studies of animal ears have accumulated worldwide, but IHC study of human ear tissue has been limited. Keithley et al. (33) studied Na/K-ATPase localization in the cochlear lateral wall of human temporal bones using archival celloidin-embedded sections and demonstrated that, unlike animal models showing a decline in the Na/K-ATPase content of the stria vascularis and spiral ligament at 6 months after the induction of hydrops, there was no decline in Na/K-ATPase content in human temporal bone sections of Menière's disease. Keithley and Tian (32) studied fibronectin immunolocalization in celloidin-embedded human temporal bone sections by using the nonheating AR-IHC method and demonstrated that unlike the diminished fibronectin immunoreactivity indicated in aged rats, fibronectin in the basilar membrane of human cochlea was not reduced with aging. Linthicum et al. (40) and Tian et al. (86) studied the contents of the human adult intraosseous endolymphatic sac using archival human temporal bone sections with the nonheating AR method and demonstrated the localization of carbohydrates and protein-containing substances in the human endolymphatic sac in a more accurate fashion, revealing different amounts of the various identified substances in sacs from patients with Menière's disease, patients with labyrinthine fibrosis, and controls. Human temporal bone collection is an irreplaceable resource for study of the pathology of ear diseases, as emphasized recently by Nadol (50), since many disease processes in the human ear are unique conditions, with no known animal models.

Morphology-Based Molecular Biologic Analysis

The rapid development of molecular biology in recent years has dramatically changed the face of biomedical research. The current accumulation of information on viral DNA found in human temporal bone tissue (91) [gene mapping of hereditary hearing impairment and mutations in mitochondrial chromosomes associated with hearing disorders (76) and other diseases (93)] has pointed out one of the future goals of research in ear disease, i.e., discovering the related gene products and their function in both normal and pathologic conditions (76). IHC staining of human temporal bone tissue sections provides one potential approach to demonstrate a variety of alterations of protein expression, which may contribute to an understanding of various pathways of ear diseases and provide clues to possible etiology and pathogenesis for further study.

In general, there are two approaches to studying pathogenesis based on molecular biology, the classical and reverse approaches (Figure 8). Based on morphology, the classical approach has been applied successfully in otopathology. For example, the discovery of measles virus in otosclerotic tissue was initially demonstrated by electron microscopy (42), while an IHC method readily demonstrates virus antigenicity in the tissue (7). Molecular biologic methods were subsequently employed to examine this possible etiology of otosclerosis (51,92). Classical morphology still remains the starting point of an investigation, and many would still argue that no natural science that is

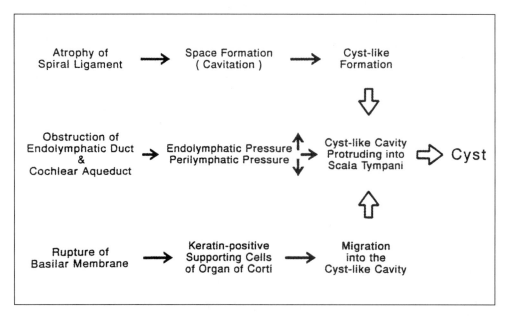

Figure 7. Diagram of possible cyst mechanism in the scala tympani demonstrated by AR-IHC using a monoclonal antibody to keratin from a case of otosclerosis (see text for details). Reprinted with permission from Reference 74a.

clinically relevant can exist without direct observation of natural phenomena in the context of tissues, and ultimately patients (25,29,60). The unique advantage of morphology is its sharp localization of natural phenomena, normal or abnormal, in the exact compartment of cells or tissues, providing insight into studies of cell and tissue functions, as well as an understanding of the mechanisms of disease. From this point of view, the morphologic approach may not soon be replaced by other methods.

For example, Lim et al. (37) did an IHC study of human otosclerotic tissue, based on their careful morphologic studies of otosclerosis, and pointed out the possible immune mechanisms of otosclerosis. Paparella (52) studied the pathogenesis and pathophysiology of Menière's disease based on many years of his careful observation of both clinical patients and human temporal bone morphology. His conclusions on the etiopathogenesis of Meniere's disease is critical for further study using molecular biology techniques. The concept of morphology-based molecular biologic analysis has been applied in numerous biomedical research studies. As a good example, Chuong and co-workers (14,87,95) studied the morphogenesis of chicken feathers using this morphology based molecular biology approach, starting from morphologic observation of epithelial-mesenchymal interactions that may initiate functional tissue morphogenesis. The ongoing search for factors that initiate or influence this epithelial-mesenchymal interaction is based on molecular biologic techniques com-

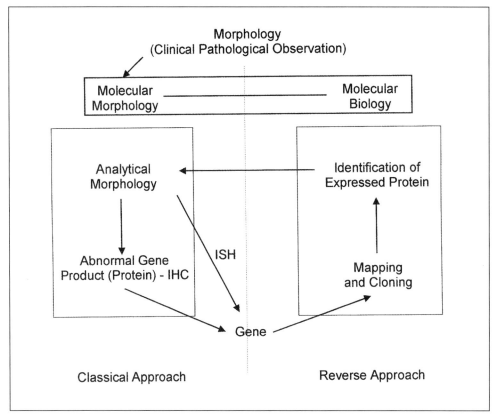

Figure 8. Diagram of two research approaches in studying pathogenesis based on molecular biology. Note that morphology is always the starting point of study and is important for both approaches. IHC, immunohistochemistry; ISH, in situ hybridization. Reprinted with permission from Reference 74a.

bined with a morphology-based approach. Chuong's recent data concerning sonic hedgehog (Shh) in feather morphogenesis (87) emphasize the significance of accurate localization of Shh in epithelial compartments during early and late developmental stages using IHC and in situ hybridization. In general, future studies of human temporal bone collections may continue to follow the way of functional morphology on the basis of molecular biology, i.e., molecular morphology.

REMODELING CELLOIDIN-EMBEDDED TISSUE SECTIONS

A critical issue for future AR-IHC study is the use of remodeled celloidin-embedded human temporal bone sections. Thick celloidin sections should be remodeled into thinner sections for several reasons: *(i)* thick sections (20 μm) cannot provide satisfactory color differentiation, particularly for nuclear or cell surface immunostaining; *(ii)* valuable human temporal bone collections are less rapidly depleted when thin sections are employed; *(iii)* it is difficult to mount thick celloidin sections on the slides, even after complicated procedures as described above; *(iv)* it is difficult to use heating methods for celloidin sections; and *(v)* thick sections require elongated incubation times and large amounts of immunostaining reagents.

In 1988, Schuknecht (59) documented a method of remodeling celloidin-embedded human temporal bone section for electron microscopy using clove oil to remove celloidin from the section. Subsequently, Portmann et al. (53) developed a similar method to dissect the area of interest from celloidin section and remove the celloidin using clove oil. We designed a simpler method for remodeling celloidin-embedded human temporal bone section, as follows:

1. Dissect the area of interest for IHC staining, keeping the remainder of the section for other studies.

2. Following the protocol for embedding tissue in JB-4 (glycol methacrylate; Polysciences, Warrington, PA, USA), embed the dissected celloidin section in JB-4.

3. Cut a 1-μm section of a JB-4-embedded celloidin section, mount on charged or coated slides as mentioned above, after drawing a circle around the tiny tissue using a diamond pen, and dry at 60°C for 1 hour.

4. Following the nonheating AR protocol, immerse the thin section in 1:5 diluted NaOH-methanol solution for a short time (a few minutes; the exact time may be monitored by using microscopy, to retain good morphology).

5. If necessary, the heating AR method may be applied before nonheating treatment (step 4) as a combined AR method. The combined AR technique has been successfully employed using Epon-embedded archival tissue for electron microscopy (77,96).

We also tried semithin (1 μm) sections of routinely processed Epon-embedded tissue sections for AR-IHC staining using the protocol introduced above and obtained satisfactory positive staining of keratin in the organ of Corti (unpublished data).

Other approaches to modified human temporal bone tissue section may also be helpful in the future. Formalin-fixed, acid-decalcified, paraffin-embedded human temporal bone sections (including some surgical specimens of the human ear) have been adapted for IHC staining (27,41,44). Paraffin-embedded tissue sections have the advantages of being thinner and more suited for IHC staining, yielding results comparable with diagnostic surgical pathology in both morphology and IHC. Michaels et al. (45) created an interesting technique for human temporal bone collection using a special saw to slice temporal bones at a thickness of 2 to 3 mm without prior decalcification. This procedure is based on the principle of specimen examination usually followed in surgical pathology. First, the sections are viewed by the naked eye, equivalent to the gross examination. Second, microscopic examination allows selection of areas of interest and appropriate procedures, such as embedding in paraffin or celloidin, with decalcification for light microscopy, or alternatively embedding in Epon for electron microscopy. In the recent study of Michaels et al. (46) of human temporal bone of patients with the acquired immunodeficiency syndrome, IHC staining was used in an attempt to demonstrate the existence of cytomegalovirus; the use of AR pretreatment may be helpful in enhancing the success of this approach.

CONCLUSION

AR-IHC used for human temporal bone study is an important approach toward an understanding of the pathogenesis and etiology of ear diseases. Ongoing research using AR-IHC can be expected to provide valuable information by combining the features of traditional morpholgy with IHC and molecular biology. To achieve the best results while saving the irreplaceable human temporal bone collection for more studies in the future, it is advisable to remodel traditional thick celloidin sections where possible.

ACKNOWLEDGMENTS

Part of this chapter and Figures 1, 2, 7, and 8 have been reproduced with permission from Reference 74a. Figures 3–6 are reproduced with permission from Reference 74. Authors want to express sincere appreciation to Dr. Linthicum at the House Ear Institute for his kind help in human temporal bone study.

REFERENCES

1. **Allam, A.F.** 1970. Pathology of the human spiral ligament. J. Laryngol. Otol. *84*:765-779.
2. **Altermatt, H.J., J.-O. Gebbers, C. Muller, J. Laissue, and W. Arnold.** 1992. Immunohistochemical characterization of the human endolymphatic sac and its associated cell populations. Acta Otolaryngol. (Stockh) *112*:299-305.
3. **Altschuler, R.A., M.H. Parakkal, and J. Fex.** 1983. Localization of enkephalin-like immunoreactivity in acetylcholinesterase-positive cells in the guinea pig lateral superior olivary complex that project to the cochlea. Neuroscience *9*:621-630.
4. **Anniko, M., L.-E. Thornell, and I. Virtanen.** 1987. Cytoskeletal organization of the human inner ear. II. Characterization of intermediate filaments in the cochlea. Acta Otolaryngol. (Stockh) (Suppl. *437*):29-54.
5. **Anniko, M. and W. Arnold.** 1990. Cytoskeletal network of intermediate filament proteins in the adult human vestibular labyrinth. Acta Otolaryngol (Stockh) (Suppl. *470*):40-50.
6. **Anniko, M. and W. Arnold.** 1991. Acetylcholine receptor localization in human adult cochlear and vestibular hair cells. Acta Otolaryngol (Stockh) *111*:491-499.
7. **Arnold, W. and I. Friedmann.** 1987. Presence of viral specific antigens (measles, rubella) around the active otosclerotic focus. Ann. Otol. Rhinol. Laryngol. *66*:167-171.
8. **Arnold, W. and I. Friedmann.** 1990. Immunohistochemistry of otosclerosis. Acta Otolaryngol. (Stockh) (Suppl. *470*):124-129.
9. **Battifora, H.** 1994. p53 immunohistochemistry: a word of caution (editorial). Hum. Pathol. *25*:435-437.
10. **Bauwens, L.J.J.M., J.E. Veldman, and E.H. Huizing.** 1990. Progress in temporal bone histopathology. III. An improved technique for immunohistochemical investigation of the adult human inner ear. Acta Otolaryngol. (Stockh) (Suppl. *470*):34-39.
11. **Bauwens, L.J.J.M. (Ed.).** 1991. Intermediate Filament Proteins in The Human Audio-Vestibular Organ. An Immunohistochemical Study, p. 15-57. L.J.J.M. Bauwens, The Netherlands.

12. **Bluestone, C.D. and R.F. Naunton.** 1989. Human temporal bone research workshop report. Ann. Otol. Rhinol. Laryngol. (Suppl. *143*):3-56.

13. **Bui, H.T., F.H. Linthicum, F.M. Hofman, C.A. Bowman, and W.F. House.** 1989. An immunohistochemical study of the endolymphatic sac in patients with acoustic tumors. Laryngoscope *99*:775-778.

14. **Chuong, C.-M. and G.M. Edelman.** 1985. Expression of cell-adhesion molecules in embryonic induction. I. Morphogenesis of nestling feathers. J. Cell Biol. *101*:1009-1026.

15. **Cote, R.J. and C.R. Taylor.** 1996. Immunohistochemistry and related marking techniques, p. 136-175. *In* I. Damjanov and J. Linder (Eds.), Anderson's Pathology. 10th ed. Mosby, St. Louis.

16. **Davis, G.L., G.J. Spector, M. Strauss, and J.N. Middlekamp.** 1977. Cytomegalovirus endolabyrinthitis. Arch. Pathol. Lab. Med. *101*:118-121.

17. **Fex, J. and R.A. Altschuler.** 1986. Neurotransmitter-related immunocytochemistry of the organ of Corti. Hear. Res. *22*:249-263.

18. **Flock, A., A. Bretscher, and K. Weber.** 1982. Immunohistochemical localization of several cytoskeletal proteins in inner ear sensory and supporting cells. Hear. Res. *6*:75-89.

19. **Fraenkel-Conrat, H., B.A. Brandon, and H.S. Olcott.** 1947. The reaction of formaldehyde with proteins. IV. Participation of indole groups. Gramicidin. J. Biol. Chem. *168*:99-118.

20. **Fraenkel-Conrat, H. and H.S. Olcott.** 1948. Reaction of formaldehyde with proteins. VI. Cross-linking of amino groups with phenol, imidazole, or indole groups. J. Biol. Chem. *174*:827-843.

21. **Fraenkel-Conrat, H. and H.S. Olcott.** 1948. The reaction of formaldehyde with proteins. V. Cross-linking between amino and primary amide or guanidyl groups. J. Am. Chem. Soc. *70*:2673-2684.

22. **Futaki, T., Y. Nagao, and S. Kikuchi.** 1988. Immunohistochemical analysis of the lateral wall of the endolymphatic sac in Meniere's patients. Adv. Oto-Rhino-Laryng. *42*:129-134.

23. **Ganbo, T., I. Sando, C.D. Balaban, C. Suzuki, and M. Sudo.** 1997. Immunohistochemistry of lymphocytes and macrophages in human celloidin-embedded temporal bone sections with acute otitis media. Ann. Otol. Rhinol. Laryngol. *106*:662-668.

24. **Guiter, G.E., P.W. Kwan, and R.A. DeLellis.** 1995. Unwanted tissue immunoreactivities following microwave antigen retrieval: a critical analysis. Lab. Invest. *72*:165A.

25. **Holbrook, K.A.** 1989. Biologic structure and function: perspectives on morphologic approaches to the study of the granular layer keratinocyte. J. Invest. Dermatol. (Suppl. *92*):84S-104S.

26. **Huang, C.-C.** 1987. Bone resorption in experimental otosclerosis in rats. Am. J. Otolaryngol. *8*:332-341.

27. **Ichimiya, I., J.C. Adams, and R.S. Kimura.** 1994. Changes in immunostaining of cochleas with experimentally induced endolymphatic hydrops. Ann. Otol. Rhinol. Laryngol. *103*:457-468.

28. **Ishiyama, A., I. Lopez, and P.A. Wackym.** 1994. Choline acetyltransferase immunoractivity in the human vestibular end-organs. Cell Biol. Int. *18*:979-984.

29. **Iurato, S.** 1988. Cochlear morphology from Wurzburg (1951) to Turin (1987): old and new aspects. Acta Otolaryngol. (Stockh) *105*:389-391.

30. **Johnsson, L.-G., J.E. Hawkins, and F.H. Linthicum.** 1978. Cochlear and vestibular lesions in capsular otosclerosis as seen in microdissection. Ann. Otol. Rhinol. Laryngol. *87*(2Pt3):1-40.

31. **Kawauchi, H., I. Ichimiya, N. Kaneda, and G. Mogi.** 1992. Distribution of immunocompetent cells in the endolymphatic sac. Ann. Otol. Rhinol. Laryngol. *101*:39-47.

32. **Keithley, E.M. and Q. Tian.** 1994. Fibronectin-like immunoreactivity of the basilar membrane of celloidin-embedded human temporal bone sections. Acta Otolaryngol. (Stockh) *114*:613-619.

33. **Keithley, E.M., S. Horowitz, and M.J. Ruckenstein.** 1995. Na, K-ATPase in the cochlear lateral wall of human temporal bones with endolymphatic hydrops. Ann. Otol. Rhinol. Laryngol. *104*:858-863.

34. **Kelemen, G. and F.H. Linthicum.** 1969. Labyrinthine otosclerosis. Acta Otolaryngol. (Stockh) (Suppl. *253*):5-68.

35. **Kuijpers, W., E.L.G.M. Tonnaer, T.A. Peters, and F.C.S. Ramaekers.** 1992. Developmentally-regulated coexpression of vimentin and cytokeratins in the rat inner ear. Hear. Res. *62*:1-10.

36. **Kumagami, H., S. Nakajima, and K. Mizukoshi.** 1991. Scanning electron microscopy and immunoglobulins of the endolymphatic sac in Meniere's disease. Acta Otolaryngol. (Stockh) (Suppl. *481*):170-175.

37. **Lim, D.J.** 1985. Pathogenesis and pathology of otosclerosis: a review, p. 43-57. *In* Y. Nomura (Ed.), Hearing Loss and Dizziness. Igaku-Shoin, Tokyo.

38. **Lim, D.J., Y.S. Liu, and H. Birck.** 1976. Secretory lysozyme of the human middle ear mucosa—immunocytochemical localization. Ann. Otol. Rhinol. Laryngol. *85*:50-60.

39. **Lim, D.J., M. Robinson, and W.H. Saunders.** 1987. Morphologic and immunohistochemical observation of otosclerotic stapes: a preliminary study. Am. J. Otolaryngol. *8*:282-295.

40. **Linthicum, F.H., Q. Tian, and M. Milicic.** 1995. Constituents of the endolymphatic tubules as demonstrated by three-dimensional morphometry. Acta Otolaryngol. (Stockh) *115*:246-250.

41. **Matsune, S., T. Shima, M. Ohyama, K. Sakamoto, and H. Tsurumaru.** 1995. Immunohistochemical study on temporal bone of autopsy cases with mycobacterium leprae infection. J. Otolaryngol. Jpn. *98*:1881-1886 (in Japanese).

42. **McKenna, M.J., G.B. Mills, F.R. Galey, and F.H. Linthicum.** 1986. Filamentous structures morphologically similar to viral nucleocapsids in otosclerotic lesions in two patients. Am. J. Otol. *7*:25-28.

43. **McKenna, M.J. and B.G. Mills.** 1989. Immunohistochemical evidence of measles virus antigens in active oto-

sclerosis. Otolaryngol. Head Neck Surg. *101*:415-421.

44. **Megerian, C.A., B.Z. Pilch, A.K. Bhan, and M.J. McKenna.** 1997. Differential expression of transthyretin in papillary tumors of the endolymphatic sac and choroid plexus. Laryngoscope *107*:216-221.

45. **Michaels, L., M. Wells, and A. Frohlich.** 1983. A new technique for the study of temporal bone pathology. Clin. Otolaryngol. *8*:77-85.

46. **Michaels, L., S. Soucek, and J. Liang.** 1994. The ear in the acquired immunodeficiency syndrome: I. Temporal bone histopathologic study. Am. J. Otol. *15*:515-522.

47. **Mighell, A.J., P.A. Robinson, and W.J. Hume.** 1995. Patterns of immunoreactivity to an anti-fibronectin polyclonal antibody in formalin-fixed, paraffin-embedded oral tissues are dependent on methods of antigen retrieval. J. Histochem. Cytochem. *43*:1107-1114.

48. **Moore, J.K., Y.-L. Guan, and S.-R. Shi.** 1996. Prenatal maturation of dendrites in human brainstem auditory nuclei (abstr). Assoc. Res. Otolaryngol. *19*:86.

49. **Moore, J.K., Y.-L. Guan, and S.-R. Shi.** 1997. Axogenesis in the human fetal auditory system, demonstrated by neurofilament immunohistochemistry. Anat. Embryol. *195*:15-30.

50. **Nadol, J.B.** 1996. Techniques for human temporal bone removal: information for the scientific community. Otolaryngol. Head Neck Surg. *115*:298-305.

51. **Niedermeyer, H.P. and W. Arnold.** 1995. Otosclerosis: a measles virus associated inflammatory disease. Acta Otolaryngol. (Stockh) *115*:300-303.

52. **Paparella, M.M.** 1991. Pathogenesis and pathophysiology of Meniere's Disease. Acta Otolaryngol. (Stockh) (Suppl. *485*):26-35.

53. **Portmann, D., J. Fayad, F.H. Linthicum, and H. Rask-Andersen.** 1990. Transmission electron microscopy of previously embedded celloidin sections. Acta Otolaryngol. (Stockh) (Suppl. *470*):7-12.

54. **Raphael, Y., G. Marshak, A. Barash, and B. Geiger.** 1987. Modulation of intermediate-filament expression in developing cochlear epithelium. Differentiation *35*:151-162.

55. **Rask-Andersen, H., J. Stahle, and H. Wilbrand.** 1977. Human cochlear aqueduct and its accessory canals. Ann. Otol. Rhinol. Laryngol. *86*(5Pt.2):1-16.

56. **Schrader, M., J. Poppendieck, and B. Weber.** 1990. Immunohistologic findings in otosclerosis. Ann. Otol. Rhinol. Laryngol. *99*:349-352.

57. **Schuknecht, H.F. (Ed.).** 1974. Pathology of the Ear. 1st ed., p. 351-373. Harvard University Press, Cambridge, MA.

58. **Schuknecht, H.F.** 1987. Temporal bone collections in Europe and the United States. Observations on a productive laboratory, pathologic findings of clinical relevance, and recommendations. Ann. Otol. Rhinol. Laryngol. 96(Suppl. *130*):3-19.

59. **Schuknecht, H.F.** 1989. Light and electron microscopy on the same temporal bone. Ann. Otol. Rhinol. Laryngol. 98(Suppl. *143*):40.

60. **Schuknecht, H.F. (Ed.).** 1993. Pathology of the Ear. 2nd ed. Lea & Febiger, Philadelphia.

61. **Schuknecht, H.F. and C.W. Gross.** 1966. Otosclerosis and the inner ear. Ann. Otol. Rhinol. Laryngol. *75*:423-435.

62. **Schulte, B.A. and J.C. Adams.** 1989. Immunohistochemical localization of vimentin in the gerbil inner ear. J. Histochem. Cytochem. *37*:1787-1797.

63. **Sebenik, M. and R. Wieczorek.** 1995. Nonspecific nuclear staining (NNS) after antigen retrieval (AR). Lab. Invest. *72*:168A.

64. **Shi, S.-R. and S.K. Juhn.** 1985. Immunohistochemical study of cochlear cells using monoclonal keratin antibody AE1, p. 314-316. *In* E. Myers, (Ed.), New Dimensions in Otorhinolaryngology—Head and Neck Surgery, Vol. 2. Excerpta Medica, Amsterdam.

65. **Shi, S.-R., M. Kobari, I. Ohtani, and T. Aikawa.** 1990. Immuno-electron microscopic study of keratin distribution in the cochlea using monoclonal antibody. Ann. Otol. Rhinol. Laryngol. *99*:817-826.

66. **Shi, S.-R., M.E. Key, and K.L. Kalra.** 1991. Antigen retrieval in formalin-fixed, paraffin-embedded tissues: an enhancement method for immunohistochemical staining based on microwave oven heating of tissue sections. J. Histochem. Cytochem. *39*:741-748.

67. **Shi, S.-R., C. Cote, K.L. Kalra, C.R. Taylor, and A.K. Tandon.** 1992. A technique for retrieving antigens in formalin-fixed, routinely acid-decalcified, celloidin-embedded human temporal bone sections for immunohistochemistry. J. Histochem. Cytochem. *40*:787-792.

68. **Shi, S.-R., A.K. Tandon, C. Cote, and K.L. Kalra.** 1992. S-100 protein in human inner ear: use of a novel immunohistochemical technique on routinely processed, celloidin-embedded human temporal bone sections. Laryngoscope *102*:734-738.

69. **Shi, S.-R., A.K. Tandon, R.R.M. Haussmann, K.L. Kalra, and C.R. Taylor.** 1993. Immunohistochemical study of intermediate filament proteins on routinely processed, celloidin-embedded human temporal bone sections by using a new technique for antigen retrieval. Acta Otolaryngol. (Stockh) *113*:48-54.

70. **Shi, S.-R. and Q. Tian.** 1993. Development of an antigen retrieval technique for immunohistochemistry on archival celloidin-embedded sections. J. Histochem. Cytochem. *41*:1121.

71. **Shi, S.-R., J. Gu, K.L. Kalra, T. Chen, R.J. Cote, and C.R. Taylor.** 1995. Antigen retrieval technique: a novel approach to immunohistochemistry on routinely processed tissue sections (review). Cell Vision 2:6-22.

306

72. **Shi, S.-R., R.J. Cote, and C.R. Taylor.** 1997. Antigen retrieval immunohistochemistry: past, present, and future. J. Histochem. Cytochem. *45*:327-343.

73. **Shi, S.-R., R.J. Cote, L.L. Young, and C.R. Taylor.** 1997. Antigen retrieval immunohistochemistry: practice and development. J. Histotechnol. *20*:145-154.

74. **Shi, S.-R. and F.H. Linthicum.** 1997. Inner ear membrane ruptures demonstrated with keratin immunohisto-chemistry. Otolaryngol. Head Neck Surg. *117*:S195-S198.

74a. **Shi, S.-R., R.J. Cote, and C.R. Taylor.** 1998. Antigen retrieval immunuhistochemistry used for routinely processed celloidin-embedded human temporal bone sections: standardization and development (review). Auris Nasus Larynx. *25*:425-443.

75. **Slepecky, N. and S.C. Chamberlain.** 1986. Correlative immuno-electron-microscopic and immuno-fluorescent localization of actin in sensory and supporting cells of the inner ear by use of a low-temperature embedding resin. Cell Tissue Res. *245*:229-235.

76. **Snow, J.B.** 1997. News from the National Institute on Deafness and Other Communication Disorders. Am. J. Otol. *18*:285-287.

77. **Stirling, J.W. and P.S. Graff.** 1995. Antigen unmasking for immunoelectron microscopy: labeling is improved by treating with sodium ethoxide or sodium metaperiodate, then heating on retrieval medium. J. Histochem. Cytochem. *43*:115-123.

78. **Swanson, P.E.** 1997. HIERanarchy: the state of the art in immunohistochemistry (editorial). Am. J. Clin. Pathol. *107*:139-140.

79. **Takahashi, M. and J.P. Harris.** 1988. Anatomic distribution and localization of immunocompetent cells in nor-mal mouse endolymphatic sac. Acta Otolaryngol. (Stockh) *106*:409-416.

80. **Taylor, C.R.** 1994. The current role of immunohistochemistry in diagnostic pathology. Adv. Pathol. Lab. Med. *7*:59-105.

81. **Taylor, C.R. and R.J. Cote (Eds.).** 1994. Immunomicroscopy: A Diagnostic Tool for the Surgical Pathologist. 2nd ed., p. 1-70. W.B. Saunders, Philadelphia.

82. **Taylor, C.R., S.-R. Shi, B. Chaiwun, L. Young, S.A. Imam, and R.J. Cote.** 1994. Strategies for improving the immunohistochemical staining of various intranuclear prognostic markers in formalin-paraffin sections: androgen receptor, estrogen receptor, progesterone receptor, p53 protein, proliferating cell nuclear antigen, and Ki-67 anti-gen revealed by antigen retrieval technique. Hum. Pathol. *25*:263-270.

83. **Taylor, C.R., S.-R. Shi, B. Chaiwun, L. Young, S.A. Imam, and R.J. Cote.** 1994. Standardization and repro-ducibility in diagnostic immunohistochemistry (correspondence). Hum. Pathol. *25*:1107-1109.

84. **Taylor, C.R., S.-R. Shi, C. Chen, L. Young, C. Yang, and R.J. Cote.** 1996. Comparative study of antigen retrieval heating methods: microwave, microwave and pressure cooker, autoclave, and steamer. Biotech. His-tochem. *71*:263-270.

85. **Taylor, C.R., S.-R. Shi, and R.J. Cote.** 1996. Antigen retrieval for immunohistochemistry. Status and need for greater standardization. Appl. Immunohistochem. *4*:144-166.

86. **Tian, Q., H. Rask-Andersen, and F.H. Linthicum.** 1994. Identification of substances in the endolymphatic sac. Acta Otolaryngol. (Stockh) *114*:632-636.

87. **Ting-Berreth, S.A. and C.-M. Chuong.** 1996. Sonic hedgehog in feather morphogenesis: inducton of mes-enchymal condensarion and association with cell death. Dev. Dynamics *207*:157-170.

88. **Usami, S., M. Igarashi, and G.C. Thompson.** 1987. GABA-like immunoreactivity in the chick basilar papilla and the lagenar macula. Hear. Res. *30*:19-22.

89. **Usami, S., M. Igarashi, and G.C. Thompson.** 1988. Light- and electron-microscopic study of gamma-aminobu-tyric-acid-like immunoreactivity in the guinea pig organ of Corti. ORL *50*:162-169.

90. **Veldman, J.E., F. Meeuwsen, M. van Dijik, Q. Key, and E.H. Huizing.** 1985. Progress in temporal bone histopathology. II. Immunotechnology applied to the temporal bone. Acta Otolaryngol. (Stockh) (Suppl. *423*):29-35.

91. **Wackym, P.A.** 1997. Perspectives on the future of temporal bone research (editorial). Am. J. Otol. *18*:693-696.

92. **Wackym, P.A.** 1997. Molecular temporal bone pathology: I. Historical foundation. Laryngoscope *107*:1156-1164.

93. **Wackym, P.A.** 1997. Molecular temporal bone pathology: II. Ramsay Hunt Syndrome (Herpes Zoster Oticus). Laryngoscope *107*:1165-1175.

94. **Wackym, P.A., P.E. Micevych, and P.H. Ward.** 1990. Immunoelectron microscopy of the human inner ear. Laryngoscope *100*:447-454.

95. **Widelitz, R.B., T.-X. Jiang, A. Noveen, S.A. Ting-Berreth, E. Yin, and C.-M. Chuong.** 1997. Molecular his-tology in skin appendage morphogenesis. Microsc. Res. Tech. *38*:452-465.

96. **Wilson, D.F., D.-J. Jiang, A.M. Pierce, and O.W. Wiebkin.** 1996. Antigen retrieval for electron microscopy using a microwave technique for epithelial and basal lamina antigens. Appl. Immunohistochem. *4*:66-71.

97. **Wright, J.L. and H.F. Schuknecht.** 1972. Atrophy of the spiral ligament. Arch. Otolaryngol. *96*:16-21.

98. **Yamane, H., Y. Nakai, and M. Igarashi.** 1987. The endolymphatic sac and its free-floating cells, p. 125-131. *In* M.D. Graham and J.L. Kemink (Eds.), The Vestibular System: Neurophysiologyc and Clinical Research. Raven Press, New York.

Appendix

Appendix:
Antigen Retrieval Technique

Shan-Rong Shi, Richard J. Cote, Yan Shi, and Clive R. Taylor

Department of Pathology, University of Southern California Keck School of Medicine, Los Angeles, CA, USA

INTRODUCTION

In this appendix, use of the term antigen retrieval (AR) technique is confined to high-temperature heating of deparaffinized tissue sections in a water solution to achieve a stronger intensity of immunohistochemical staining. This heating AR technique is very simple: the tissue sections are boiled in the retrieval solution for 10 minutes or more (for a few antigens, shorter heating times are effective). That the method is effective and reliable for retrieval of a variety of antigens that have been masked by formalin fixation is evident from an abundance of publications worldwide (11,14,88, 90,91,93,94,112). Several modifications of the heating methods and the AR solutions (defined as certain solutions used for immersing the slides during the heating process) have been developed and applied in clinical and research laboratories, without any consensus as to a standard method (105). The lack of a uniform approach is particularly important in quantitative or semiquatitative immunohistochemistry (IHC), as emphasized by Taylor et al. (112) in a call for greater standardization for the AR technique. Any attempt to standardize AR should take into account the following principles: major factors that influence the effectiveness of AR-IHC; control tissues, including fresh frozen tissue, to confirm the results; and clinical evaluation of the results.

Effectiveness Factors

All the major factors that influence the effectiveness of AR-IHC (see Chapter 2) are critical issues in attempts to standardize the AR technique. The goal is to establish an optimal AR protocol for maximal retrieval of routinely processed paraffin tissue sections that have been fixed in formalin with a variable time schedule (92). Based on two major factors, the heating conditions (heating temperature × heating time) and

Antigen Retrieval Techniques
Edited by Shan-Rong Shi, Jiang Gu, and Clive R. Taylor
©2000 Eaton Publishing, Natick, MA

the pH value of the AR solution, a test battery approach has been employed for a number of antibodies and has yielded optimal protocols for many of the more commonly used antibodies (see Chapter 2).

Controls

Control tissues including fresh frozen tissue are necessary to confirm the results. Detailed principles regarding immunostaining controls can be found in recent publications (8,108). In most cases, a negative control slide treated under AR-equivalent conditions is essential to demonstrate the validity of the immunostaining result. Although most studies report satisfactory results without false positivity, care must be taken when performing AR-IHC to rule out any false positivity or spurious alteration of the immunostaining pattern (7,90,91,105,112). For example, we found that weakly positive nuclear staining may be seen when using a low-pH AR solution for the monoclonal antibody to MIB-1 (Ki-67) (88,90,91,109,112). Other articles have reported nonspecific staining or unwanted immunoreactivity with AR-IHC (36,64,82). Thus, for any antibody tested, knowledge of immunolocalization of the antigen in fresh frozen tissue is valuable as a gold standard. When establishing the AR process for an antibody new to the laboratory, it is advisable that frozen tissue sections be stained simultaneously to validate the immunolocalization obtained in paraffin sections by using AR-IHC.

In some circumstances, it is necessary to employ matched pairs of frozen and paraffin tissue sections from the same case to demonstrate the exact immunostaining pattern for certain antigens characterized by heterogeneous expression in a tissue (89). For example, using the test battery approach, we developed an AR-IHC protocol for the monoclonal antibody to thrombospondin (TSP), but we observed discrepant staining patterns in bladder and prostate tissues. To clarify this discrepancy, 10 matched pairs of frozen and paraffin tissue sections were tested to compare the TSP-immunolocalization patterns, using the same AR protocol for paraffin sections. The results in frozen sections mirrored those obtained in paraffin sections, thereby discounting technical artifacts consequent on fixation as a cause of the discrepancies and confirming that the AR-IHC protocol using a low-pH solution for TSP is optimal for routinely processed paraffin tissue sections. It is notable that variable immunostaining patterns of TSP have also been reported by others (42).

There is, however, the interesting question as to the universal validity of frozen section as a gold standard: it has become clear that some antigens are lost by diffusion, degradation, or fixation extraction in frozen sections. Indeed, for some antibody/antigen combinations the formalin paraffin section is now the gold standard. For example, the use of AR with ER-1D5 on routine paraffin sections has achieved much improved staining, in both intensity and number of positive cells. Results with the previously employed estrogen receptor-immunocytochemical assay (ER-ICA) using the monoclonal antibody H222 (Abbott, North Chicago, IL, USA) on paraffin sections have been equaled or surpassed, as have the results obtained in frozen sections. Our studies indicate that the intensity and number of positive cells for ER-1D5 with AR-IHC are maximized by using the AR solution at low pH (86). One explanation for the stronger intensity of ER-1D5 on paraffin sections after AR-IHC, compared with frozen section, may be that some receptor molecules or epitopes are lost in the frozen sections by autolysis, by diffusion, or due to extraction by the fixative employed. Pertschuk and Axiotis have discussed this issue in detail in Chapter 9. The major question raised here is: which of these approaches gives the right answer? Battifora (6,7) published two editorial articles analyzing this issue with respect to AR-IHC of ER and p53. Studies have shown that the increased sensitivity achieved using an ER-1D5 antibody in paraffin sections after AR-IHC provides a better correlation with overall survival and disease-free survival than does the dextran-coated charcoal (DCC) cytosol assay or ER-ICA with antibody H222. Thus, in the context of predicting prognosis and therapy, the AR-IHC method for ER using ER-1D5 is preferred (see Chapter 9).

Battifora (6) also posed the question as to whether the time has arrived to abandon the cytosol- and frozen- section-based receptor assays altogether in favor of paraffin-based ICA (6). We would answer in the affirmative: the time has come, providing that an effective AR procedure is employed (107).

Other similar examples representing increased IHC staining signals in paraffin sections (using AR treatment) compared with frozen sections include staining with antibodies to retinoblastoma (Rb), p53, etc. We recently demonstrated significantly increased immunoreactivity for a monoclonal antibody to prostate stem cell antigen (PSCA, clone #3E6 IgG 3k, provided by the University of California at Los Angeles); a reproducible cell membrane staining pattern could only be revealed in paraffin sections using the AR treatment, in contrast to negative membrane immunostaining in frozen sections. Further studies using nonfixed frozen tissue sections may be necessary to clarify whether the immunostaining result of paraffin section after AR is valid (Thu et al., unpublished data). Possible reasons for the stronger immunostaining signals for some antibodies on archival paraffin sections achieved by AR-IHC, compared with frozen sections, may be that some molecules are lost in the frozen sections by autolysis, diffusion, or the fixation employed, as evidenced by the immunohistochemical detection of estradiol that can be obtained by formalin-fixed, paraffin-embedded tissue sections, but not by frozen sections (described in Chapter 1).

Clinical Evaluation on the Basis of Follow-up Data

Studies based on evaluation of the intensity of AR-IHC with reference to clinical follow-up data have demonstrated that standardization of AR-IHC should be based on correlation with clinical outcome. This concept has been well exemplified in the ER immunocytochemical studies conducted by Pertschuk et al. (see Chapter 9).

PROTOCOLS

High-temperature heating is the most important factor for the AR technique. Different heating methods may yield similar results if heating conditions are adjusted appropriately (111). For most antibodies tested to date, boiling temperature for 10 minutes will provide satisfactory results. Currently, the microwave (MW) oven, autoclave, pressure cooker, microwave with pressure cooker, conventional heating such as a water bath, and steamer have been used, principally with regard to duration of heating, as evidenced in the following protocols.

Protocols for special applications such as immunogold electron microscopy (IEM), in situ hybridization, terminal deoxynucleotidyl transferase (TdT)-mediated dUTP nick-end labeling (TUNEL), multiple immunostaining, archival cervical smears, brain tissues, nonheating AR methods, and animal tissues are described in other chapters in this book.

Materials and Reagents

- MW oven. Various kinds of domestic MW ovens with an output power around 1000 W have been widely applied. In our hands, the model R-4A46 from Sharp (900 W, 2450 MHz; Memphis, TN, USA) with multiple sequence power settings has provided an easier way to run some of the protocols mentioned below. Several laboratory microwave ovens have been designed with controlled temperature and other conditions that can then be measured accurately during the heating process, such as the H2550 Laboratory Microwave Processor (EBS, Agawam, MA, USA) as well as other modern ultrarapid microwave processors manufactured in Italy (see Chapter 12).
- Other heating equipment. An autoclave used for sterilization is used, allowing superheating at 120°C. A domestic pressure cooker with an operating pressure of 103 kPa/15 psi can also be used for superheating. A plastic steamer designed by Ventana Biotek Systems (Newport Beach, CA, USA) may be employed for convenient use of the autostainer from the same manufacturer. Hot plates and water baths are available for conventional heating methods at boiling or other desired temperatures.
- Slide container. A plastic Coplin jar is commonly used for AR heating sections. Any other larger plastic containers may be employed to contain slides and solution. Note that loosening the cover is important to avoid increased pressure during boiling.
- A plastic pressure cooker (Nordicware, MN, USA). This can be set in a microwave oven to reach a superheating condition.
- AR solutions. See below and other chapters for details.

Treatment of Routinely Formalin-Fixed, Paraffin-Embedded Tissue Sections before Antigen Retrieval Treatment

1. Mount the tissue sections on slides coated with either poly-L-lysine or 3-aminopropyltriethoxysilane (APES) or charged slides provided by Fisher Scientific (Pittsburgh, PA, USA), and dry the slides at 60°C for at least 1 hour to promote adherence of the tissue sections to the slides. Overnight incubation produces optimal adhesion.

2. Deparaffinize by using a routine Histoclear or xyline procedure. Rehydrate by graded alcohols, blocking the endogenous peroxidase with an H_2O_2-methanol solution. Routine deparaffinization may be omitted if you are using high-temperature heating as the AR treatment. This simple modification was reported by Yorukoglu and Cingoz (115), based on the fact that high-temperature heating itself can remove the wax; thus heating may replace the routine deparaffinization step. After heating the paraffin-embedded tissue sections in the first jar as in the AR procedure described below, immediately transfer slides to the second jar containing buffer solution for a second heating cycle. It may be better to heat the two (or three) jars containing solution simultaneously, to maintain same temperature.

3. Rinse the slides in three changes of distilled water for 15 minutes prior to AR treatment.

Microwave Heating Method (83)

1. Place the slides in plastic Coplin jars containing an AR solution such as distilled

water, buffer solution, metal salt solution, urea, glycine-HCl, pH 3.5, EDTA-NaCl solution of pH 8.0, etc.

2. Cover the jars with loose-fitting screw caps and heat in the MW oven for 10 minutes. The 10-minute heating time is divided into two 5-minute cycles with an interval of 1 minute between cycles to check the fluid level in the jars. If necessary, more AR solution is added after the first 5 minutes to avoid drying out the tissue sections. Standardization of heating time by beginning to count the time only after the solution has reached boiling is recommended, to avoid discrepancies between different laboratories when using various MW ovens.

3. After completion of the heating phase, remove the Coplin jars from the oven, and allow to cool for 15 minutes.

4. Slides are then rinsed twice in distilled water and in phosphate-buffered saline (PBS) for 5 minutes and are ready for IHC staining.

H2550 Laboratory Microwave Processor (88,112)

1. This MW processor is available with continuous temperature readouts. Its power output is regulated by a temperature feedback mechanism and a timer, which is capable of monitoring both temperature and heating time.

2. Fix a Coplin jar on a thick board or plastic plate and set it in the center portion of the turntable, filling the jar with distilled or tap water. Set the temperature probe into the Coplin jar through a hole in the cap to measure the temperature.

3. Set all test jars around the central probe jar as close as possible.

4. Turn on the MW processor. Set the required time and temperature.

5. Turn on the turntable, making sure the jars are not moved by the probe and the table.

6. Start the MW heating; the timer is automatically controlled.

7. For heating at 100°C, divide the heating time into 5-minute cycles, as mentioned above.

8. This MW processor is particularly useful for a test battery when lower temperature heating is required (see below).

Calibration Technique for the Microwave Oven (106)

1. Turn on the MW at high power (800 W) for 2 to 3 minutes until the solution comes to a rapid boil, and then turn off the oven. Note the exact time the solution to boiled.

2. Set the oven power at 3 to 4 (30%–40% power or 250 + 50 W) or at defrost (low power). Heat for 7 to 10 minutes. (If using a 500-W oven, set power level at 5–6 or 50%–60%, i.e., 250 W). Adjust the setting so that the oven cycles on and off every 20 to 30 seconds and the solution boils for about 5 to 10 seconds in each cycle.

3. The following formula can be used to determine the power setting: $S = 250/P \times 10$, where S = the MW power setting for AR, and P = the output power of the individual MW oven. For example, if a MW oven output power is 800 W, then the power setting for AR (S) is: $S = 250/800 \times 10 = 3.1$. Therefore, it should be set at 3 and heated for 7 to 10 minutes.

Autoclave Heating Method (4,96)

1. Set the slides in Coplin jars or other kinds of containers filled with AR solutions. Fix the covers in place with a special tape designed for the autoclave.
2. Set the jars with slides in the center portion of the autoclave.
3. Tightly close the door of the autoclave as required by the instructions.
4. Set the temperature to 120°C for 10 minutes.
5. Allow a cool-down period of 20 to 30 minutes after heating.
6. For IHC staining, follow the same procedure as for MW heating.

Pressure Cooker Method (65,71)

1. A domestic cooker with an operating pressure of 103 kPa/15 psi is filled with one-third of the AR solution and heated by hot plate to boiling.
2. Slides suspended in metal slide racks are placed quickly into the AR solution, and the pressure lid is tightly replaced.
3. The timer starts when the pressure indicator valve reaches the maximum (around 4 min). The optimal period of pressurized boiling is 1 to 2 minutes.
4. After heating, the cooker is depressurized and cooled under running water, the lid is then removed. Cold tap water is added to replace the hot AR solution. A 15- to 20-minute cooling time may be required as in the MW heating method.

Microwave + Plastic Pressure Cooker (76,111)

1. Fill three plastic staining jars containing as many as 25 slides with AR solution and place into a plastic pressure cooker (Nordicware). Add approximately 600 mL of distilled water to the pressure cooker to reach one-half of the volume, making sure that all three jars stand in the water at a stable position.
2. Place the plastic pressure cooker containing three staining jars with tissue slides as described above in the MW oven (a Sharp carousel MW oven, model R-4A46, with multiple sequence cooking, which can switch from one power level setting to another automatically). Set the oven at maximum power (900 W, 2450 MHz) for 15 minutes to boil the water, followed by a 40% power setting for another 15 minutes (simmer) to maintain boiling.
3. Cool down for 15 to 20 minutes, and follow with the procedure for the regular MW AR method.

Steam Heating AR (111)

1. Use Steam HIER (heat-induced epitope retrieval) provided by Ventana Biotek Systems (Newport Beach, CA, USA) for convenient use of the BioTek autostainer.
2. Set the slides in the TechMate slide holder in the regular face-to-face orientation maintaining the capillary gap.
3. Fill the steamer with distilled water to the top line and heat to boiling point. Turn the dial to 30 minutes and proceed to the next step.
4. Add 10 mL to each of the 10-well trays in the gray tile provided by BioTek, and place the slide holder on the gray tile with the tips of the slide pairs in the AR solution located in the 10-well trays. Then place the gray tile with the slide holder into the center of the steam chamber.

5. Place the whole steam chamber base on the steamer while boiling vigorously for 20 minutes.

6. After cooling the heated slides for 15 minutes, the remaining procedure for IHC is similar to the MW heating method.

Flow Cytometry

AR Heating Treatment Prior to Enzyme Digestion (56)

1. Cut two 50-μm-thick tissue sections and put them into a glass tube. Carry out routine paraffinization.

2. Immerse deparaffinized sections in cold citrate solution (2 mg citric acid/mL of distilled water, pH 6.0) and set in a water bath at 80°C for 2 hours.

3. After a 15-minute cooling period at room temperature, wash the sections in PBS, followed by enzyme digestion in pepsin solution (1 mg/mL) in 0.1 N HCl at 37°C for 15 minutes.

4. Filter the sample by a 50-μm mesh nylon filter.

5. Wash the pellet to clean pepsin using centrifugation at 400× g and resuspend the pellet in PBS/bovine serum albumin (BSA).

6. Follow by immunostaining or other staining method to detect DNA.

Perform enzyme digestion followed by heating treatment (81)

1. Cut paraffin-embedded tissue sections 50 μm thick and deparaffinize routinely.

2. Perform enzyme digestion of the deparaffinized tissue sections with pepsin (0.05% in normal saline, pH 1.65) for 60 minutes in a water bath at 37°C.

3. After 60 minutes of incubation, vortex samples every 5 minutes for an additional 30 minutes. Terminate enzyme digestion by adding chilled 10% fetal bovine serum in PBS.

4. Filter the sample using 40-μm nylon mesh, wash in PBS, and centrifuge at 800× g for 10 minutes. Resuspend the pellet in 0.01 mol/L citrate buffer, pH 6.0.

5. Heat the sample in citrate buffer using a 600-W microwave oven for one or two cycles of 60 seconds each.

6. Follow by the immunohistochemical staining procedure.

Extraction of Proteins from Archival Paraffin-Embedded Tissue Sections (40)

1. Cut paraffin-embedded tissue sections 50 μm thick and mount on plain glass slides.

2. Perform routine deparaffinization, immerse in distilled water, and air-dry.

3. Perform microdissection according to the morphologic findings observed by a hematoxylin and eosin-stained slide to collect 5 mm^2 cancer tissue from the deparaffinized thick section. The average dry weight of such a 5 mm^2 × 50-μm-thick section of cancer tissue is 0.74 mg (range 0.56–1.11 mg).

4. Cut the dissected tissues into small pieces, and put them into an Eppendorf tube. Add 200 μL of RIPA buffer, pH 7.6 (1 mol/L sodium dihydrogen phosphate, 10 mmol/L disodium hydrogen phosphate, 154 mmol/L sodium chloride, 1% Triton® X-100, 12 mmol/L sodium deoxycholate, 0.2% sodium azide, 0.95 mmol/L fluoride, 2 mmol/L phenylmethylsulfonyl fluoride, 50 mg/mL aprotinin, 50 mmol/L leupeptin),

containing 2% sodium dodecyl sulfate (SDS) to the sample tube.

5. Incubate the sample at 100°C for 20 minutes followed by 60°C for 2 hours. This may achieve the best results, in that 121.5 μg of protein may be extracted from a 5 mm^2 × 50-μm-thick section of cancer tissue.

6. After incubation, centrifuge the tissue lysate at 15 000× g for 20 minutes at 4°C. Collect the supernatants, and store at -80°C until used for protein assay.

COMPARISON OF ANTIGEN RETRIEVAL HEATING METHODS

Taylor et al. (111) reported a comparative study of AR heating methods including microwave, microwave and pressure cooker, autoclave, and steamer using 21 antibodies on archival formalin-fixed, paraffin-embedded sections. The study demonstrated only minor differences among the heating methods for AR when the optimal concentration of primary antibody for the immunostaining procedure was used. In conclusion, different heating methods can yield similar intensities of AR immunostaining if the heating conditions (temperature and time) are adjusted appropriately. For example, a comparable intensity of AR-IHC for retinoblastoma protein (pRB) was achieved by using autoclave heating at 120°C for 10 minutes and equally by MW heating at 100°C for 60 minutes when the same AR solution (Tris-HCl buffer, pH 10.0) was used (89). In studies comparing different heating methods, false conclusions may be reached if the heating conditions (temperature × time) are not comparable, as in the case of MW heating at 100°C for 10 minutes versus autoclave or pressure cooker at 120°C for 10 minutes. The fact that several heating devices may provide similar results permits the use of different AR heating methods according to the equipment available. Various advantages have been noted with respect to the different heating methods currently employed (Table 1).

ANTIGEN RETRIEVAL SOLUTIONS

As discussed previously in Chapters 1 and 2, recent research achievements have demonstrated that among all components of the AR solution, the pH value is the most critical factor that may significantly influence the efficiency of AR-IHC (86). The chemical composition of the AR solution may also play a role. The use of metal salts in the AR solution was based on earlier studies that used zinc formalin fixation of tissue for better preservation of antigenicity (44). We originally speculated that metal salt solutions might play a role in refixation of the retrieved antigens, because salt solutions gave slightly better retrieval effects than pure water for some antibodies (83). Improved AR-IHC staining using metal solutions was subsequently demonstrated by numerous studies (28,32–35,48,58,62,66,75,95,98,101–104,110). Siitonen et al. (98) compared AR-IHC staining with other antigen unmasking methods, using monoclonal antibodies to proliferate cell nuclear antigen (PCNA; 19A2 and PC10) on archival paraffin sections of 109 cases of breast carcinoma. They concluded that the best immunostaining results were achieved using saturated lead thiocyanate with the 19A2 antibody. However, it has subsequently been shown that metal salts are not an essential component of the AR buffer. Furthermore, the toxic effect of metal salts, particularly lead salts, is a major drawback.

To avoid potential toxicity, several alternative AR solutions such as citrate, Tris and

Table 1. Advantages and Disadvantages of Five Heating Methods for Antigen Retrieval

Method	Advantages	Disadvantages	Time[a] (min)
Microwave, 5 min × 2	Shortest time, simple instrument, widely available and inexpensive	Must check solution level, difficult to standardize with large batches of slides; may be hot or cold spots	25
5 min × 4	Simple instrument, widely available and inexpensive	Requires attention for 20 min to check solution level; may be hot or cold spots; difficult to standardize with large batches of slides	35
Microwave with pressure cooker	Simple, inexpensive; load many slides each time; high-intensity stain; larger container eliminates cold spots	Requires slightly longer time than simple microwave	45
Steam HIER	No loading and unloading of slides into carrier for automated use; conserves AR solution; inexpensive; no cold spots	Preheated steam; originally designed for autostainer; can be used manually	35
Autoclave	High-intensity stain; load many slides each time; no cold spots	Expensive, may not be available in small laboratory; careful handling due to the pressure in autoclave	45

[a]Total period required including set-up or preheating, the retrieval process itself, and cool-down.

Reprinted with permission from Reference 111.

other buffer solutions and urea were subsequently developed (18,29,30,49,57,84, 85,110); EDTA or EGTA (69), glycine-HCl buffer (41), and others (88,90,91,112) were also used. Pileri et al. (78) conducted a comparative study using three different AR solutions: 0.01 mol/L citrate buffer (pH 6.0), 0.1 mol/L Tris-HCl (pH 8.0), and 1 mmol/L EDTA-NaOH solution (pH 8.0), using the pressure cooking heating method (for 1–2 min). They found that EDTA appeared to be best, while citrate buffer often produced the poorest results. Tris-HCl buffer was intermediate in terms of both intensity and number of positive cells. A recent study in our laboratory reached a similar conclusion. We confirmed that Tris-HCl buffer at pH 10.0 yielded intense staining, as reported previously (86); however, subsequent immunostaining was often more difficult, because of detached tissue sections and apparent loss of surface tension. (Drops of reagent spread rapidly across the whole slide and dry quickly.) These findings support the growing opinion that EDTA-NaOH at pH 8.0 may be the preferred AR solution for most antibodies used in surgical pathology.

Although the chemical component of the AR solution may play a role as a possible cofactor in the heating procedure, no single component is both essential and best for AR. Morgan et al. (69) observed that calcium has an adverse effect on AR-IHC, at least for the monoclonal antibody MIB-1. Other unpredictable effects also occur,

Table 2. Test Battery Suggested for Screening an Optimal Antigen Retrieval Protocol

	Tris-HCl buffer (pH)		
	1.0–2.0 (Slide #)[a]	7.0–8.0 (Slide #)[a]	10.0–11.0 (Slide #)[a]
Super-high (120°C)[b]	#1	#4	#7
High (100°C), 10 min	#2	#5	#8
Mid-high (90°C), 10 min[c]	#3	#6	#9

[a]One more slide may be used for control without AR treatment. Citrate buffer of pH 6.0 may be used to replace Tris-HCl buffer, pH 7.0 to 8.0, as the results are the same.

[b]The temperature of super-high at 120°C may be reached by either autoclaving or microwave heating at a longer time.

[c]The temperature of mid-high at 90°C may be obtained by either a water bath or a microwave oven monitored with a thermometer.

Reprinted with permission from Reference 90.

making choice of the AR solution difficult. To determine the ideal AR solution, we recommend a test battery, because different antigens may require different conditions for retrieval (26,86,88,109,112). It may be possible to obtain an equivalent intensity of staining with several different AR solutions, if the pH value of the AR solution and the heating conditions are optimized, using the test battery method, as discussed just below. For example, Katoh and Breier (47) found that equally good results of p53 immunostaining by the AR-IHC method were obtained with normal saline, citrate buffer, or distilled water. Similarly, Hazelbag et al. (38) tested a broad panel of monoclonal antibodies against a variety of keratins on formalin-fixed, paraffin-embedded tissues with different AR solutions. They concluded that MW heating in either Target Unmasking Fluid (TUF; Dianova, Hamburg, Germany) or a simple detergent, DET, in a 0.05% solution, yielded similar results. [DET contains anionogenic (15%–30%) and nonionogenic (5%–15%) surfactants (Dish Clean, Bosman Chemie, Heijningen, The Netherlands).] Based on our study of AR-IHC and pH (86), three categories of antigens were identified based on pH values of AR solutions, a finding supported by recent studies concerning protein stucture indicating that the complexity of protein structure may be analyzed by grouping it into several categories based on its functional units (114). Therefore, it is possible to establish several optimal AR protocols for several corresponding antigens by using the test battery.

TEST BATTERY APPROACH

A test battery may be defined as a preliminary test of AR technique examining two major factors, heating condition ($T \times t$) and pH value. It is performed to establish an optimal protocol for the antigen tested.

Typically, three levels of heating conditions and pH values (low, moderate, and high) may be applied to screen for a potentially optimal AR-IHC protocol for a particular antigen of interest, as indicated in Table 2. The test battery method can also be performed in two sequential steps. In the first step, we tested three AR solutions at different pH values as listed above in Table 2, with one standard temperature (100°C for 10 min) to find the optimal value. In the second step, we tested optimal heating conditions based on the established pH value.

We have demonstrated that different heating methods, including MW, MW and pressure cooker, steam, and autoclave (111), can be evaluated in a similar fashion and adjusted to yield similar satisfactory AR-IHC staining intensity. Nevertheless, there may be some unpredictable correlations between heating condition and certain pH values. In our preliminary studies, when using a middle or high pH solution, the higher the temperature, the better the staining for most nuclear and cytoplasmic antibodies tested. In contrast, when using a low pH solution, overly intense heating (such as in a pressure cooker) may yield a poor result. For example, the strongest intensity of MIB-1 or pRB on archival paraffin sections was achieved either with regular MW heating and a low pH solution, or a high pH solution with intense heating (pressure cooker or elongated regular MW heating method). A low pH with intense heating gave poor results (89).

The test battery thus serves as a rapid screening approach to identify an optimal protocol for each antibody/antigen to be tested. The goal is to establish the maximal retrieval level for formalin-masked antigens with a variety of fixation times, to standardize immunostaining results. In one study of 14 antibodies using the test battery method, we demonstrated that the strongest intensity of AR-IHC for most antibodies tested was achieved either using low pH buffer solution with regular MW heating conditions or high pH buffer with intense heating conditions (such as autoclave heating or MW heating for elongated heating time) (87,89). In addition, a test battery may identify some false-negative AR-IHC staining, as indicated in Figure 1.

TECHNICAL NOTES AND TROUBLESHOOTING

Applications in Special Fields

Flow Cytometry of Archival Paraffin-Embedded Tissue

The MW heating AR method has been successfully applied to archival paraffin-embedded tissues to enhance the detection efficiency of flow cytometry (FCM) (54,56,73,81). Two different protocols have been documented:

1. Heating treatment prior to enzyme digestion was recommended by Leers et al. (56). They demonstrated that this method allows high-resolution DNA analysis of routinely processed paraffin-embedded tissues with double efficiency of recovery of single cells compared with the standard method without heating. In addition, the keratin-positive fraction and the fluorescence intensity were increased compared with that of the cells obtained from the fresh tissue.

2. Enzyme digestion followed by heating treatment was adopted to achieve enhancement of FCM on paraffin-embedded tissue sections as exemplified by Redkar and Krishan (81). They demonstrated a successful result for FCM analysis of estrogen and progesterone receptors in formalin-fixed, paraffin-embedded human breast cancers. However, the heating time must be adjusted to obtain reasonable DNA histograms when using their protocol.

Diagnostic Cytology

Boon et al. (12) demonstrated that the MW AR technique could be applied to cervical smears initially stained by the Papanicolaou method, with satisfactory results for MIB-1 nuclear staining, to screen the positive diagnostic cells using the PAPNET computer system (NSI, Suffern, NY, USA).

Plastic-Embedded Tissue Thin Sections: Epoxy, Epon, or Methyl Methacrylate Resin

Numerous articles have been published since Suurmeijer and Boon (103) documented the application of AR in plastic tissue sections in 1993. AR-IHC is readily adapted to bone marrow samples, with the advantages of clear background and intense signal for reliable, high-quality IHC. This improved stain quality is particularly desirable for demonstration of neoplastic cells in regenerative marrow after chemotherapy, as well as the detection of residual disease after treatment. AR-IHC is also suitable for formalin-fixed, acid-decalcified tissues (5,10,52,100). Brorson (13) described a comparative study to demonstrate how AR affects the yield of immunogold labeling on epoxy sections embedded with different amounts of accelerator, leading to the conclusion that the combination of an increased amount of accelerator during tissue processing for epoxy embedding, together with the AR heating method,

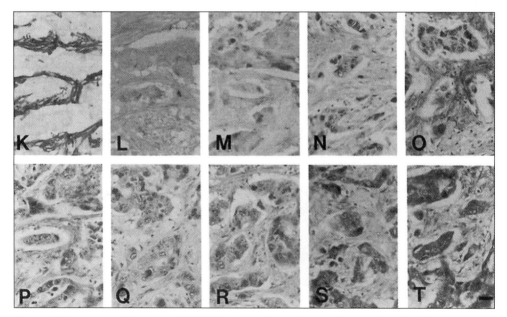

Figure 1. Comparison of intensity of AR-IHC by using the test battery for monoclonal antibody to thrombospondin (TSP) on sections of bladder carcinoma. The AR protocols used are arranged in the following order: pH 1.0, 100°C, 20 min (K); pH 1.0, 100°C, 10 min (L); pH 1.0, 90°C, 10 min (M); pH 6.0, 100°C, 20 min (N); pH 6.0, 100°C, 10 min (O); pH 6.0, 90°C, 10 min (P); pH 10.0, 100°C, 20 min (Q); pH 10.0, 100°C, 10 min (R); pH 10.0, 90°C, 10 min (S); no AR pretreatment (T). The strongest extracellular labeling of TSP was found by using an AR solution at pH 1.0, as shown in K. Under lower heating conditions (L, M), the intensity was decreased progressively (K > L > M). Other protocols using pH 6.0 or 10.0 gave poor results, similar to a lack of pretreatment (T). Diaminobenzidine (DAB) was used as the chromogen, with hematoxylin counterstaining. Original magnification 100×. Scale bar = 50 μm. Reprinted with permission from Reference 90. **(See color plate A12).**

provides enhancement of IHC staining on epoxy sections. In our experience, Epon-embedded tissue sections benefit from a de-Epon procedure using NaOH-ethanol or methanol after AR heating. Under these conditions, a shorter heating time and/or lower heating temperature may be possible for some antibodies tested, resulting in superior morphologic detail (93). Recently, Hand and Church (37) documented a successful AR protocol using a pressure cooker for 3 minutes at 121°C for methyl methacrylate-embedded semithin sections (2 µm) of tonsil. For better immunostaining of CD3, they pretreated slides with 0.1% trypsin at 37°C for 20 minutes, followed by an AR heating protocol in a pressure cooker.

Immunfluorescence

D'Ambra-Cabry et al. (22) reported the use of AR as a potential option in retrospective studies of skin diseases such as bullous pemphigoid and eosinophilic dermatitis by direct immunofluorescence (IF), based on a comparative study of fresh frozen tissue and archival paraffin-embedded tissue. Fariss et al. (27) reported excellent immunolocalization of the tissue inhibitor of metalloproteinases-3 (TIMP-3) in formalin-paraffin sections of retina/choroid of adult human eyes using AR with sodium phosphate/citrate buffer, pH 3.5, and immunofluorescence. However, in spite of these successes, two major issues must be solved before AR-IF can be performed routinely on archival tissues: (*i*) the sensitivity obtained by AR-IF on fixed paraffin sections is lower than that of frozen section; and (*ii*) possible altered AR-IF-staining patterns may be found. For example, Al-Rifai et al. (2) demonstrated spurious intercellular staining within the epidermis, which was not found in frozen section, when combining heating AR and 0.3% trypsin digestion. There are preliminary indications that improved results may be obtained by combining AR with low antibody concentration and a signal amplification system (63).

In Situ Hybridization

Following earlier studies concerning application of high-temperature pretreatment for in situ hybridization (ISH) (55,61,97), Oliver et al. (72) conducted a quantitative comparison of several pretreatment regimens, including MW heating, autoclave heating at 100°C or above, conventional heating at 90°C, and proteinase K treatment for ISH. The sensitivity of the six pretreatments was evaluated by densitometric analysis of ISH signal on autoradiographs, based on the same experimental conditions. The strongest ISH signal was achieved by the MW heating RNA retrieval procedure, which showed identical results for frozen and paraffin sections. Enzymatic digestion yielded 50% intensity compared with frozen sections. Both the autoclave, and heating at 90°C yielded a weaker signal, around 10%, compared with the frozen sections. In this study the protocol of MW heating pretreatment involved immersing sections in 10 mmol/L citrate buffer, pH 6.0, and microwaving at full power in an 800-W microwave oven for three 5-minute periods, with washes in diethyl pyrocarbonate (DEPC)-treated water.

Protein Extraction

Ikeda et al. (40) developed a protocol for extraction of diagnostically useful proteins from formalin-fixed, paraffin-embedded tissue sections. By heating the deparaffinized tissue sections at 100°C for 20 minutes before incubation at 60°C for 2 hours in RIPA solution, 121.5 µg of protein may be extracted from 5 mm^2 × 50-µm-thick tissue. They successfully detected a variety of membrane-bound cytosolic and nuclear proteins in archival paraffin-embedded tissues to obtain valuable information for molecular biology.

Nonspecific Staining after Antigen Retrieval Treatment

Most studies have reported satisfactory results without false positivity for most antibodies tested (14,19,23,30,57,83,88,90,91,93,94,103,112). Recently, Baas et al. (3) reported that a potential false-positive result might be obtained after extreme AR treatment when using the monoclonal antibody DO7 (anti-p53), and there have been sporadic reports of unexpected staining problems with other antibodies. However, further investigation is needed, correlating AR findings with both frozen section and molecular assays. The current consensus is that the immunolocalization of p53 in paraffin sections after AR treatment is comparable with the pattern obtained in frozen sections, as evidenced by a number of studies demonstrating that AR pretreatment significantly increased the immunostaining intensity using the antibody DO-7 but did not alter the pattern of immunoreactivity for p53 (9,21,60).

Binks et al. (9) compared the staining of DO-7 obtained with and without AR, comparing paraffin sections and direct smears of specimens from pulmonary non-small cell carcinomas, and were not able to find evidence of false positivity. Nevertheless, some studies have reported spurious nonspecific staining following use of a broad panel of antibodies, particularly when using different heating conditions and/or different AR solutions with a variety of pH values. For example, weak positive nuclear staining was found when a low-pH AR solution was used for monoclonal antibody to MIB-1 (86). Sebenik et al. (82) attributed nonspecific nuclear staining after AR to the secondary antibody, suggesting that retitration of the second antibody may be necessary if nonspecific staining occurs when using AR-IHC. Wieczorek et al. (113) concluded that the problem resides with the primary antibody, based on a study employing three AR solutions, 1% zinc sulfate (pH 4.9), 0.01 mol/L citrate buffer (pH 6.0), and 0.01 mol/L Tris buffer (pH 9.0), with careful control groups to exclude potential false-positive staining caused by endogenous biotin or electrostatic binding of immunoglobulins. These authors concluded that nuclear positivity is nonspecific and is easily eliminated by retitration of the primary antibody to a higher dilution. In another study, focal keratin staining was observed in archival paraffin sections of malignant melanoma and plasma cell tumors when using heating AR, possibly resulting from detection of low levels of keratins in these tumors (36).

One potential cause of increased background after AR heating may be the unmasking of endogenous biotin, which accounts for some positive staining in frozen tissue sections, particularly for liver, kidney, adrenal cortex, and thyroid tissues (15,45). In this instance, the cytoplasmic biotin reaction appears as a fine granular staining pattern in the cytoplasm. Kashima et al. (45) found a high incidence (93 of 208) of this form of positive cytoplasmic biotin staining in thyroid lesions, with the highest incidence in papillary carcinoma. This effect can be avoided by using a routine blocking procedure or a detection system free of avidin-biotin complex. It is important to keep in mind that any background staining that may be observed in frozen tissue sections may also be found in MW-heated archival paraffin sections.

Caution must be used when testing new antibodies using different AR protocols, as emphasized recently by Swanson (105). Indeed, variable immunostaining patterns have been reported when using different AR protocols (64). The incorporation of frozen sections into a test battery used to select an optimal AR protocol is extremely helpful in identifying any false positivity or unexpected change of staining pattern, as exemplified by the TSP immunolocalization in the prostate and bladder mentioned above.

Detached Tissue Sections after the Antigen Retrieval Heating Process

Pretreated slides, either commercially charged or poly-L-lysine coated, are recommended prior to heat treatment to protect tissue sections from detachment. We found that thinner tissue sections adhere more firmly than thicker sections, but that different types of tissue vary in adhesiveness to glass slides. In our experience, tissues with more fat detach more readily. Baking the paraffin sections in a 60°C oven overnight appears to increase adhesion. In a few difficult cases, the use of heating at lower temperature (90°C) for extended heating times may reduce tissue damage and detachment while achieving a similar AR result.

To improve adhesion, a postadhesive method was designed by Pateraki and Kontogeorgos (74) for stored paraffin sections that were already mounted on regular plain slides (without treatment for adhesion) but required heating by AR pretreatment. The reported protocol is as follows: place paraffin sections in an oven at 58°C for 3 hours. After 2 to 3 dips in acetone, immerse the slides in a Coplin jar containing Vectabond glue (Vector, Burlingame, CA, USA) for 30 minutes, cover the jar, follow with three washes in distilled water, and dry in the oven overnight. To ensure safety, the process of using acetone and Vectabond glue should be done under a hood. We tried this postadhesion method in our laboratory recently and achieved satisfactory results. In our experience, for some difficult cases, commercially charged slides may be additionally coated with chemicals such as poly-L-lysine, APES, or albumin with gelatine to enhance adhesion. Mote et al. (70) summarized their experience in maximal tissue retention by using positively charged slides coated with Mayer albumin adhesive. To reduce background staining due to APES-coated slides when using the immunogold-silver staining method, Krenacs and Krenacs (53) found that washing slides in a buffer containing 0.1% detergent after heat treatment may yield clean background and sharp contrast for both paraffin- and resin-embedded tissue sections.

Counterstaining after Antigen Retrieval

Hematoxylin used for counterstaining after AR-IHC staining is satisfactory in most situations, except when an AR solution at low pH is used. After heating the tissue section in a low pH solution, nuclear staining for hematoxylin may be compromised. Since a low pH AR solution is preferable for some antigens, it is necessary to find a way to correct this acid-induced defect of counterstaining. Recently, we found that dropping 1 N NaOH solution on slides for 10 minutes may improve hematoxylin counterstaining following low pH AR; otherwise, other nuclear stains should be employed.

Inconsistent Results

Although inconsistency is becoming less of a problem in larger laboratories where many slides are processed routinely every day, irregular results may be expected in both clinical and research laboratories when technicians or research staff are not familiar with the AR process. Possible causes include the following.

Inconsistency of the Treatment Itself

The AR treatment itself may be inconsistent, such as variable heating temperatures resulting from using different MW ovens, nonuniform Coplin jars or other containers of different sizes, variability in the total numbers of containers placed in the oven, location of Coplin jars at different sites in the oven, or allowing drying of the slides during heating due to loss of the AR solution during boiling.

Unanticipated Reactions

The AR solution contains a mixture of chemicals that may undergo unanticipated reactions, a problem that occurs when heating different buffer solutions together at high temperature, or combining various metal salt solutions, particularly calcium salts.

Incorrect Performance

The immunohistochemical staining procedure may be performed incorrectly. One particular pitfall is that following successful AR, it is frequently necessary to retitrate primary and secondary antibodies to higher dilutions reflective of the greater availability of antigen (effectively gives increased sensitivity). Sections that were previously negative may then stain positively.

Stored Slides

A decrease in the intensity of IHC may occur in cut sections on slides stored for protracted periods. This phenomenon is not well understood and is not uniform or predictable for different antigens or different storage tissues or conditions. We have compared our own experience for common antibodies such as p53 and p27 with that in the literature (31,43,46,80). We performed IHC staining of 23 cases of bladder cancer bearing demonstrable p53 gene mutations by molecular analysis, using stored slides and freshly cut paraffin sections. Of the 23 cases, p53-positive immunostaining was found in 9 of 23 (39%) and 18 of 23 (78%) of stored and nonstored slides, respectively, when AR was not used. When AR was employed on additional slides from these cases, p53-positive staining was significantly increased, to 18 of 23 (78%) and 19 of 23 (83%) of stored and nonstored slides, respectively (Stein et al., unpublished data).

In short, AR levels the playing field for storage conditions, just as it does for fixation conditions. Similar conclusions have been documented in literature (31,46). For example, Grabau et al. (31) carefully compared the influence of stored tumor tissue paraffin sections in temperatures at -80°, 4°, or 20°C, or unmounted at 4°C for 3 years using eight antibodies for IHC staining. They concluded that the IHC intensity was decreased with increasing storage temperature, but that immunoreactivity could be restored by an efficient AR protocol. In our hands, the monoclonal antibody to p27 (clone DCS-72.F6; Neomarkers, Fremont, CA, USA) requires fresh cut tissue sections to achieve the strongest intensity of staining even with our regular AR protocol (20). Preliminary studies suggest that a combination of an AR heating protocol with signal amplification may be needed to reach a satisfactory intensity of staining for p27.

Different Fixatives

Several formalin substitutes have been used in pathology, in attempts to preserve better antigenicity for IHC. An AR protocol that is optimal for routinely formalin-fixed, paraffin-embedded tissue sections may be invalid for tissues exposed to other fixatives. Prento and Lyon (79) compared the performance of six commercial fixatives, proposed as formalin substitutes, with that of formalin and concluded that the best immunostaining was achieved by combining formalin fixation with AR, and further, that none of the six commercial formalin substitutes was adequate for histology. Zhang et al. (116) compared the efficiency of AR-IHC between tissues fixed in formalin or in Lillie's fixative (formalin-alcohol-acetic acid). They demonstrated that 14 of the 15 antibodies tested showed decreased immunoreactivity in tissue fixed by Lillie's fixative, particularly for nuclear immunostaining. The use of multitissue blocks made of alcohol-stored tissues should not be expected to perform in a similar fashion to formalin-fixed tissues and may yield different IHC results from those previously documented for routine formalin-paraffin sections (68,91). p53 immunostaining following MW heating of alcohol-fixed tissue sections has been reported to produce false-positive and unexpected staining patterns in some tissue components (1). Note that improperly fixed tissues, partially exposed to formalin, due to large size or inadequate formalin solution, are in essence fixed in alcohol during later stages of processing; such tissues show irregular results by AR, not surprisingly.

Low-Temperature Heating Method

As previously described, the heating condition is the most important factor influencing the effectiveness of the AR technique. Studies in our laboratories with multiple antigen/antibody combinations repeatedly confirmed the existence of a reverse correlation between heating temperature (T) and heating time (t), or, to state it another way, the effectiveness of AR heating treatment equals the product of $T \times t$. For example, in one study a comparable maximal intensity of staining for MIB-1 was achieved by the following heating conditions ($T \times t$): 100°C x 20 min, 90°C × 30 min, 80°C × 50 min, and 70°C × 10 h (90,92). In summary, the effectiveness of heating AR-IHC is heat dependent: the higher the temperature of heating, the shorter the period of heating and vice versa.

For most antigens tested, higher temperatures yield stronger AR-IHC intensity (11,88,90,91,93,94). In our laboratory, very few antigens, such as p16 (unpublished data) and collagen type III, yield optimal results at lower temperatures. This is also the experience of others (17,25,51,77). Igarashi et al. (39) found that overnight heating at a lower temperature (60°C) was better for muscle actin (HHF35) and smooth-muscle actin (CCG 7) antigens. Elias and Margiotta (25) reported on a low-temperature AR method using a water bath at 80°C for 2 hours in citrate buffer, pH 6.0, claiming an effectiveness equivalent to the standard method for antibodies to steroid hormone receptor. Recently, Koopal and colleagues (51) reported on low-temperature (80°C) heating overnight with Tris-HCl buffer, pH 9.0, using 16 antibodies; they obtained satisfactory results. Other investigators have reported that, for ER, superior results are achieved by a low-temperature heating (60°C overnight) with acetic acid at pH 7.0 to 8.0, or 0.2 mol/L boric acid at pH 7.0 (77). It has been proposed, and is generally agreed, that lower temperatures may have advantages for better preservation of morphology and may reduce the risk of detachment of sections from the slides

(17,25,51,77). In any event, if temperatures are reduced then the heating time must usually be extended to achieve satisfactory results, based on the principle of $T \times t$.

Combining Use of Antigen Retrieval and Other Unmasking Methods

Although the AR heating technique enhances the staining of many antibodies for routinely processed paraffin sections, some antigens, particularly cell surface markers, are still not readily demonstrable in archival tissues. If successful immunostaining is not obtained using regular heating methods, lower or higher temperatures and extended heating periods may be employed, or AR may be combined with enzymatic digestion or signal amplification methods. Malisius et al. (59) reported combining the use of heating AR and a tyramide amplification method for immunostaining of CD2, CD3, CD4, and CD5 in archival paraffin sections. Subsequently, Butmarc et al. (16) adopted a combined AR-IHC protocol with biotinylated tyramine enhancement for monoclonal antibody to CD5 (Leu-1, clone L17F12; Becton Dickinson, San Jose, CA, USA) and obtained satisfactory results in 75% of cases of chronic lymphocytic leukemia, 86% of mantle cell lymphoma cases, and 100% of T-cell lymphoma cases. Successful staining of paraffin sections for CD5 has now been repeated by several authors (24,94,99). Kawai and Osamura (50) studied the efficiency of AR and tyramide signal amplification on archival praffin sections and demonstrated that while amplification alone may enhance the intensity for some antibodies, it may also be significantly improved by the AR heating method. For some antibodies, such as MIB-1, amplification alone will not suffice, but must be preceded by AR. Other strategies remain to be explored, exemplified by the sequential use of reducing agents (mercaptoethanol or sodium hydrosulfite) followed by the AR heating procedure, an approach that restored vimentin reactivity in some spindle cell tumors that otherwise were falsely negative (67).

ACKNOWLEDGMENTS

Part of this chapter adapted with permission from references 91 and 93a.

REFERENCES

1. **Allison, R.T. and T. Best.** 1998. p53, PCNA and Ki-67 expression in oral squamous-cell carcinomas—the vagaries of fixation and microwave enhancement of immunocytochemistry. J. Oral. Pathol. Med. 27:434-440.
2. **Al-Rifai, I., J. Kanitakis, M. Faure, and A. Claudy.** 1997. Immunofluorescence diagnosis of bullous dermatoses on formalin-fixed tissue sections after antigen retrieval. Am. J. Dermatopathol. 19:103-104.
3. **Baas, I.O., F.M. van den Berg, J.-W.R. Mulder, M.J. Clement, S.J.C. Slebos, S.R. Hamilton, and F.J.A. Offerhaus.** 1996. Potential false-positive results with antigen enhancement for immunohistochemistry of the p53 gene product in colorectal neoplasms. J. Pathol. 178:264-267.
4. **Bankfalvi, A., H. Navabi, B. Bier, W. Bocker, B. Jasani, and K.W. Schmid.** 1994. Wet autoclave pretreatment for antigen retrieval in diagnostic immunohistochemistry. J. Pathol. 174:223-228.
5. **Barou, O., N. Laroche, S. Palle, C. Alexandre, and M.H. Lafage-Proust.** 1997. Pre-osteoblastic proliferation assessed with BrdU in undecalcified, epon-embedded adult rat trabecular bone. J. Histochem. Cytochem. 45:1189-1195.
6. **Battifora, H.** 1994. Immunocytochemistry of hormone receptors in routinely processed tissues (editorial). Appl. Immunohistochem. 2:143-145.
7. **Battifora, H.** 1994. p53 immunohistochemistry: a word of caution (editorial). Hum. Pathol. 25:435-437.
8. **Bhan, A.K.** 1995. Immunoperoxidase, Ch. 38, p. 711-723. *In* R.B. Colvin, A.K. Bhan, and R.T. McCluskey (Eds.), Diagnostic Immunopathology, 2nd ed. Raven Press, New York.
9. **Binks, S., C.A. Clelland, J. Ronan, and J. Bell.** 1997. p53 gene product expression in resected non-small cell

carcinoma of the lung with studies of concurrent cytological preparations and microwave antigen retrieval. J. Clin. Pathol. *50*:320-323.

10. **Blythe, D., N.M. Hand, P. Jackson, S.L. Barrans, R.D. Bradbury, and A.S. Jack.** 1997. Use of methyl methacrylate resin for embedding bone marrow trephine biopsy specimens. J. Clin. Pathol. *50*:45-49.

11. **Boon, M.E. and L.P. Kok.** 1995. Breakthrough in pathology due to antigen retrieval. Mal. J. Med. Lab. Sci. *12*:1-9.

12. **Boon, M.E., S. Beck, and L.P. Kok.** 1995. Semiautomatic PAPNET analysis of proliferating (MiB-1-positive) cells in cervical cytology and histology. Diagn. Cytopathol. *13*:423-428.

13. **Brorson, S.H.** 1998. The combination of high-accelerator epoxy resin and antigen retrieval to obtain more intense immunolabeling on epoxy sections than on LR-white sections for large proteins. Micron *29*:89-95.

14. **Brown, R.W. and R. Chirala.** 1995. Utility of microwave-citrate antigen retrieval in diagnostic immunohisto-chemistry. Mod. Pathol. *8*:515-520.

15. **Bussolati, G., P. Gugliotta, M. Volante, M. Pace, and M. Papotti.** 1997. Retrieved endogenous biotin: a novel marker and a potential pitfall in diagnostic immunohistochemistry. Histopathology *31*:400-407.

16. **Butmarc, J.R., H.P. Kourea, E. Levi, and M.E. Kadin.** 1998. Improved detection of CD5 epitope in formalin-fixed paraffin-embedded sections of benign and neoplastic oymphoid tissues by using biotinylated tyramine enhancement after antigen retrieval. Am. J. Clin. Pathol. *109*:682-688.

17. **Carson, N.E., J. Gu, and C.D. Ianuzzo.** 1998. Detection of myosin heavy chain in skeletal muscles using mon-oclonal antibodies on formalin fixed, paraffin embedded tissue sections. J. Histotechnol. *21*:19-24.

18. **Cattoretti, G., M.H.G. Becker, G. Key, M. Duchrow, C. Schluter, J.Galle, and J.Gerdes.** 1992. Monoclonal antibodies against recombinant parts of the Ki-67 antigen (MIB 1 and MIB 3) detect proliferating cells in microwave-processed formalin-fixed paraffin sections. J. Pathol. *168*:357-363.

19. **Cattoretti,G., S. Pileri, C. Parravicini, M.H.G. Becker, S. Poggi, C. Bifulco, G. Key, L. D'Amato, E. Sabat-tini, E. Feudale, et al.** 1993. Antigen unmasking on formalin-fixed, paraffin-embedded tissue sections. J. Pathol. *171*:83-98.

20. **Cote, R.J., Y. Shi, S. Groshen, A.-C. Feng, C. Cordon-Cardo, D. Skinner, and G. Lieskovosky.** 1998. Asso-ciation of p27Kip1 levels with recurrence and survival in patients with stage C prostate carcinoma. J. Natl. Can-cer Inst. *90*:916-920.

21. **Daidone, M.G., E. Benini, S. Rao, S. Pilotti, and R. Silvestrini.** 1998. Fixation time and microwave oven irra-diation affect immunocytochemical p53 detection in formalin-fixed paraffin sections. Appl. Immunohistochem. *6*:140-144.

22. **D'Ambra-Cabry, K., D.H. Deng, K.L. Flynn, K.L. Magee, and J.S. Deng.** 1995. Antigen retrieval in immuno-fluorescent testing of bullous pemphigoid. Am. J. Dermatopathol. *17*:560-563.

23. **Dookhan, D.B., A.J. Kovatich, and M. Miettinen.** 1993. Non-enzymatic antigen retrieval in immunohisto-chemistry. Comparison between different antigen retrieval modalities and proteolytic digestion. Appl. Immuno-histochem. *1*:149-155.

24. **Dorfman, D.M. and A. Shahsafaei.** 1997. Usefulness of a new CD5 antibody for the diagnosis of T-cell and B-cell lymphoproliferative disorders in paraffin sections. Mod. Pathol. *10*:859-863.

25. **Elias, J.M. and M. Margiotta.** 1997. Low temperature antigen restoration of steroid hormone receptor proteins in routine paraffin sections. J. Histotechnol. *20*:155-158.

26. **Evers, P. and H.B.M. Uylings.** 1994. Microwave-stimulated antigen retrieval is pH and temperature dependent. J. Histochem. Cytochem. *42*:1555-1563.

27. **Fariss, R.N., S.S. Apte, B.R. Olsen, K. Iwata, and A.H. Milam.** 1997. Tissue inhibitor of metalloproteinases-3 is a component of Bruch's membrane of the eye. Am. J. Pathol. *150*:323-328.

28. **Gerasimov, G., M. Bronstein, K. Troshina, G. Alexandrova, I. Dedov, T. Jennings, B.V.S. Kallakury, R. Izquierdo, A. Boguniewicz, H. Figge, et al.** 1995. Nuclear p53 immunoreactivity in papillary thyroid cancers is associated with two established indicators of poor prognosis. Exp. Mol. Pathol. *62*:52-62.

29. **Gerdes, J., M.H.G. Becker, G. Key, and G. Cattoretti.** 1992. Immunohistological detection of tumour growth fraction (Ki-67) in formalin-fixed and routinely processed tissues. J. Pathol. *168*:85-87.

30. **Gown, A.M., N. de Wever, and H. Battifora.** 1993. Microwave-based antigenic unmasking. A revolutionary new technique for routine immunohistochemistry. Appl. Immunohistochem. *1*:256-266.

31. **Grabau, K.A., O. Nielsen, S. Hansen, M.M. Nielsen, A.-V. Lankholm, A. Knoop, and P. Pfeiffer.** 1998. Influ-ence of storage temperature and high-temperature antigen retrieval buffers on results of immunohistochemical staining in sections stored for long periods. Appl. Immunohistochem. *6*:209-213.

32. **Greenwell, A., J.F. Foley, and R.R. Maronpot.** 1991. An enhancement method for immunohistochemical stain-ing of proliferating cell nuclear antigen in archival rodent tissues. Cancer Lett. *59*:251-256.

33. **Gu, J.** 1994. Microwave in immunocytochemistry, p. 67-80. *In* J. Gu and G.W. Hacker (Eds.), Modern Methods in Analytical Morphology. Plenum Press, New York.

34. **Gu, J., M. Forte, H. Hance, N. Carson, C. Xenachis, and R. Rufner.** 1994. Microwave fixation, antigen retrieval and accelerated immunocytochemistry. Cell Vision *1*:76-77.

35. **Gu, J., M. Forte, C. Xenachis, N. Tarazona, J. Windsor, and E.C. Santoian.** 1994. Immunohistochemical demonstration of PCNA and Ki 67 positivities in stimulated myochariocytes indicates dividing potential for car-diac muscle cells in adult heart. Cell Vision *1*:91-92.

329

36.**Guiter, G.E., P.W. Kwan, and R.A. DeLellis.** 1995. Unwanted tissue immunoreactivities following microwave antigen retrieval: a critical analysis. Lab. Invest. *72*:165A.

37.**Hand, N.M. and R.J. Church.** 1998. Superheating using pressure cooking: its use and application in unmasking antigens embedded in methyl methacrylate. J. Histotechnol. *21*:231-236.

38.**Hazelbag, H.M., L.J.C. Mvd Broek, E.B.L. van Dorst, G.J.A. Offerhaus, G.J. Fleuren, and P.C.W. Hogendoorn.** 1995. Immunostaining of chain-epecific keratins on formalin-fixed, paraffin-embedded tissues: a comparison of various antigen retrieval systems using microwave heating and proteolytic pre-treatments. J. Histochem. Cytochem. *43*:429-437.

39.**Igarashi, H., H. Sugimura, K. Maruyama, Y. Kitayama, I. Ohta, M. Suzuki, M. Tanaka, Y. Dobashi, and I. Kino.** 1994. Alteration of immunoreactivity by hydrated autoclaving, microwave treatment, and simple heating of paraffin-embedded tissue sections. APMIS *102*:295-307.

40.**Ikeda, K., T. Monden, T. Kanoh, M. Tsujie, H. Izawa, A. Haba, T. Ohnishi, M. Sekimoto, N. Tomita, H. Shiozaki, and M. Monden.** 1998. Extraction and analysis of diagnostically useful proteins from formalin-fixed, paraffin-embedded tissue sections. J. Histochem. Cytochem. *46*:397-403.

41.**Imam, S.A., L. Young, B. Chaiwun, and C.R. Taylor.** 1995. Comparison of 2 microwave based antigen retrieval solutions in unmasking epitopes in formolin-fixed tissue for immunostaining. Anticancer Res. *15*:1153-1158.

42.**Iruela-Arispe, M.L., D.J. Liska, E.H. Sage, and P. Bornstein.** 1993. Differential expression of thrombospondin 1, 2, and 3 during murine development. Dev. Dyn. *197*:40-56.

43.**Jacobs, T.W., J.E. Prioleau, I.E. Stillman, and S.J. Schnitt.** 1996. Loss of tumor marker-immunostaining intensity on stored paraffin slides of breast cancer. J. Natl. Cancer Inst. *88*:1054-1059.

44.**Jones, M.D., P.M. Banks, and B.L. Caron.** 1981. Transition metal salts as adjuncts to formalin for tissue fixation. Lab. Invest. *44*:32A.

45.**Kashima, K., S. Yokoyama, T. Daa, I. Nakayama, P.A. Nickerson, and S. Noguchi.** 1997. Cytoplasmic biotin-like activity interferes with immunohstochemical analysis of thyroid lesions: a comparison of antigen retrieval methods. Mod. Pathol. *10*:515-519.

46.**Kato, J., S. Sakamaki, and Y. Niitsu.** 1995. More on p53 antigen loss in stored paraffin slides. N. Engl. J. Med. *333*:1507-1508.

47.**Katoh, A. and S. Breier.** 1994. Nonspecific antigen retrieval solutions. J. Histotechnol. *17*:378-378.

48.**Kawai, K., S. Umemura, and Y. Tsutsumi.** 1994. Antigen retrieval by heating treatment. Saibo (Cell) *26*:152-157 (in Japanese).

49.**Kawai, K., A. Serizawa, T. Hamana, and Y. Tsutsumi.** 1994. Heat-induced antigen retrieval of proliferating cell nuclear antigen and p53 protein in formalin-fixed, paraffin-embedded sections. Pathol. Int. *44*:759-764.

50.**Kawai, K. and R.Y. Osamura.** 1998. Epitope retrieval vs. amplification techniques in diagnostic immunohistochemistry. J. Histochem. Cytochem. *46*:A14.

51.**Koopal, S.A., M.I. Coma, A.T.M.G. Tiebosch, and A.J.H. Suurmeijer.** 1998. Low-temperature heating overnight in Tris-HCl buffer pH 9 is a good alternative for antigen retrieval in formalin-fixed paraffin-embedded tissue. Appl. Immunohistochem. *6*:228-233.

52.**Krenacs, T. and M. Rosendaal.** 1998. Connexin 43 gap junctions in normal, regenerating, and cultured mouse bone marrow and in human leukemias: their possible involvement in blood formation. Am. J. Pathol. *152*:851-854.

53.**Krenacs, T. and L. Krenacs.** 1999. Immunogold-silver staining (IGSS) for single and multiple antigen detection in archived tissues following antigen retrieval. AIMM *7*:93-94.

54.**Lan, H.Y., P. Hutchinson, G.H. Tesch, W. Mu, and R.C. Atkins.** 1996. A novel method of microwave treatment for detection of cytoplasmic and nuclear antigens by flow cytometry. J. Immunol. Methods *190*:1-10.

55.**Lan, H.Y., W. Mu, Y.Y. Ng, D.J. Nikolic-Paterson, and R.C. Atkins.** 1996. A simple, reliable, and sensitive method for nonradioactive in situ hybridization: use of microwave heating to improve hybridization efficiency and preserve tissue morphology. J. Histochem. Cytochem. *44*:281-287.

56.**Leers, M.P.G., B. Schutte, P.H.M.H. Theunissen, F.C.S. Ramaekers, and M. Nap.** 1999. Heat pretreatment increases resolution in DNA flow cytometry of paraffin-embedded tumor tissue. Cytometry *35*:260-266.

57.**Leong, A.S.-Y. and J. Milios.** 1993. An assessment of the efficacy of the miceowave antigen-retrieval procedure on a range of tissue antigens. Appl. Immunohistochem. *1*:267-274.

58.**Lucassen, P.J., R. Ravid, N.K. Gonatas, and D.F. Swaab.** 1993. Activation of the human supraoptic and paraventricular nucleus neurons with aging and in Alzheimer's disease as judged from increasing size of the Golgi apparatus. Brain Res. *632*:105-113.

59.**Malisius, R., H. Merz, B. Heinz E. Gafumbegete, B.U. Koch, and A.C. Feller.** 1997. Constant detection of CD2, CD3, and CD5 in fixed and paraffin-embedded tissue using the peroxidase-mediated deposition of biotin-tyramide. J. Histochem. Cytochem. *45*:1665-1672.

60.**McCluggage, G., H. McBride, P. Maxwell, and H. Bharucha.** 1997. Immunohistochemical detection of p53 and bcl-2 proteins in neoplastic and non-neolastic endocervical glandular lesions. Int. J. Gyn. Pathol. *16*:22-27.

61.**McMahon, J. and S. McQuaid.** 1996. The use of microwave irradiation as a pretreatment to in situ hybridization for the detection of measles virus and chicken anaemia virus in formalin-fixed paraffin-embedded tissue. Histochem. J. *28*:157-164.

62.**Merz, H., O. Rickers, S. Schrimel, K. Orscheschek, and A.C. Feller.** 1993. Constant detection of surface and cytoplasmic immunoglobulin heavy and light chain expression in formalin-fixed and paraffin-embedded material. J. Pathol. *170*:257-264.

63.**Merz, H., R. Malisius, S. Mannweiler, R. Zhou, W. Hartmann, K. Orscheschek, P. Moubayed, and A.C. Feller.** 1995. ImmunoMax. A maximized immunohistochemical method for the retrieval and enhancement of hidden antigens. Lab. Invest. *73*:149-156.

64.**Mighell, A.J., P.A. Robinson, and W.J. Hume.** 1995. Patterns of immunoreactivity to an anti-fibronectin polyclonal antibody in formalin-fixed, paraffin-embedded oral tissues are dependent on methods of antigen retrieval. J. Histochem. Cytochem. *43*:1107-1114.

65.**Miller, R.T. and C. Estran.** 1995. Heat-induced epitope retrieval with a pressure cooker—suggestios for optimal use. Appl. Immunohistochem. *3*:190-193.

66.**Mintze, K., N. Macon, K.E. Gould, and G.E. Sandusky.** 1995. Optimization of proliferating cell nuclear antigen (PCNA) immunohistochemical staining: a comparison of methods using three commercral antibodies, various fixation times, and antigen retrieval solution. J. Histotechnol. *18*:25-30.

67.**Moll, B. and Z. Jelveh.** 1998. Antigen recovery for vimentin immunostaining by reducing agents for two cases of spindle cell tumors. J. Histotechnol. *21*:45-48.

68.**Momose, H., P. Mehta, and H. Battifora.** 1993. Antigen retrieval by microwave irradiation in lead thiocyanate. Appl. Immunohistochem. *1*:77-82.

69.**Morgan, J.M., H. Navabi, K.W. Schimid, and B. Jasani.** 1994. Possible role of tissue-bound calcium ions in crtrate-mediated high-temperature antigen retrieval. J. Pathol. *174*:301-307.

70.**Mote, P.A., J.A. Leary, and C.L. Clarke.** 1998. Immunohistochemical detection of progesterone receptors in archival breast cancer. Biotech. Histochem. *73*:117-127.

71.**Norton, A.J., S. Jordan, and P. Yeomans.** 1994. Brief, high-temperature heat denaturation (pressure cooking): A simple and effective method of antigen retrieval for routinely processed tissues. J. Pathol. *173*:371-379.

72.**Oliver, K.R., R.P. Heavens, and D.J.S. Sirinathsinghji.** 1997. Quantitative comparison of pretreatment regimens used to sensitize in situ hybridization using oligonucleotide probes on paraffin-embedded brain tissue. J. Histochem. Cytochem. *45*:1707-1713.

73.**Overton, W.R., E. Catalano, and J.P. McCoy.** 1996. Method to make paraffin-embedded breast and lymph tissue mimic fresh tissue in DNA analysis. Cytometry *26*:166-171.

74.**Pateraki, M. and G. Kontogeorgos.** 1997. Postadhesive technique for archival paraffin sections. Biotech. Histochem. *72*:168-170.

75.**Pavelic, Z.P., L.G. Portugal, M.J. Gootee, P.J. Stambrook, C. Smith, R.E Mugge, L. Pavelic, K. Wilson, C.R. Buncher, Y.-Q. Li, et al.** 1993. Retrieval of p53 protein in paraffin-embedded head and neck tumor tissues. Arch. Otolaryngol. Head Neck Surg. *119*:1206-1209.

76.**Pertschuk, L.P., Y.-D. Kim, C.A. Axiotis, A.S. Braverman, A.C. Carter, K.B. Eisenberg, and L.V. Braithwaite.** 1994. Estrogen receptor immunocytochemistry: the promise and perils. J. Cell. Biochem. *19*(Suppl):134-137.

77.**Peston, D. and S. Shousha.** 1998. Low temperature heat mediated antigen retrieval for the demostration of oestrogen and progesterone receptors in formalin-fixed paraffin sections. J. Pathol. *186*:A21.

78.**Pileri, S.A., G. Roncador, C. Ceccarelli, M. Piccioli, A. Briskonatis, E. Sabattini, S. Ascani, D. Santini, P.P. Piccaluga, O. Leone, et al.** 1997. Antigen retrieval techniques in immunohistochemistry: comparison of different methods. J. Pathology. *183*:116-123.

79.**Prento, P. and H. Lyon.** 1997. Commercial formalin substitutes for histopathology. Biotech. Histochem. *72*:273-282.

80.**Prioleau, J. and S.I. Schnitt.** 1995. p53 antigen loss in stored paraffin slides. N. Engl. J. Med. *332*:1521-1522.

81.**Redkar, A.A. and A. Krishan.** 1999. Flow cytometric analysis of estrogen, progesterone receptor expression and DNA content in formalin-fixed, paraffin-embedded human breast tumors. Cytometry *38*:61-69.

82.**Sebenik, M. and R. Wieczorek.** 1995. Nonspecific nuclear staining (NNS) after antigen retrieval (AR). Lab. Invest. *72*:168A.

83.**Shi, S.-R., M.E. Key, and K.L. Kalra.** 1991. Antigen retrieval in formalin-fixed, paraffin-embedded tissues: an enhancement method for immunohistochemical staining based on microwave oven heating of tissue sections. J. Histochem. Cytochem. *39*:741-748.

84.**Shi, S.-R., B. Chaiwun, L. Young, R.J. Cote, and C.R. Taylor.** 1993. Antigen retrieval technique utilizing citrate buffer or urea solution for immunohistochemical demonstration of androgen receptor in formalin-fixed paraffin sections. J. Histochem. Cytochem. *41*:1599-1604.

85.**Shi, S.-R., B. Chaiwun, L. Young, A. Imam, R.J. Cote, and C.R. Taylor.** 1994. Antigen retrieval using pH 3.5 glycine-HCl buffer or urea solution for immunohistochemical localization of Ki-67. Biotech. Histochem. *69*:213-215.

86.**Shi, S.-R., A. Imam, L. Young, R.J. Cote, and C.R. Taylor.** 1995. Antigen retrieval immunohistochemistry under the influence of pH using monoclonal antibodies. J. Histochem. Cytochem. *43*:193-201.

87.**Shi, S.-R., R.J. Cote, L. Young, C. Yang, C. Chen, G.D. Grossfeld, D.A. Ginsberg, F.L. Hall, and C.R. Taylor.** 1995. Development of optimal protocols for antigen retrieval immunohistochemistry based on the effects of variation in temperature and pH: use of a 'test battery', p. 828-829. *In* G.W. Bailey, M.H. Ellisman, R.A. Hennigar, and N.J. Zaluzec (Eds.), JMSA Proceedings Microscopy and Microanalysis. Jones & Begell Publishing, New York.

88. **Shi, S.-R., J. Gu, K.L. Kalra, T. Chen, R.J. Cote, and C.R. Taylor.** 1995. Antigen retrieval technique: a novel approach to immunohistochemistry on routinely processed tissue sections (review). Cell Vision 2:6-22.

89. **Shi, S.-R., R.J. Cote, C. Yang, C. Chen, H.-J. Xu, W.F. Benedict, and C.R. Taylor.** 1996. Development of an optimal protocol for antigen retrieval: a 'test battery' approach exemplified with reference to the staining of retinoblastoma protein (pRB) in formalin-fixed paraffin sections. J. Pathol. *179*:347-352.

90. **Shi, S.-R., R.J. Cote, and C.R. Taylor.** 1997. Antigen retrieval immunohistochemistry: past, present, and future. J. Histochem. Cytochem. *45*:327-343.

91. **Shi, S.-R., R.J. Cote, L.L. Young, and C.R. Taylor.** 1997. Antigen retrieval immunohistochemistry: practice and development. J. Histotechnol. *20*:145-154.

92. **Shi, S.-R., R.J. Cote, B. Chaiwun, L.L. Young, Y. Shi, D. Hawes, T. Chen, and C.R. Taylor.** 1998. Standardization of immunohistochemistry based on antigen retrieval technique for routine formalin-fixed tissue sections. Appl. Immunohistochem. 6:89-96.

93. **Shi, S.-R., R.J. Cote, and C.R. Taylor.** 1998. Antigen retrieval immunohistochemistry used for routinely processed celloidin-embedded human temporal bone sections: standardization and development. Auris Nasus Larynx 25:425-443.

93a. **Shi, S.-R., R.J. Cote, and C.R. Taylor.** 1999. Standardization and further development of antigen retrieval immunohistochemistry: strategies and future goals. J. Histotechnol. *22*:177-192.

94. **Shi, Y., G.-D. Li, and W.-P. Liu.** 1997. Recent advances of the antigen retrieval technique. Linchuang yu Shiyan Binglixue Zazhi (J. Clin. Exp. Pathol.) *13*:265-267 (in Chinese).

95. **Shin, H.J.C., D.M. Shin, and J.Y. Ro.** 1994. Optimization of proliferating cell nuclear antigen immunohistochemical staining by microwave heating in zinc sulfate solution. Mod. Pathol. 7:242-248.

96. **Shin, R.-W., T. Iwaki, T. Kitamoto, and J. Tateishi.** 1991. Hydrated autoclave pretreatment enhances TAU immunoreactivity in formalini-fixed normal and Alzheimer's kisease brain tissues. Lab. Invest. *64*:693-702.

97. **Sibony, M., F. Commo, P. Callard, and J.-M. Gasc.** 1995. Enhancement of mRNA in situ hybridization signal by microwave heating. Lab. Invest. *73*:586-591.

98. **Siitonen, S.M., O.-P. Kallioniemi, and J.J. Isola.** 1993. Proliferating cell nuclear antigen immunohistochemistry using monoclonal antibody 19A2 and a new antigen retrieval technique has prognostic impact in archival paraffin-embedded node-negative breast cancer. Am. J. Pathol. *142*:1081-1089.

99. **Singh, N. and D.H. Wright.** 1997. The value of immunohistochemistry on paraffin wax embedded tissue sections in the differetiation of small lymphocytic and mantle cell lymphomas. J. Clin. Pathol. *50*:16-21.

100. **Sormunen, R. and A.S.-Y. Leong.** 1998. Microwave-stimulated antigen retrieval for immunohistology and immunoelectron microscopy of resin-embedded sections. Appl. Immunohistochem. 6:234-237.

101. **Spires, S.E., C.D. Jennings, E.R. Banks, D.P. Wood, D.D. Davey, and M.L. Cibull.** 1994. Proliferating cell nuclear antigen in prostatic adenocarcinoma: correlation with established prognostic indicators. Urology 43:660-666.

102. **Stieber, A., Z. Mourelatos, and N.K. Gonatas.** 1996. In Alzheimer's disease the Golgi apparatus of a population of neurons without neurofibrillary tangles is fragmented and atrophic. Am. J. Pathol. *148*:415-426.

103. **Suurmeijier, A.J.H. and M.E. Boon.** 1993. Notes on the application of microwaves for antigen retrieval in paraffin and plastic tissue sections. Eur. J. Morphol. *31*:144-150.

104. **Suurmeijier, A.J.H. and M.E. Boon.** 1993. Optimizing keratin and vimentin retrieval in formalin-fixed, paraffin-embedded tissue with the use of heat and metal salts. Appl. Immunohistochem. *1*:143-148.

105. **Swanson, P.E.** 1997. HIERanarchy: the state of the art in immunohistochemistry (editorial). Am. J. Clin. Pathol. *107*:139-140.

106. **Tacha, D.E. and T. Chen.** 1994. A modified antigen retrieval method. A calibration technique for microwave ovens. J. Histotechnol. *17*:365-366.

107. **Taylor, C.R.** 1996. Paraffin section immunocytochemistry for estrogen receptor. The time has come. Cancer 77:2419-2422.

108. **Taylor, C.R. and R.J. Cote (Eds.).** 1994. Immunomicroscopy: A Diagnostic Tool for the Surgical Pathologist. 2nd ed., p. 1-70. W.B. Saunders, Philadelphia.

109. **Taylor, C.R., S.-R. Shi, B. Chaiwun, L. Young, S.A. Imam, and R.J. Cote.** 1994. Standardization and reproducibility in diagnostic immunohistochemistry (correspondence). Hum. Pathol. *25*:1107-1109.

110. **Taylor, C.R., S.-R. Shi, B. Chaiwun, L. Young, S.A. Imam, and R.J. Cote.** 1994. Strategies for improving the immunohistochemical staining of various intranuclear prognostic markers in formalin-paraffin sections: androgen receptor, estrogen receptor, progesterone receptor, p53 protein, proliferating cell nuclear antigen, and Ki-67 antigen revealed by antigen retrieval technique. Hum. Pathol. *25*:263-270.

111. **Taylor, C.R., S.-R. Shi, C. Chen, L. Young, C. Yang, and R.J. Cote.** 1996. Comparative study of antigen retrieval heating methods: microwave, microwave and pressure cooker, autoclave, and steamer. Biotech. Histochem. *71*:263-270.

112. **Taylor, C.R., S.-R. Shi, and R.J. Cote.** 1996. Antigen retrieval for immunohistochemistry. Status and need for greater standardization. Appl. Immunohistochem. *4*:144-166.

113. **Wieczorek, R., R. Stover, and M. Sebenik.** 1997. Nonspecific nuclear immunoreactivity after antigen retrieval

using acidic and basic solutions. J. Histotechnol. *20*:139-143.

114. **Wilson, J.E.** 1991. The use of monoclonal antibodies and limited proteolysis in elucidation of structure-function relationships in proteins, p. 7-250. *In* C.H. Suelter (Ed.), Methods of Biochemical Analysis. John Wiley & Sons, New York.

115. **Yorukoglu, K. and S. Cingoz.** 1997. Epitope retrieval technique: a simple modification that reduces staining time. Appl. Immunohistochem. *5*:71.

116. **Zhang, P.J., H. Wang, E.L. Wrona, and R.T. Cheney.** 1998. Effects of tissue fixatives on antigen preservation for immunohistochemistry: a comparative study of microwave antigen retrieval on Lillie fixative and neutral buffered formalin. J. Histotechnol. *21*:101-106.

Index

A

Ab-3, 35f
ABC method, 9
  vs. ImmunoMax Method, 226, 229f, 230f
AC
  MIB-1, 63
  MIB-1-positive staining, 59–60, 59f
Acetone-methyl benzoate-xylene procedure
  cell proliferation markers, 185–186
Adenocarcinoma (AC)
  MIB-1, 63
  MIB-1-positive staining, 59–60, 59f
Adenocarcinoma in situ (AIS)
  MIB-1-positive staining, 59–60, 59f
Adhesion
  improvement, 325
AE1, 30, 43, 49
  AR-IHC, 261f
    formalin-fixed, paraffin-embedded tissues, 259
  pH, 188, 197
AIS
  MIB-1-positive staining, 59–60, 59f
Alcohol
  vs. formalin, 20
Alcohol-based reagents
  cell proliferation markers, 185–186
Alcohol groups, 22
Aldehydes
  chemistry, 20–22
Alkaline phosphatase (AP), 129
Aluminum chloride
  high-temperature heating method, 106t
Alzheimer's disease
  tau immunostaining
    autoclaves, 198
  TUNEL, 82f
Amides, 22
Amines
  primary, 22
Amplification techniques
  vs. AR
    diagnostic immunohistochemistry,

249–252
Androgen receptors (AnR)
  historical perspective, 159–160
  immunohistochemistry
    image analysis, 160–161
  prostate cancer, 159–161
Anti-BCL-6 rabbit polyclonal antibody, 170f
Antibodies
  anti-PCNA, 184
  cross-reactivity
    blockage, 130
  diagnostic
    mouse experimental pathology, 172–173
  Ki-S1, 185
  monoclonal. *See* Monoclonal antibodies (mAbs)
  murine formalin-fixed, paraffin-embedded tissues, 174t
  polyclonal, 166
    anti-BCL-6 rabbit, 170f
    rat, 167
  primary, 212t
  validation, 169–170
Antigenicity
  loss, 27
Antigen matrix model, 269–270
Antigen retrieval
  heat-induced. *See* Heat-induced antigen retrieval
Antigen retrieval (AR), 1–4
  artifacts, 224–225
  development, 17–36
    formalin fixation, 20–28
    Fraenkel-Conrat, 28–31
    high-temperature heating method, 29
    modifications, 30–31
    nonheating method, 29
  effect mechanism, 31–34
  future, 34–36
  pH, 44–46
    patterns, 46f
  pitfalls, 224–225
  pre-antigen retrieval treatment, 48–49
  protocol

MIB-1-positive staining, 59

L

Labyrinthine fibrosis, 301
Lead salts
  disadvantages, 47
Lectin, 173
Ligand-binding assays
  ER, 154
Light microscopic immunolabeling. *See*
  Microscopic immunolabeling
Light microscopy (LM), 93
  protocols
    plastic-embedded tissue, 102t–104t
Lillie's fixative, 327
Linear markers
  double immunostaining, 170f
Literature review
  MIB-1, 57–58
  in situ hybridization, 118t–119t
LM, 93
  protocols
    plastic-embedded tissue, 102t–104t
Low-pH
  microscopic immunolabeling, 280
Low-temperature heating, 327–328
LSAB2 kit, 265
Lymph nodes
  PNA, 175f
  proliferating cells
    Ki-67, 169f
Lymphoid cells
  MIB-1-positive staining, 59–60, 59f
Lysine, 22
  cross-linking, 26f
Lysine/formaldehyde reaction, 26f

M

MAbs. *See* Monoclonal antibodies
Magnesium chloride
  in situ hybridization, 121
Mannich reaction, 21, 22, 23f, 29
Masking effect, 27
Masking of the tissue antigen, 139
MEDLINE search

MIB-1, 57–58
Medulloblastomas, 147
Megalin
  protein A-gold, 281f
Melanoma cells
  MIB-1, 202f
Menière's disease, 301, 302
Metallothioneins
  CIN, 58
Metal salts
  disadvantages, 47
Metaphase
  ultrasensitive FISH, 243
Methacarn
  cell proliferation markers, 185–186
Methanol, 291
Methylene glycol, 24
Methyl methacrylate
  plastic-embedded tissue sections,
    322–323
MIB-1, 35f
  AR-IHC
    formalin-fixed, paraffin-embedded
      tissues, 259
  AR-IHC protocols, 260t
  autoclaves, 198
  cervical cytology, 57–59
  citrate buffer, 147
  EDTA-NaOH solution, 197
  formaldehyde-fixed tissues
    calcium, 203
  grading, 64–66, 65f
  heat-induced AR with TSA
    amplification, 251f, 252
  67-kDa laminin receptor, 58
  MEDLINE search, 57–58
  melanoma cells, 202f
  p53, 58
  pH, 197
  pKi-67, 201
  proliferating endocervical cells, 63
  proliferating reserve cells, 61–63
  Tris-HCl, 146
  unsatisfactory smears, 64
    upgrading, 66, 66t
  vs. other prognosticators, 58, 58t
MIB-1-positive cells

345

Protease digestion
microscopic immunolabeling, 275
Protein A-gold
megalin, 281f
Protein cross-linkages
formalin fixation, 19–20
Protein extraction, 317–318, 323–324
Proteolytic enzyme digestion, 11
cell proliferation markers, 186
with heat-induced AR
cell proliferation markers, 187
Proteolytic enzyme pretreatment, 10
PSA, 30
PTEN, 211
PubMed search
MIB-1, 57–58

Q

Quantitative immunohistochemistry
(QIHC), 256, 266–269
antigen measurement, 267–268
Her-2/neu, 268
image analysis systems, 266–267
Ki-67, 268
manual method, 266–267
Midwestern assay, 268
p53, 268
stereology based-systemic random
sampling method, 266
Quicgel method, 268, 270

R

RAG-1
staining, 173f
RAG-2
staining, 173f
Rat monoclonal antibodies, 167
Rat polyclonal antibodies
Ki-67, 167
Rat prostate
apoptotic cells
microwave-enhanced in situ
end-labeling, 72, 81f, 84
R-banding
fluorescence

ultrasensitive FISH, 244
Rb gene, 207, 208
Reagents
experimental pathology, 165–169
Renaturation, 32
Repair cells
PAPNET scanning, 67
Reserve cells
benign
MIB-1-positive staining, 59–60, 59f
chromatin pattern, 62
cytologic presentation, 62–63
identification, 61
nuclei deformation, 61–62
Resin etching
immunoelectron microscopy, 96
Reticular cells
mouse IgG1 monoclonal antibody,
171f
Retrieval solution
microwave-stimulated antigen
retrieval, 142–143

S

SAB
protocol, 61
vs. TSA, 250
Scala tympani
epithelial cell-line cyst, 295, 301f
SCC
p53
MIB-1, 58
Schiff bases, 21, 22
formation, 26f
Serine, 22
with lysine
cross-linking, 26f
Serine/formaldehyde interaction, 22
Serine/formaldehyde reaction, 25f
Signal amplification
classification
IHC, 263
simplification
IHC, 262–266
Signal amplification techniques
immunoelectron microscopy, 95

Unmasking
  antigens, 139–140
  biotin, 324
  enzyme, 96
  physical, 96
  sodium metaperiodate
    deosmication, 107
URM, 187–188, 198–199

V

Validation
  antibodies, 169–170
Vimentin, 30, 43
Virchow, Rudolf, 17

W

Western Regional Research Laboratory,
  28–29

Z

Zenker's solution
  cell proliferation markers, 185–186